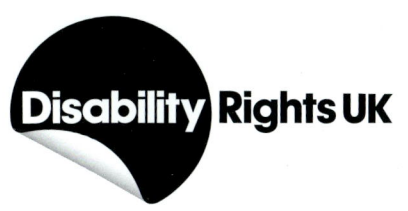

Holidays
in the British Isles
A guide for disabled people

© Disability Rights UK

Holidays in the British Isles
A guide for disabled people

ISBN 978-1-903335-62-8
© Disability Rights UK 2013

Published by Disability Rights UK.
Registered Charity No. 1138585

All rights reserved. No part of this publication may be reproduced, stored in a retrieval system or transmitted in any form by any means, electronic, mechanical, photocopying, recording or otherwise, without the prior permission in writing of the publishers.

Disability Rights UK does not endorse any commercial organisations. Acceptance of commercial advertising or sponsorship or editorial reference should not be interpreted as an endorsement of the commercial firms involved.

All information is provided in good faith but Disability Rights UK cannot be held responsible for any omissions, inaccuracies or complaint arising from editorial or advertising matter.

Design: © Anderson Fraser Partnership, London
Printed & bound by: Stephens & George Print Group, Merthyr Tydfil

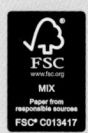

Disability Rights UK
12 City Forum, 250 City Road,
London EC1V 8AF
Tel: 020 7250 3222
Fax: 020 7250 0212
www.disabilityrightsuk.org

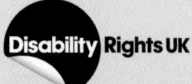

Editor:
Sarah Cosby

Author:
Sarah Cosby
Deb Kamofsky

Contributors:
Lesley Baliga
Mary Convill
Ian Greaves
Ben Kersey
John Stanford
Friederike Traiser

Production:
Anderson Fraser: Deb Kamofsky,
Paul McKenzie and Humphrey Weightman

Photographs:
VisitBritain/Pawel Libera
Motability
Jersey Tourism Image Library
Paul McKenzie
Shutterstock

Thanks to:
To the tourist boards of the Channel Islands, England, the Isle of Man, Scotland and Wales for their information and co-operation.

Tourism For All for the investment they make into ensuring accessible travel and holidays for all. We wish them all the best with the launch of the new Open Britain site www.openbritain.net

Special thanks to VisitEngland for providing information about their register of accommodation that meets the standards of their National Accessible Scheme.

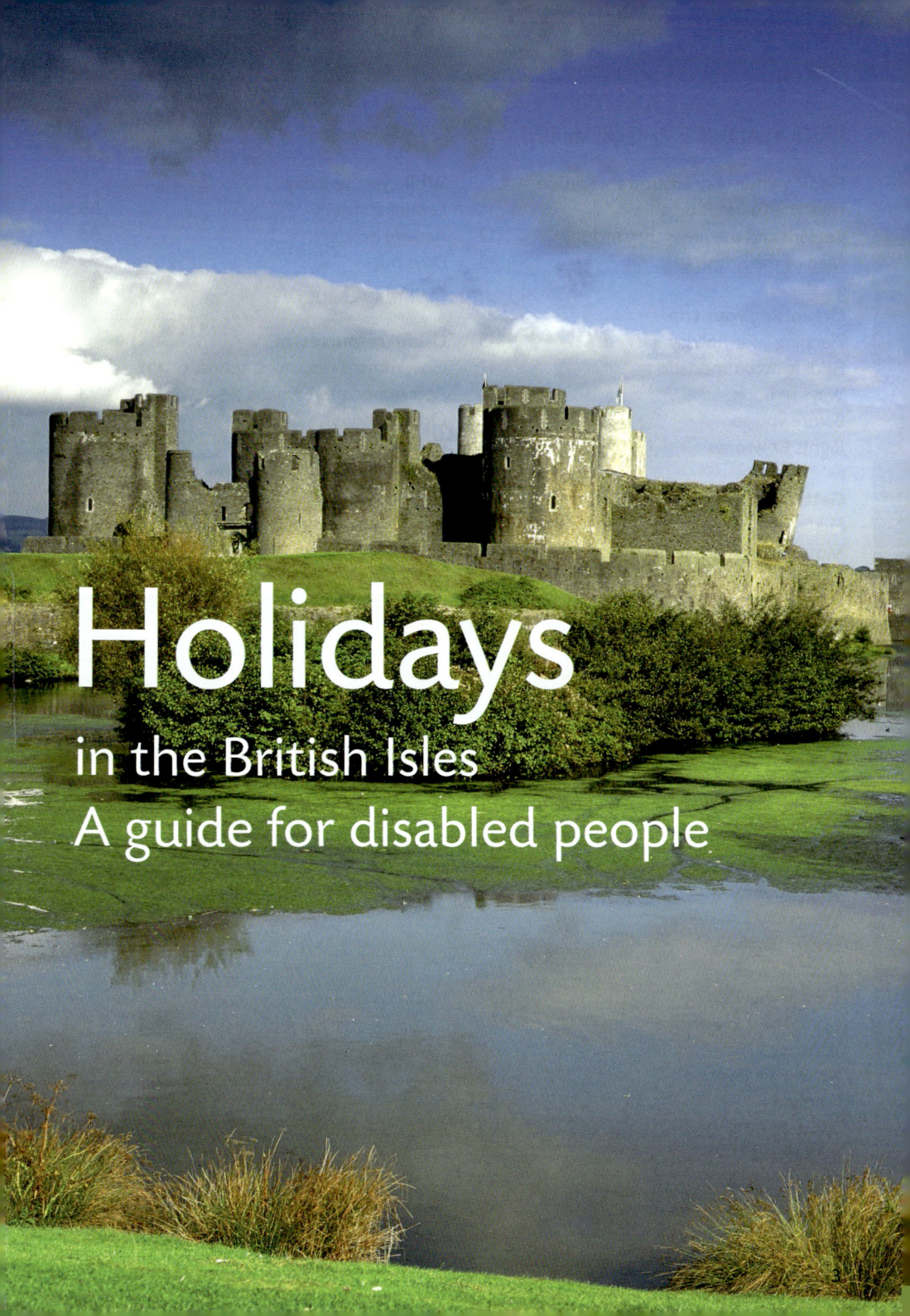

Holidays
in the British Isles
A guide for disabled people

INTRODUCTION

OPEN BRITAIN

THE PREMIER ACCESSIBLE TOURISM WEBSITE

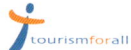 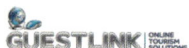

Feature on the 2013 website, App and partner publications – www.openbritain.net

OpenBritain is relaunching on 19th March 2013 promoting tourism businesses with detailed accessibility information. As recommended by VisitEngland:

"Research by VisitEngland in 2012 revealed the importance of specialist websites for disabled travellers. VisitEngland supports the ambitions of the new OpenBritain website to connect disabled travellers with a wealth of accessible tourism businesses, including those rated by the National Accessible Scheme."

Ross Calladine

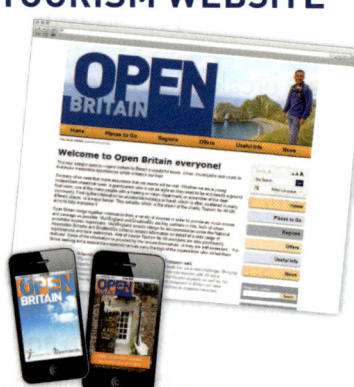

REACH MORE VISITORS...

- **The definitive source – Powered by Guestlink** – The OpenBritain data hub will hold information from thousands of accommodation, attraction and event businesses – reaching visitors via our website, App and partner publications
- **NEW 2013 Website – Easy to use, search and book**[1] – includingw all quality assessed tourism businesses providing up-to-date accessibility information www.openbritain.net
- **New App** – for i-Phone, i-Pad and Android – Find and check accessibility information (live Summer 2013)
- **Membership to Tourism for All**[2] – the UK voice for accessible tourism, providing businesses with the use of logos, access to training, monthly e-newsletter, assistance with access statements and discounts on business support

JOIN TODAY – OPENBRITAIN IS FREE

Quality assessed businesses providing up-to-date accessibility information (using Guestlink) can have a FREE basic entry on the OpenBritain website and data hub

Raise your profile with a Enhanced or Enhanced with gallery entry – from just £60 + VAT a year – Priority listing, more images, online booking and Tourism for All membership

Complete the order form on the following page and click email to book or call me for more information

Alternatively, CALL or EMAIL our friendly team today
Tel: 01733 296913 or email: OB@hudsons-media.co.uk
If you would like to print and post this booking form, please send to:
OpenBritain, Hudson's Media Ltd, 35 Thorpe Road, Peterborough, PE3 6AG

Finding your way around this Guide

The book is divided into two parts. Part 1 provides general advice and guidance to help you organise your trip and includes a list of organisations and resources you may find useful. Part 2 offers you an armchair tour around the British Isles, to help you decide where you might want to go and let you know about some of the local resources available to you in each region.

1: Advice and guidance

Organising your trip
This section helps you think about choosing a destination, understand how accommodation is graded and assessed and finally, book your holiday.

Getting there and travelling around
This section offers advice to help with travel planning, public transport, motoring and parking.

While you're away
This section includes ideas on how to spend your leisure time while away. Because an important part of your freedom on holiday is finding accessible public toilets, we've included details of the National Key Scheme.

Useful resources
A list of organisations that cover the British Isles including those involved with tourism, holiday provision, equipment and vehicle hire, and some helpful publications and websites.

2: Around the British Isles

About each region
A region-by-region tour, including a brief introduction to the area and its tourist attractions, a map, and a list of local resources including tourist boards, transport, sources of local information and advice and local equipment hire companies.

New this year, we are featuring a number of accessible 'Things to see or do' in each region.

You will also find a selection of places to stay, including accommodation assessed under VisitEngland's National Accessible Scheme (NAS). An index of all properties listed can be found at the back of this Guide.

For more comprehensive and detailed accommodation listings, visit the new, Open Britain website at:
Ⓦ www.openbritain.net

FINDING YOUR WAY AROUND THIS GUIDE

Regions and the areas they include

- **Greater London**
  The London boroughs of Greater London and a Central London area, (roughly that within the Congestion Charge area) including the City of London and parts of Camden, Islington, Lambeth, Southwark and Westminster.

- **South East England**
  East Sussex, Kent, Surrey and West Sussex.

- **Southern England**
  Berkshire, Buckinghamshire, Hampshire, the Isle of Wight and Oxfordshire.

- **West Country**
  Gloucestershire, Somerset, Wiltshire, Dorset and the area around Bristol.

- **Devon & Cornwall**

- **Eastern England**
  Bedfordshire, Cambridgeshire, Essex, Hertfordshire, Norfolk and Suffolk.

- **East Midlands**
  Derbyshire, Leicestershire, Lincolnshire, Northamptonshire and Nottinghamshire and the southern part of the area that used to form Humberside.

- **West Midlands**
  Herefordshire, Shropshire, Staffordshire, Warwickshire, West Midlands and Worcestershire.

- **North West England**
  Cheshire, Cumbria, Greater Manchester, Lancashire and Merseyside.

- **Yorkshire**
  North, South and West Yorkshire and the East Riding of Yorkshire and Kingston-upon-Hull districts.

- **North East England**
  Durham, Northumberland and Tyne & Wear and the Tees Valley.

- **South East Scotland**
  Edinburgh, Falkirk, the Lothians and the Scottish Borders.

- **South West Scotland**
  Ayrshire, Dumfries & Galloway, Dunbartonshire, Lanarkshire, Renfrewshire and Glasgow.

- **East Scotland**
  Aberdeenshire, Angus, Clackmannan, Fife, Perth & Kinross and Stirling.

- **Highlands & Islands of Scotland**
  Argyle & Bute, Highlands, Moray, Orkney, Shetland and the Western Isles.

- **North Wales**
  Anglesey, Conwy, Denbighshire, Flintshire and Gwynedd.

- **Mid & West Wales**
  Carmarthenshire, Ceredigion, Pembrokeshire and Powys.

- **South Wales**
  The area that formed the counties of Glamorgan and Gwent including Cardiff and Swansea.

- **Northern Ireland**

- **Republic of Ireland**

- **Channel Islands**

- **Isle of Man**

FINDING YOUR WAY AROUND THIS GUIDE

These regions do not necessarily correspond to official administrative areas but were originally devised for the convenience of Radar National Key Scheme keyholders.

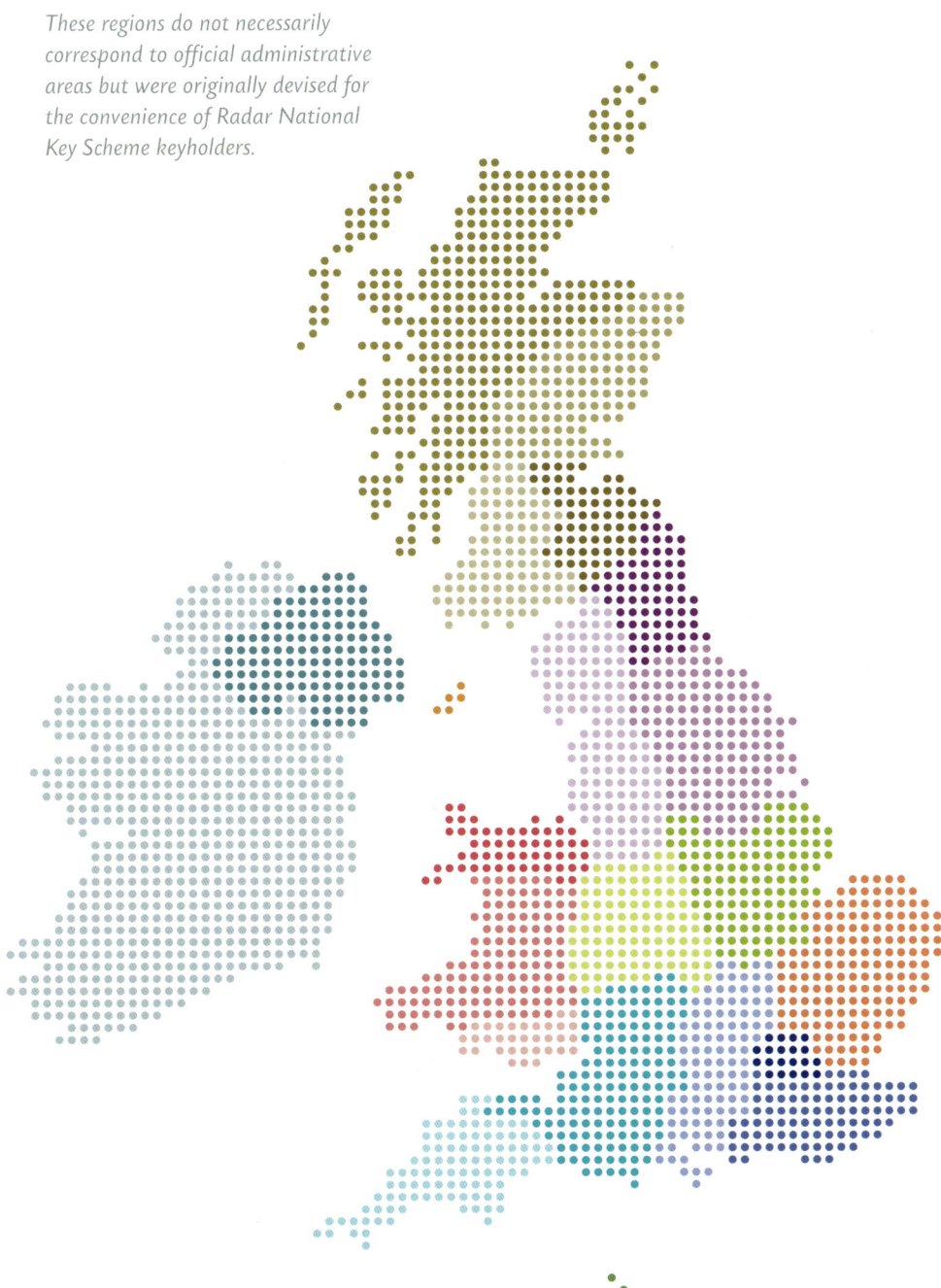

HOLIDAYS IN THE BRITISH ISLES

ADVICE & GUIDANCE

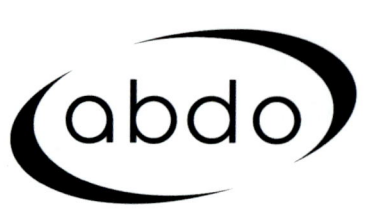

Association of British Dispensing Opticians

ArjoWiggins

Supported by
Arjo Wiggins
Fine Papers
Limited

With best wishes from

A T Graphics Ltd
4 Milnyard Square
Orton Southgate
Peterborough
Cambridgeshire
PE2 6GX

North West Trading Co

Buyers and suppliers of marine and offshore equipment

69 Portsoy Crescent, Ellon,
Aberdeenshire, AB41 8AL

Tel: 01358 729884
Fax: 01358 729885

Email: nwtandco@btconnect.com
Web: www.nwtandco.com

Polux Limited
High temperature cables

Manufacture of high temperature cables and other high temperature products including threads, yarns and fabrics.

● **www.polux.co.uk**

Quartis Ltd

Is pleased to support
Disability Rights UK

ORGANISING YOUR TRIP

Planning your holiday

Holiday brochures often say little about what is available for people with a disability or health condition. However, many providers of holiday-related services do have facilities available and some are committed to providing a comfortable and welcoming experience. So how do you choose where to go and where to stay?

What type of holiday?

Whether you are thinking of a city break to shop and visit art galleries, a peaceful relaxing rest in the countryside or a fun-filled time at the seaside, there will be many destinations in the British Isles to choose from.

Finding inspiration

Holiday brochures and travel magazines are a great source of holiday ideas. Have a look at the travel sections of national newspapers or their online versions. Lots of people write travel and holiday blogs on the internet. For interesting travel tips and ideas, try the Lonely Planet blog or TravelPod.

Where to go?

Finding information

Find out as much as you can about the area you are thinking of visiting. This Guide provides an overview about each region around the British Isles and lists some of the places you can visit when you get there, but it is worth doing more research.

Take a look at our suggested websites and publications for inspiration.

You can get help, advice and ideas from tourist information centres and travel companies. Call in to speak to them in person or get in touch by email or telephone.

Where to stay?

Do you want to be pampered in a five-star hotel, self-cater in a countryside cottage, have fun in a holiday park or are you looking for a respite break?

Your questions will be similar. What kind of accommodation shall I stay in? How do I look at the choices? How will I know that it is the quality I expected? Will it have the facilities or nearby resources that I want? How can I find out whether it will meet my requirements if I have an accessibility need?

HOLIDAYS IN THE BRITISH ISLES

ADVICE & GUIDANCE

Would you like a hotel with a swimming pool? Somewhere you can bring a pet? Holiday providers, guidebooks and tourist boards use slightly different symbols to represent facilities at premises or leisure facilities. They should let you see at a glance whether the hotel has the general facilities you want.

> **TOP TIP**
>
> Remember you can only do so much by email. Talking to the people who run the accommodation can be helpful. It is always worth asking what they can do to help you out. A large hotel chain may have someone specifically responsible for accessibility.
>
> Ask as many questions as you need and find out as much as you can about the accommodation before you book. When you have decided, try to book accommodation well in advance.

Grading systems for accommodation quality are quite consistent. When you find accommodation of the right quality, within your price range, check the facilities directly with the provider. Some places will have all the facilities you want. Others may seem less well equipped but if you talk to them in advance, they may be able to arrange for the support or equipment you need.

ORGANISING YOUR TRIP

Finding accommodation

So how do you find the right kind of accommodation of the right quality that will also meet your accessibility needs? You have the right and should ask hotels to provide you with their 'Access Statement'. You can also research online or look for hotels that have been assessed under the National Accessible Scheme.

Checking accessibility

Accessible accommodation can be enjoyed by everyone, including people with access needs. This includes people with hearing and visual impairments, wheelchair users, older and less mobile people and people with pushchairs.

Some hotels include accessibility information on their websites. You can also find details via national and local tourist board websites or at:
- www.openbritain.net
- www.disabledgo.com

Look for symbols which show that the accommodation has been assessed or audited by DisabledGo or under the National Accessible Scheme (NAS). Check that the information is still up to date by contacting the hotel directly and ask about their facilities and rooms specifically designed for disabled people.

Ask for their Access Statement: This is an explanation of how access and facilities for disabled people have been addressed in their particular accommodation. If you are considering booking, it's a good idea to make any access requests in writing as you will then have a record that you asked about these services. The last thing you want to do is arrive and find out that the person on duty has no record of the things you need.

If you have mobility problems you may want to ask for a room on the lowest floor so that you're not dependent on lifts in an emergency. Every place that offers accommodation should have a clear plan and instructions about what to do if there is a fire or other emergency when you need to get out safely.

If you use a wheelchair, let the hotel know how wide it is. Ask them to confirm door widths and make sure there is space to move your wheelchair around comfortably. If the room has a roll-in shower, ask if they have an adapted shower wheelchair you can use. Think about the additional equipment that you use at home.

HOLIDAYS IN THE BRITISH ISLES

ADVICE & GUIDANCE

Assessing accessibility

ENGLAND
National Accessible Scheme (NAS)
The National Accessible Scheme, run by VisitEngland is a nationally recognised rating of the accessibility of visitor accommodation to enable you to know which accommodation providers are best for you. Their standards cover mobility, visual and hearing impairments.

Accommodation that has been assessed as meeting NAS standards can display one or more of the symbols on the right.

You can find out more about the Scheme on the VisitEngland website at:
 www.visitengland.com/accessforall

At the back of this Guide you will find an index showing all accommodation listed in each region, with its relevant NAS symbol.

For a full list of NAS assessed properties, visit:
 www.openbritain.net

Mobility Impairment Logos

Older and less mobile guests
If you can climb a flight of stairs, but banisters or grip handles would make this easier, look out for this logo.

Part-time wheelchair users
If you have problems walking or can walk a maximum of 3 steps, or need to use a wheelchair some of the time, look out for this logo.

Independent wheelchair users
Similar to the international logo for independent wheelchair users. If you're a wheelchair user and travel independently, look out for this logo.

Assisted wheelchair users
If you're a wheelchair user and travel with a friend or family member who helps you with everyday tasks, this logo applies to you.

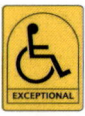
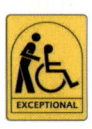

Access Exceptional
Achieves the standards above for either independent wheelchair users or assisted wheelchair users and fulfils additional, more demanding requirements with reference to the British Standard BS 8300.

ORGANISING YOUR TRIP

Visual Impairment Logos

Visually impaired and blind people (1)
If you have difficulty reading small print, are registered blind, have poor sight or a visual impairment, accommodation with this logo is suitable for you.

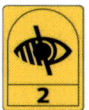

Visually impaired and blind people (2)
An exceptional level of facilities and services that would be suitable for anyone with a visual impairment from mild sight loss to having no sight at all.

Hearing Impairment Logos

Hearing impaired and deaf people (1)
If you have a slight hearing difficulty, are deaf, wear a hearing aid or have a hearing impairment, look out for accommodation displaying this logo.

Hearing impaired and deaf people (2)
An exceptional level of facilities and services that would be suitable for anyone with a hearing impairment from mild hearing loss to profound deafness.

SCOTLAND
Accessibility categories

As part of the VisitScotland grading scheme, properties are inspected and graded by Quality Advisors using criteria drawn up in co-operation with wheelchair users. Where a property holds one of the awards below, at least one bedroom in a hotel, guesthouse, B&B or hostel is accessible to the level given.

They are awarded one or more of the following gradings:

Category 1: Wheelchair access without assistance. Accessible to a wheelchair user travelling independently.

Category 2: Wheelchair access with assistance. Accessible to a wheelchair user travelling with assistance.

Category 3: Access for those with mobility impairment. Accessible to a wheelchair user able to walk a few paces and up a maximum of three steps.

You can find detailed descriptions of each category online or get more information by calling:
- 0845 859 1006
- www.visitscotland.com

HOLIDAYS IN THE BRITISH ISLES

ADVICE & GUIDANCE

And search facilities to locate appropriate accommodation at:
- www.visitscotland/accommodation/accessible

WALES
You can search for accommodation on the VisitWales website and can filter your search for suitability according to mobility, hearing or visual impairment.
- www.visitwales.co.uk

REPUBLIC OF IRELAND
By law, to comply with the Disability Act, Fáilte Ireland (the Irish national tourism authority) must make its buildings, services and information accessible to people with disabilities. The Fáilte Ireland Access Officer can be contacted to arrange help or information for people with disabilities to access the services and information it provides.
- 01 8847781
- accessibility@failteireland.ie

LONDON
Direct Enquiries has carried out access audits of selected hotels around the UK. Their resource is particularly helpful for hotels in London. They use a system with 18 basic and 11 additional disabled access symbols to represent specific access resources.

Directory Enquiries also run Inclusive London; an online nationwide access register of buildings, venues and services. Inclusive London's listings are compiled from Access Audits, guided telephone access assessments and information supplied by the businesses listed and user-contributed information.

Find out more at:
- www.directenquiries.com
- www.inclusivelondon.com

Visit London provide the *Official London Tourist Guide* and this contains a wide range of information on access.
- www.visitlondon.com

Assessing quality

STAR RATINGS

Each assessing body works to very similar criteria and awards a number of stars from one to five, to reflect facilities and overall quality. The more stars awarded, the higher the level of quality. If you see a quality assessment logo displayed next to your chosen accommodation, it means an official assessor has visited, and rated.

How is accommodation graded?

The star rating system covers all kinds of accommodation including:
- Hotel (country house, small hotel, town house and metro hotel);
- Guest house, B&B, farmhouse, inn, restaurant with rooms;
- Self-catering, campus accommodation, serviced apartments;
- Touring park, campsite, caravan park, timber lodge or chalet.

Different types of accommodation offer different facilities so each type of accommodation is assessed in different ways and different criteria apply according to the market's expectation of that kind of accommodation.

For details about quality assessments in Britain, visit the relevant tourist board website for each country you are thinking of visiting. You can also find details of accommodation definitions and quality ratings at:

AA
- www.theaa.com/travel/accommodation_restaurants_grading.html

England
- www.qualityintourism.com

Scotland
- www.visitscotland.com/quality-assurance

Wales
- www.visitwales.co.uk/holiday-accommodation-in-wales/grading-visit-wales-tourist

Northern Ireland
- www.discovernorthernireland.com/Accommodation-Rating-System-A1592

The Republic of Ireland
- www.discoverireland.ie/shamrock
- www.discoverireland.ie/Where-To-Stay/Accommodation-Guide

Some of these sites also have online search and booking systems to help you identify and contact accommodation with the specific facilities you need.

ADVICE & GUIDANCE

AWARD SCHEMES

England

VisitEngland gives awards to hotels and guest accommodation (Gold only for Self-Catering and Caravan Parks) that provide exceptional quality in all areas.

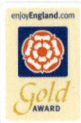

Gold award: This award is given to Hotels, Guest Accommodation, Self-Catering properties and Caravan Parks. It reflects a very high level of quality. Properties achieving the Gold award have exceptional levels of quality, comfort and cleanliness in bedrooms and bathrooms, and outstanding levels of customer care and food.

Silver award: This award is given to Hotels and Guest Accommodation. It reflects a high level of quality, comfort and cleanliness in bedrooms and bathrooms with very good levels of customer care and food provision.

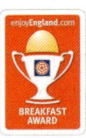

Breakfast award: Sponsored by Kellogg's, this award recognises those hotels and B&Bs that offer their guests a quality and choice of breakfast, service and hospitality that exceeds what would be expected at their star rating.

Scotland

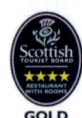

Gold award: In Scotland the Gold award recognises serviced accommodation which consistently achieves the highest levels of excellence within their VisitScotland star grading. Scotland's equivalent of England's Caravan Parks Gold award is the Thistle award.

Wales

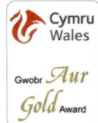

Gold award: Recognises outstanding quality, exceptional comfort and unfailing hospitality.

HOLIDAYS IN THE BRITISH ISLES

ORGANISING YOUR TRIP

Ways to book

You can book your holiday in a number of ways. You can use a travel agent, a tour operator, go direct to an accommodation or travel provider or book online, although there may be limits to booking accessible accommodation via mainstream websites.

Booking through an agent

Some tour operators and holiday services specialise in holidays for disabled people. Whether you choose a specialist or go to a general provider, it is sensible to book holidays through travel agents or tour operators that are members of the Association of British Travel Agents (ABTA). Their booking conditions will meet ABTA's code of conduct. And, if the company runs into financial difficulties ABTA can help you to get money back. They also run an arbitration scheme to deal with complaints about their members.

Association of British Travel Agents (ABTA)
30 Park Street, London SE1 9EQ
☎ 0901 201 5050
🌐 www.abta.com

Booking on the internet

The internet has changed the process of booking travel and holidays and it is a good way to compare prices and find last-minute deals.

To get the best deals you may need to be flexible about dates and/or the place you want to go. If you have specific requirements, you will need to balance these against possible cost savings.

To get the best deal, you will need to do plenty of research so leave yourself good time. There are lots of websites that can help, with some specialising in flights and others in accommodation. Booking flights and hotels separately can save money, but bundles or package deals are often cheaper.

Travel
Specialist websites like Skyscanner or Cheapflights.co.uk are useful for flights. Recently, Kayak.com has emerged as an up-and-coming favourite but a quick Google search will bring up lots of alternatives. It is worth trying several different sites as each collates information about available flights in different ways.

Plan rail ticket purchases 12 weeks before your travel date. This is usually when advance tickets (generally the cheapest fares) become available.

HOLIDAYS IN THE BRITISH ISLES

ADVICE & GUIDANCE

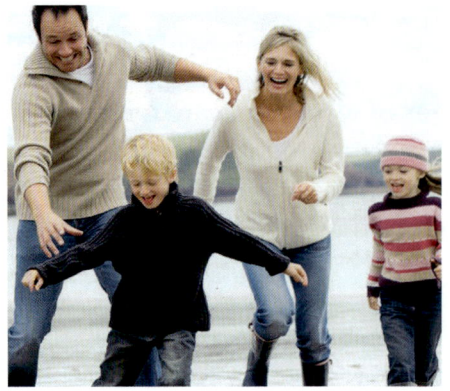

The Trainline offers an email alert system which lets you know when advance tickets for a specific journey come on sale.
 www.thetrainline.com

Hotels
Once you've arranged your travel, you will need a place to stay. You can book online through websites like Hotels.com, LateRooms and Trivago. Once you've located some suitable accommodation, you can sort results in terms of price, star rating or criteria such as distance from the airport or city centre.

Take the time to look carefully at what is included in the price. Sometimes the total booking price doesn't cover breakfast, towels, VAT or internet use.

Packages
While some websites specialise in either travel or accommodation, others focus on package deals. Examples include lastminute.com, Expedia and TravelSupermarket.com.

Most holiday sites – including those specialising in flights, hotels or travel to particular regions – now offer holiday options as a bundle. This is more common with flights abroad but it can also work with UK destinations and holidays too. Planning your whole trip on one website can often save you money.

Explore all of the different options available to you if you're looking for a bargain.

FINDING THE BEST DEAL
Comparison websites are useful when you know where you want to go and have specific dates for travel in mind. If you're someone who's always on the lookout for a fantastic holiday deal, the web has other very handy resources:

The travel agent's website
The cheapest holidays are sometimes available directly from travel agents. For example, Thomson and MyTravel put their latest offers in a special section of the site. Bookmarking them on your computer and checking back regularly could be one way to find a great deal.

Travelzoo
When you sign-up for free at Travelzoo you'll receive a weekly email newsletter filled with the site's current most popular holiday deals. To take advantage of a deal, you'll need to purchase an online voucher, which can be redeemed once you've decided when to travel.
 www.travelzoo.com

ORGANISING YOUR TRIP

Review websites
Booking a last-minute holiday can be risky but it doesn't always have to be the case. It is always worth looking at user reviews on websites such as TripAdvisor. If you can, send in your own reviews of places you have stayed and the services you have received as a disabled person.

Booking directly

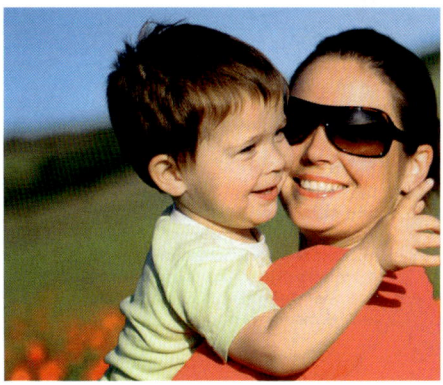

If you prefer, you can telephone or email to book directly with your chosen accommodation or holiday provider.

Describe any facilities or adjustments you need when you make the booking. If you need help to get to and from the place you are staying, then make sure you tell the provider when you book.

It is helpful to confirm by email so you can write down everything you need. If you book with a travel agent, they should let you contact a venue directly, particularly if you need to find out about equipment or support.

Your disability or health condition
You will need to decide how much you want to say about your disability when you make enquiries and bookings. The more information you can give the better, but the decision about how much you disclose is up to you. You might want to keep things private or ask them to be discreet. The most important information to share is about the adjustments you need.

Some accommodation providers might assume things about you if you are disabled. But remember that it is never OK for anyone to discriminate against you because of your disability or health condition.

TOP TIP
When comparing holidays, look carefully at what the price includes. Paying less for something that doesn't meet your requirements might be a false economy. Read the full terms and conditions before booking. There are sometimes extra costs, which could see you paying more than you thought.

ADVICE & GUIDANCE

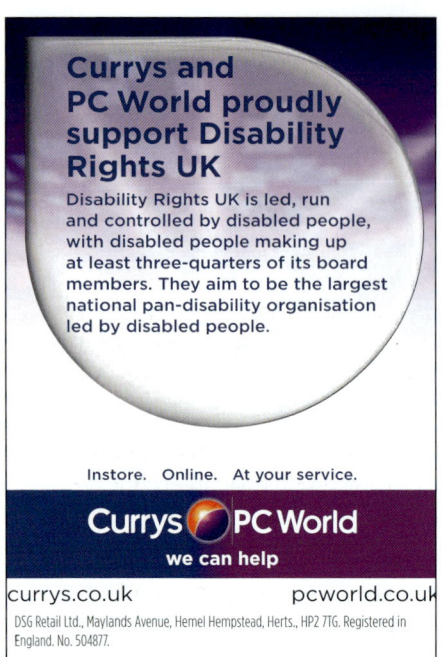

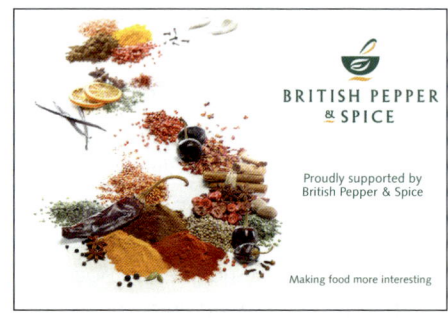

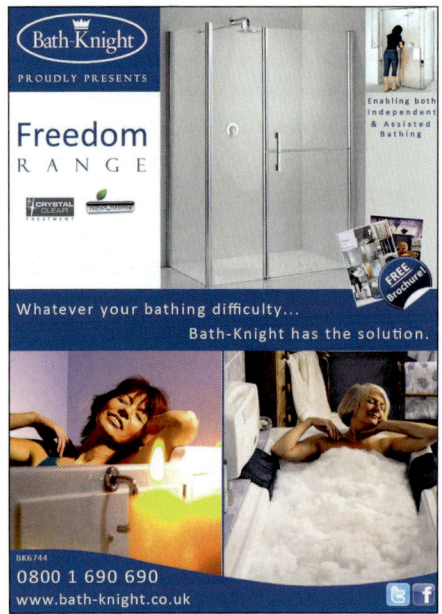

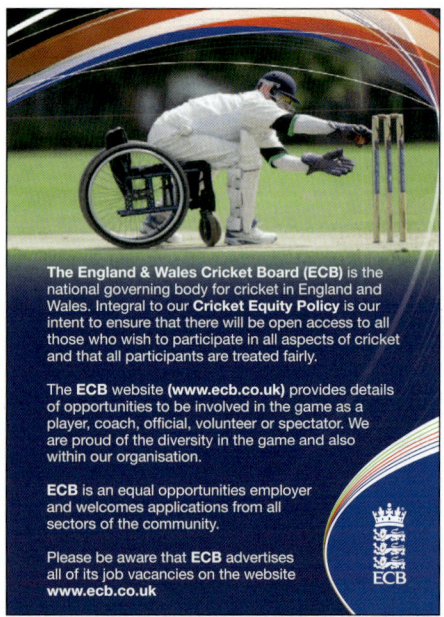

Before you go

There are key things everyone should check before going away on holiday. As a disabled person, there may be additional things you need to organise before you go.

Key things to check

The list below will give you some idea of the things you may wish to check before setting off on your holiday:
- Double check that all your holiday arrangements are in place;
- Make a list of any extra equipment you might need to take with you;
- If you need medicines, take more than you may need and take a written prescription for more, in case you lose them or run out. If you have to go through any security checks, it is helpful to have documentation that explains what your medicines are.

INSURANCE

Everyone should get insurance before they travel. You never know if your trip might get cancelled or you might be ill and not able to go. If you have no insurance, then there is little you can do to get your money back.

Make sure you get appropriate insurance for your type of holiday. You might need a specific type of insurance, particularly if you are travelling or going on an activity holiday.

If you already have a policy, check what it says before you go. You might need to get in touch with them and change it.

Your rights as a disabled person

All companies have a legal duty to make sure that they do not treat you, as a disabled customer, in a less favourable way than they would treat other customers. The Equality Act (2010) places duties on service providers, which includes insurance and travel companies providing services within the UK. For example, a company must not refuse to provide a service to a disabled person that they offer to other members of the public unless this can be justified (see below). In addition, they must not provide the service on terms or standards that are worse than those they would give to any other consumer.

However, the law does allow insurers to apply special conditions or extra charges to disabled people in certain circumstances. They can charge a disabled person a higher premium, if they can show that we are at a greater risk and therefore more likely to make a claim.

ADVICE & GUIDANCE

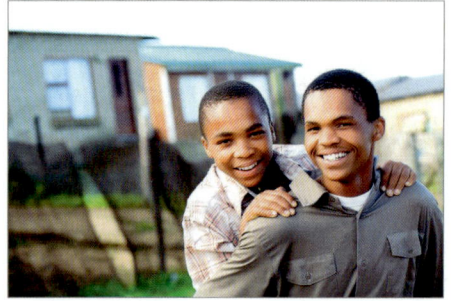

An insurance company can only justify a difference of treatment of a disabled person if:
- the decision is based on information which is relevant to the assessment of the risk being insured against;
- the information (such as statistical data, or a medical report) is from a source on which it is reasonable to rely;
- the less favourable treatment is reasonable when this information and all other relevant factors are taken into account.

It is worth checking whether any standard policy offered by a travel company meets your individual situation, including that of any equipment that has to be taken. Some voluntary organisations can assist their members, or people with the condition with which they are concerned, to obtain appropriate insurance cover which would otherwise be difficult.

Some companies with insurance packages designed specifically for disabled people are:

All Clear Travel Insurance
All Clear House, 1 Redwing Court, Ashton Road, Romford, Essex RM3 8QQ
- 0845 250 5350
- info@allcleartravel.co.uk
- www.allcleartravel.co.uk

Chartwell Insurance
Chartwell Insurance Services, East Winch Hall, East Winch, King's Lynn, Norfolk PE32 1HN
- 0844 888 5222
- info@chartwellinsurance.co.uk
- www.chartwellinsurance.co.uk

En Route Insurance
5th Floor, Cavendish House, Breeds Place, Hastings, East Sussex TN34 3AA
- 0800 783 7245
- info@enrouteinsurance.co.uk
- www.enrouteinsurance.co.uk

Fogg Travel Insurance Services Ltd
Crow Hill Drive, Mansfield, Nottinghamshire NG19 7AE
- 01623 631331
- sales@fogginsure.co.uk
- www.fogginsure.co.uk

Free Spirit
Stansted House, Rowlands Castle, Hampshire PO9 6DX
- 0845 230 5000
- contact@freespirittravelinsurance.com
- www.freespirittravelinsurance.com

Rights & wrongs

You've done your research, arranged the facilities you need and completed all your checks. You should have a hassle-free and successful holiday. But sometimes, despite best-laid plans, things go wrong. A holiday provider might not understand your needs or the standard of accommodation you expected. Here we explain our rights as disabled people, the treatment we should expect and what to do if something does go wrong.

Your rights

THE LAW

Under the Equality Act 2010, service providers in the UK must make 'reasonable adjustments' to make sure disabled people are not discriminated against. Service providers include organisations that provide:
- holiday accommodation
- tourist attractions
- restaurants and places to eat
- transport and ways to get around (please note, air travel is covered by other regulations, see below)

They cannot refuse to serve you or provide a lower standard of service because of your disability.

You cannot be treated unfavourably because of something connected with your disability, unless they can show, in a reasonable way, why they cannot change things for you.

What is a 'reasonable adjustment'?
When a disabled person wants to access or use a service, the service provider has to make 'reasonable adjustments' to any aspect of their service that would put a disabled person at a substantial disadvantage compared to a non-disabled person.

Under the Equality Act 2010, service providers only need to make changes that are 'reasonable'. These might include simple changes to layout, improved signage and staff training to improve accessibility for disabled customers. It might be something as simple as changing check-out times to accommodate your needs.

It's about what is practical in each individual situation and what resources the provider has. They will not be required to make changes that are impractical or beyond their means.

ADVICE & GUIDANCE

Reasonable adjustments can include:
- using large print for registration and guest information;
- ensuring that at least one copy of a menu is in Braille;
- providing phones with large buttons;
- providing portable vibrating alarms for guests who will not be able to hear an audible fire alarm;
- where a low reception desk is not available, providing an alternative low desk for wheelchair users.

In the UK, information produced by travel agents, tour operators, airports and airlines should be clear and simple to use. They should also take reasonable steps to make sure that their information services are accessible to disabled people. It should be available in accessible formats, such as Braille, large print or on audiotape but you may need to ask specifically and give them time to provide it.

Civil Aviation Authority Regulations for air travel

Any passenger in the UK that faces difficulty travelling within an airport or on board an aircraft through disability, injury, age or any other reason, is entitled to help from the airport or airline. Your rights as a disabled passenger apply across the EU and the UK Civil Aviation Authority (CAA) is responsible for enforcing them here in the UK.

CAA took over responsibility for handling air travel complaints from disabled people from the Equality and Human Rights Commission in 2012. If you are unhappy with the service you receive when travelling, you should first contact the airport or airline you used to complain. If you don't receive a satisfactory response, the CAA can then take up the case on your behalf.

> The CAA has now set up the 'Disability advisory group' – a forum where disability groups, consumer groups, the Department for Transport and the CAA can share data on the issues of most concern.

It is always worth getting in touch with your airline and/or airport at least 48 hours before you fly to let them know of any needs you have as this can help improve the level of support you receive.

Your responsibilities

Remember that service providers may have conditions they ask you to meet in order that they can provide you with appropriate facilities or support. Telling them your requirements is a good way to help them meet yours.

Communicating your needs

Make sure you explain your particular requirements clearly, particularly if your impairment or condition is not obvious or if you are booking by phone, post or

ORGANISING YOUR TRIP

over the internet. Don't expect staff at travel agents, travel offices or airports automatically to know or understand your needs.

If you are in a hotel or guesthouse and it will take you longer than most people to get ready in the morning, ask if you can check out slightly later. Sometimes just asking will prompt a hotel to offer an adjustment that can make all the difference to the comfort of your stay.

Your feedback after your holiday
We are often encouraged to give feedback about a holiday or accommodation. Giving your comments to the holiday provider or making comments online can reward good providers with positive marketing and encourage poor providers to improve.

What if things go wrong?

Good service providers know that making their services more accessible will benefit disabled people and could result in recommendations and return visits. If a problem arises, try to deal with it in a way that encourages them to treat you the same as any customer whose business they want to keep.

Try to sort things out amicably at the time they happen: Often problems can be solved if you tell the provider straight away.

Experiencing discrimination or a provider refusing to make adjustments for your needs: If this happens then you have legal rights under the Equality Act (2010) which requires service providers not to discriminate and to make adjustments that are reasonable. Reminding a holiday provider of this can prompt them to be more flexible and sort things out for you. If you think you may have experienced discrimination you should get in touch with the Equality Advisory Support Service (EASS) – you can find their contact details in the 'Useful resources' section of this Guide.

Complaints to do with where you are staying that are not to do with disability: If general standards in the accommodation are not what you were expecting then you should complain. Holiday providers should have a way for you to do this. For example, you might need to go to the tourist body that runs the provider or to the organisation awarding the quality rating.

Complain as soon as possible after discovering the problem. If the problem arose while you were on holiday it will help if you can show you complained at the time. Write to the holiday or accommodation provider you are complaining to, even if you have already made the complaint in person or by phone.

HOLIDAYS IN THE BRITISH ISLES

ADVICE & GUIDANCE

If your complaint is not resolved or you need some help making the complaint, contact your local Citizens Advice Bureau. Citizens Advice produce a factsheet on making a complaint about your holiday (dowloadable from their website).

Find out if the tour operator or agent you booked with is a member of a trade association such as the Association of British Travel Agents (ABTA). ABTA have some useful publications about complaints in the 'Consumer Zone' of their website. They also operate an arbitration and conciliation service to resolve disputes but you will have to pay a fee for this. If your accommodation or holiday provider is not a member of ABTA, contact the Citizens Advice Consumer Helpline.

Association of British Travel Agents
30 Park Street, London SE1 9EQ
- 0901 2015050
- www.abta.com

Citizens Advice Consumer Helpline
- 08454 040506
  08454 040505 Welsh language line
- www.adviceguide.org.uk

Offers information and advice on problems with goods and services, energy and post.

In Northern Ireland:
Consumerline
- 0300 123 6262
- www.consumerline.org.uk

GETTING THERE & TRAVELLING AROUND

Public transport

In the past, public transport was developed with little or no regard to the needs of disabled people. Thankfully this has changed – particularly as transport regulations under various pieces of both UK and EC law come into effect. However, progress still needs to be made both geographically and with various forms of transport.

Travel planning

It makes sense to plan your journey in advance. If you think you might need assistance at any point in the journey, let the people running the services know about what help you need.

In most of England, county and unitary councils have responsibilities for public transport and have a Public Transport Information Officer. Some publish specific information for disabled passengers. Elsewhere, in larger towns and cities, this responsibility is carried out by Passenger Transport Executives (PTEs) and in London, by Transport for London. Contact details for the relevant regional organisations are listed here.

> You will find even more information on transport in Disability Rights UK's self-help guide *If only I'd known that* – an information-packed guide to services, welfare rights and facilities, it covers all ages from childhood to later years. Visit www.disabilityrightsuk.org.

Centro/Network West Midlands
Centro House, 16 Summer Lane, Birmingham B19 3SD
- 0121 200 2700
  Textphone 0121 214 2787
- www.cento.org.uk

Transport for Greater Manchester
2 Piccadilly Place, Manchester M1 3BG
- 0161 244 1000
- www.tfgm.com

MerseyTravel
PO BOX 1976, Liverpool L69 3HN
- 0151 227 5181
  Textphone 0151 330 1087
- www.merseytravel.gov.uk

Metro – Public transport for West Yorkshire
Wellington House, 40-50 Wellington Street, Leeds LS1 2DE
- 0113 245 7676
- www.wymetro.com

ADVICE & GUIDANCE

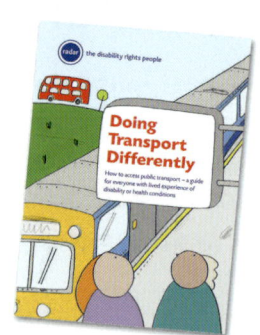

Make the most of your holiday

Asking the right questions when you're booking a holiday can make a real difference to your experience and enjoyment of your time away. ABTA provides expert guidance and advice for disabled and less mobile travellers on its website to help you get the most out of your holiday, including a checklist of questions to ask your travel agent or tour operator.

www.abta.com

ABTA The Travel Association

Doing Transport Differently

This guide includes information and travellers' tales to help and inspire people with lived experience of disability or health conditions to use public transport.

Available to order from our online shop
www.disabilityrightsuk.org

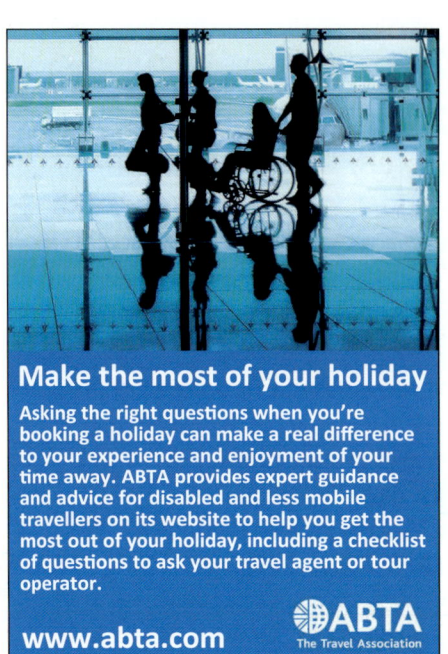

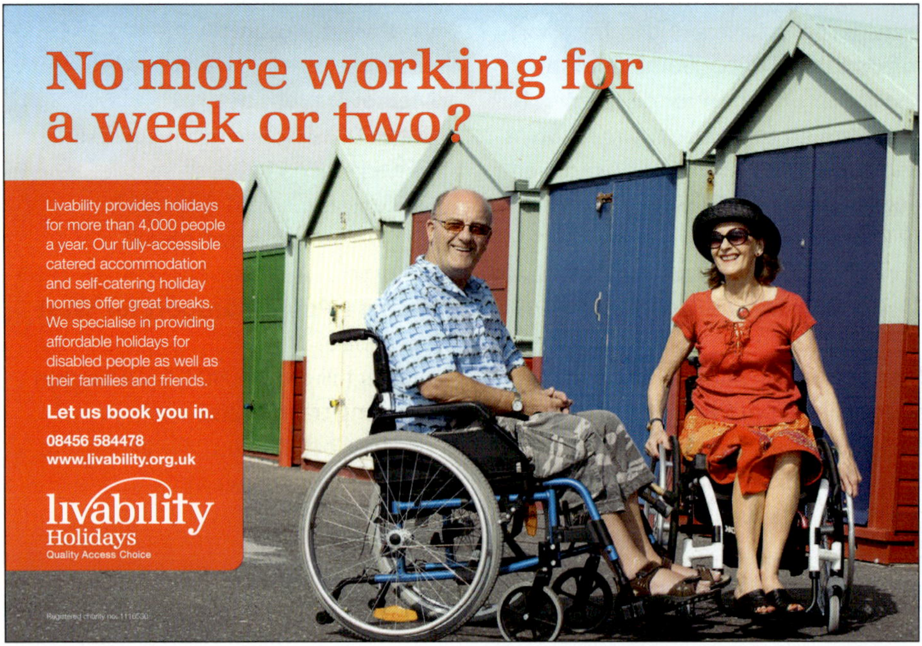

No more working for a week or two?

Livability provides holidays for more than 4,000 people a year. Our fully-accessible catered accommodation and self-catering holiday homes offer great breaks. We specialise in providing affordable holidays for disabled people as well as their families and friends.

Let us book you in.
08456 584478
www.livability.org.uk

livability Holidays
Quality Access Choice

HOLIDAYS IN THE BRITISH ISLES

GETTING THERE & TRAVELLING AROUND

Nexus – Travel in Tyne and Wear
Grainger Chambers, Hood Street,
Newcastle upon Tyne NE1 6JQ
- ☎ 0191 202 0747
  Textphone 0191 202 0501
- 🌐 www.nexus.org.uk

South Yorkshire Passenger Transport Executive
11 Broad Street West, Sheffield S1 2BQ
- ☎ 0114 276 7575
- 🌐 www.sypte.co.uk

Transport for London
Travel Information, 55 Broadway,
London SW1H 0BD
- ☎ 020 7222 1234
  Textphone 020 7918 3015
- ✉ travinfo@tfl.gov.uk
- 🌐 www.tfl.gov.uk

In Northern Ireland, rail and bus services are overseen by:

Translink
Central Station, Belfast BT1 3PB
- ☎ 028 9066 6630
  Textphone 028 9035 4007
- 🌐 www.translink.co.uk

In Scotland, the national transport agency liaises with Regional Transport Partnerships and has a range of executive functions including administering fare concessions and the Blue Badge Scheme.

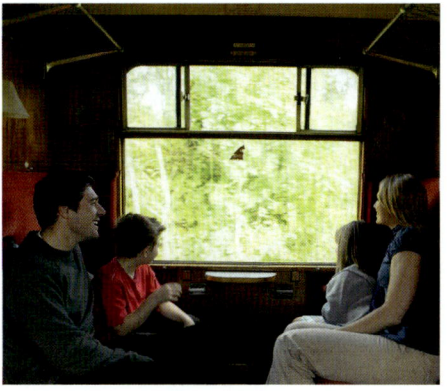

Transport Scotland
Buchanan House, 58 Portdundas Road,
Glasgow G4 0HF
- ☎ 0141 272 7100
- 🌐 www.transportscotland.gov.uk

> Disability Rights UK produce *Doing Transport Differently,* a publication that lets people with any kind of disability – learning difficulties, mental health conditions, visual impairments, hearing impairments, wheelchair users, mobility impairments and more – know what kind of access is out there, how to plan your journey, and what to do if things go wrong. The guide is written by and for disabled people and is full of travellers' experiences of using trains, buses, coaches, undergrounds, light railways, ferries and more. To download your free copy visit www.disabilityrightsuk.org

ADVICE & GUIDANCE

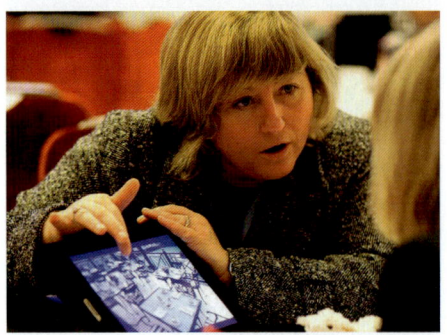

In Wales transport planning is undertaken by four Regional Transport Consortia:

For South East Wales
SEWTA
www.sewta.gov.uk

For South West Wales
SWWITCH
www.swwitch.net

For North Wales
Taith
www.taith.gov.uk

For Mid Wales
TraCC
www.tracc.gov.uk

Nationally, general information on transport services and timetables is available through:

Traveline
0871 200 2233
Text service 84268
www.traveline.org.uk

You can also find information at:

www.transportdirect.info
A transport planning website that includes options for using all types of public transport and private motoring for point-to-point journeys in Great Britain.

Ricability is an independent consumer research charity offering free, practical and unbiased reports for older and disabled people. Ricability published a report called *Wheels Within Wheels* – a guide to using a wheelchair on public transport. To find out more, visit www.ricability.org.uk or write to: Unit G03, Wenlock Business Centre, 50-56 Wharf Road, London N1 7EU. Telephone 020 7427 2460 Textphone 020 7427 2469.

TRAVEL TRAINING
In some areas, travel training is available to help disabled people use buses and other forms of public transport independently. This sort of training can help you gain confidence, particularly if you are more used to using specialist transport.

TRAVEL IN LONDON
Public transport in London is becoming more accessible, even more so due to the legacy left by the London 2012 Olympic and Paralympic Games. Buses, taxis, the Docklands Light Railway and London Tramlink all provide accessible services.

In addition many private hire (minicab) firms operate wheelchair accessible vehicles.

If you are older or disabled and public transport is not always accessible to you, assisted transport services may be the answer. You can find out more about assisted travel options including Dial-a-Ride, Taxicard and Capital Call, as well as community transport schemes on the Transport for London website:
 www.tfl.gov.uk

You can use assisted travel to go shopping, visit friends or family, go to the library, or for other recreational purposes. However, you cannot use these services for work or hospital appointments. You can read more about getting around and accessible things to do in London in the London section of this guide.

Air travel

Under new European law, if you are disabled or have difficulty moving around you can receive assistance when you fly to and from Europe, including domestic flights.

You do not need to be permanently or physically disabled to benefit from this service. In fact, anyone who has difficulty moving around, for example, because of their disability, age or a temporary injury, can receive help when they fly.

Remember that air travel is an international industry. This means that if you fly outside of the UK then you may encounter different attitudes and practices towards disability.

Things that can make air travel more complicated for disabled passengers can arise from security requirements, design and safety features of aircraft, the size of airports, and for many people, unfamiliarity with the environment.

Under EC Regulation 1107/2006 it is illegal for an airline, travel agent or tour operator to refuse a booking solely on the grounds of disability. Note however that for certain, non stable medical conditions associated with your disability, you may need medical clearance before being allowed to fly. Airport managers are required to organise the provision of the services necessary to enable disabled passengers to board, disembark and ensure a safe transit between flights. Each airline is responsible for services onboard its aircraft and should not charge extra for giving support or making an adjustment. This is against the law.

In Britain, if you are refused boarding on the grounds of disability or reduced mobility or do not get the services you have requested and need you should contact the Equality Advisory Support Service, further details can be found in the 'Useful resources' section of this Guide.

ADVICE & GUIDANCE

They will advise you on your rights and may have to refer the matter to the Civil Aviation Authority (CAA). The CAA has the power to prosecute. An airline found guilty of discrimination could face an unlimited fine.

Here are some tips that you can use when travelling by plane:

1. Before you fly
Consider the kind of assistance you may need, and check the airline's safety rules.

2. Booking your flight
Always tell your airline, travel agent or tour operator at least 48 hours in advance if you need special assistance.

3. Arriving at the airport
Find out in advance about the layout and facilities at your chosen airport. If you have asked for assistance, then airport staff should be expecting you when you arrive.

4. At the check in desk
Remember to confirm any pre-booked assistance when you check in. Seats with extra legroom are always in demand, so if you need one, explain why.

5. Moving through the airport
Airports must provide free assistance to get disabled and less mobile passengers to their flight.

6. Boarding the flight
Disabled and less mobile passengers will usually be called for boarding first. All staff who deal with customers must have disability awareness training.

7. On board
Airlines must make all reasonable efforts to arrange suitable seating for you. You can take up to two items of mobility equipment onto the aircraft.

8. Leaving the plane
Unless you're in a hurry, you will usually be the last to leave as it's easier to move around in an empty cabin.

GETTING HELP
Equality Advisory Support Service
FREEPOST Equality Advisory Support Service FPN4431
☎ 0800 444 205
  Textphone 0800 444 206
  Opening hours:
  09:00 to 20:00 Monday to Friday
  10:00 to 14:00 Saturday
  Closed Sundays and Bank Holidays

This new service replaces the helpline run by the Equality and Human Rights Commission. The Helpline is for individuals who think they may have experienced discrimination, including when travelling by air. The service aims to support individuals referred from local organisations, advisory groups, faith based organisations and other groups working within the community that support people experiencing discrimination.

Assistance for disabled passengers
Airlines generally have established procedures for assisting disabled passengers. Most disabled people, particularly those with permanent

GETTING THERE & TRAVELLING AROUND

and stable conditions, won't require medical clearance before travelling. However, the rules vary between airlines. For certain conditions you will generally need clearance for flying even if you don't normally need treatment. It is important to check when you book what, if any, medical information will be required.

Most airports are accessible and many have introduced facilities and services to make it easier for disabled people to use them. However, many airport terminals are large, complex premises so finding facilities and assistance may be difficult. Some people, who normally manage independently, may need assistance. Airports often have information for disabled people on their website and some publish access guides.

Wheelchair users should be able to use their own wheelchairs until boarding. Other people may be given wheelchair assistance to reach the aircraft door. Depending on the airline and the size of the aircraft there may be an on-board wheelchair to help you transfer to your seat.

You may be able to request a seat in a particular area, say near a toilet or with extra legroom. However, for safety reasons airlines allocate seats beside emergency exits (which do have more space) to people who are perceived as having the necessary dexterity and strength to open the doors.

Most pieces of equipment required by a disabled passenger are carried free of charge. Larger items (including wheelchairs) are carried in the hold, but smaller items can be taken into the cabin.

You should ask the airline about carriage of equipment – particularly if you may need it during the flight and, especially if you intend on carrying liquid medicine on board.

You may need to ask in advance for any assistance or service that you might need in connection with your flight. Air travel often involves more organisations than other forms of transport, particularly if the flight is by a charter aircraft as part of a holiday package. Usually requested arrangements work out well but when things do go wrong it is often the result of a failure in the communication chain. It is therefore advisable to check that appropriate messages have been passed on. You may need to emphasise the importance of the requests.

> More detailed information is included in *Your Rights to Fly – What you need to know* issued by the Equality & Human Rights Commission in 2009. The booklet can be downloaded from www.equalityhumanrights.com and is available in Easy Read format.

ADVICE & GUIDANCE

FURTHER INFORMATION ON FLYING AND THE LAW

Information from the EHRC

EC Regulation 1107/2006 affects the whole of the air travel process, not just the flight itself. It also covers booking your flights, arriving at the airport, checking in, getting on and off the plane and leaving the airport. For more information see the step-by-step guide on your rights to fly – you can find this on the EHRC website (see link above). The regulation applies to tour operators and travel agents as well as to airports and airlines. This means that tour operators and travel agents must pass on your needs to the airlines, and they in turn must inform the airports of the individual services required.

If you have a complaint you can get in touch with the Equality Advisory Support Service for further, initial advice.

Bus & coach travel

For many years, bus travel was among the least accessible forms of public transport for disabled people but things are now changing. Buses and coaches are becoming increasingly accessible to disabled people, especially wheelchair users.

Regulations now require all new buses to be equipped with lifts or ramps with a level access to a space to carry a passenger using a wheelchair. They also incorporate features such as colour-contrasted handrails and easy to operate bell-pushes. Older vehicles will however continue to be in use until 2020 when all coach companies must ensure their vehicles are accessible.

Information on routes normally served by accessible buses should be available from a Public Transport Information Office (PTE) or from the individual bus company. The boarding features of a modern bus generally work well at bus stations or other dedicated bus stands. But there can be problems at roadside bus stops if there isn't a footpath, or if the vehicle does not pull in sufficiently close to the footpath, because of road works or badly parked cars.

There has been slower progress in making scheduled long-distance coach travel accessible to wheelchair users, although since 2005 new coaches have had to be equipped with lifts.

ACCESSIBILITY OF BUSES AND COACHES

New buses and coaches designed to carry more than 22 passengers on local or scheduled services must comply with Public Service Vehicles Accessibility Regulations (PSVAR). All buses and coaches, both old and new, need to comply by the following dates:
- 1 January 2017 – all buses
- 1 January 2020 – all coaches

Regulations for England, Scotland and Wales

The PSVAR ensure public service vehicles are accessible to disabled people. They are the responsibility of the Department for Transport's Buses and Taxis Division. You can read more at
W www.gov.uk

Regulations for Northern Ireland

Northern Ireland has separate regulations by the Department for Regional Development.
W www.drdni.gov.uk

Wheelchairs on buses and coaches

By 1 January 2017 most wheelchair users will be able to travel on buses. And most wheelchair users will be able to travel on coaches by 1 January 2020. But you may find you can't if:
- your chair is very heavy or very big (taking up a space – when you are in it – of more than 700 mm wide or 1200 mm long)
- you need to travel with your legs fully extended or the backrest reclined

Before you travel: Make sure that your wheelchair is in a safe condition to travel. This means making sure that it is properly maintained and in good condition. If you have a power assisted chair you must ensure that the battery is secure. If your chair has adjustable kerb climbers, you should check that they are set not to catch on the ramp.

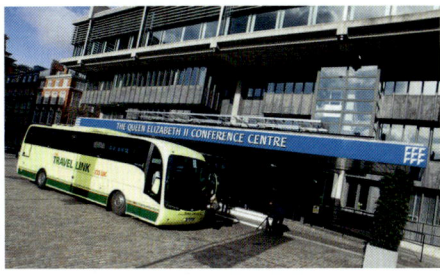

The bus or coach operator has the right to refuse to let you travel if they believe that your wheelchair is not in a safe condition. It is important to check whether your wheelchair can be carried the operator before you travel.

Further advice on taking a wheelchair on public transport can be found at:
W www.ricability.org.uk

While you are travelling: You must make sure your wheelchair brakes are on. If you use a power assisted wheelchair then you should make sure the power is switched off.

By January 2017, there will be a designated space for wheelchair users on buses, and on coaches by 1 January 2020. As a result, all buses and coaches will require:
- a forward facing wheelchair space fitted with a wheelchair restraint system and;
- a wheelchair user restraint.

On buses designed to carry standing passengers the wheelchair space may be a rearward facing protected area. This will be fitted with a padded head

ADVICE & GUIDANCE

and back restraint. The area will also have a vertical stanchion or retractable arm to prevent the wheelchair from slewing into the gangway.

Mobility Scooters
You should contact your local operator to find out whether or not your scooter is transportable on their buses and coaches before you travel.

FREE OFF-PEAK TRAVEL
Eligible older and disabled people are entitled to free off-peak travel on local buses anywhere in England. Similar concessions are available across Wales, Scotland and Northern Ireland.

If you're eligible for a free bus pass, you can use it anywhere in England during 'off-peak' times. Off-peak is:
- between 9.30 am and 11.00 pm Monday to Friday
- all day at weekends and on public holidays.

How to get free off-peak travel
If you live in England, you will be entitled to a bus pass giving free off-peak travel on local buses when you reach 'eligible age'. If you were born after 5 April 1950, the age you become eligible is tied to changes in the State Pension age for women. This affects both men and women.

You're eligible for a disabled person's pass if you live in England and are 'eligible disabled'. This means you:

- are blind or partially sighted
- are profoundly or severely deaf
- are without speech
- have a disability, or have suffered an injury, which has a substantial and long-term effect on your ability to walk
- do not have arms or have long-term loss of the use of both arms
- have a learning disability.

You're also eligible disabled if your application for a driving licence would be refused under section 92 of the Road Traffic Act 1988 (physical fitness). However, you won't be eligible if you were refused because of persistent misuse of drugs or alcohol.

Services outside England
The England bus pass only covers travel in England. It does not give you free bus travel in Wales, Scotland or Northern Ireland. If you live outside England, you'll need to apply for a different pass from your local council.

COACH AND STATION FACILITIES
If you need assistance at the coach station, contact either the station or the coach company before you travel. Let them know what you will need.

Assistance from coach drivers and other staff
Bus and coach drivers are required by law to provide reasonable assistance to disabled people. In particular to help them get on and off the bus or coach.

GETTING THERE & TRAVELLING AROUND

This does not extend to physically lifting passengers or heavy mobility equipment. If you need help to get on and off a coach, you should make a request when you book your ticket.

Induction loops
Many ticket office windows have induction loops to help people who have a hearing aid. These windows are clearly marked. Phones at many stations are also fitted with devices to help people who have a hearing aid.

Support and assistance dogs
You can take support and assistance dogs into station buffets and restaurants, and onto coaches.

Accessible toilets
Many coach stations have accessible toilets. Some operate under the National Key Scheme (NKS), which enables disabled people to use accessible public toilets independently with their own Radar key. You can buy a Radar key from Disability Rights UK. Visit www.disabilityrightsuk.org. Some coaches have toilets on board. If you can't access the toilet on a long-distance coach journey, if for instance, the toilet is situated down some steps, the driver should stop at coach stations so that you can use the toilets. You can find out more about accessible toilets later on in this section.

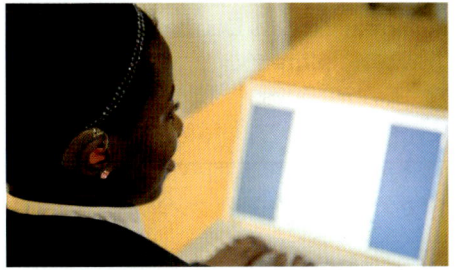

BUS AND COACH COMPANIES
Goldline, the express coach service between towns and cities in Northern Ireland, uses wheelchair accessible coaches on many of its services.

Megabus has some vehicles with a wheelchair lift. Wheelchair users should phone to make a booking so that a bus with a lift or ramp is made available.
☎ 0141 332 9841.

National Express has introduced a new vehicle in which a lift is incorporated at the main entrance and which has a space for a passenger using a wheelchair. This type of vehicle should be in use across their entire network well before 2020, when the legal obligation will be placed upon them. On other services, folded manual wheelchairs can be carried and if you give advance notice, you can get help to manage the entrance steps. National Express request that if you need assistance or the use of one of their new vehicles, you let them know 24-hours prior to travelling so that they can put assistance in place and ensure an accessible coach is put on the relevant route.

ADVICE & GUIDANCE

National Express Disabled Persons Travel Helpline
- 08717 818179
  Textphone 0121 455 0086
- dpth@nationalexpress.com
- www.nationalexpress.com

Oxford Tube, which runs regular, scheduled services between Oxford and London, has introduced 26 new low floor buses each of which has one space for a passenger using a wheelchair.
- 01865 772250
- www.oxfordtube.com

Scottish Citylink has wheelchair accessible coaches on its regular service between Edinburgh and Glasgow and its services, run in partnership with Megabus, between Glasgow and London.
- 0871 266 3333
- www.citylink.co.uk

Victoria Coach Station – This is the terminus for most coach services in and out of London and an important place at which connections can be made. There is a mobility lounge where disabled people can wait and from which assistance can be provided. To book assistance call:
- 020 7027 2520
- www.tfl.gov.uk

Door-to-door and community transport

Some localities have special transport schemes for people who are not able to use public transport. They include: 'dial-a-ride' and 'ring-and-ride'. This sort of service allows you to book an adapted vehicle to carry you on a door-to-door journey.

Demand for these services is likely to exceed the resources available so you may find a variety of restrictions in place, for example limits on the number of journeys you can book in any given period and travel may be restricted to a particular area.

> Information on firms with accessible coaches available for private hire, for group trips and other purposes, should be available from a Public Transport Information Office or PTE.

More general community transport schemes exist where no public transport is available, often, but not exclusively in rural areas. Vehicles used for community transport will often be accessible to disabled passengers.

Special transport schemes are locally run according to local priorities. You should be able to get information on what's available in your area from the relevant Public Transport Information Office.

HOLIDAYS IN THE BRITISH ISLES

GETTING THERE & TRAVELLING AROUND

Community Transport Association UK (CTA UK)
Highbank, Halton Street, Hyde, Cheshire SK14 2NY
☎ 0870 774 3586
🌐 www.ctauk.org

CTA UK gives advice and support on establishing and improving community transport schemes and provides travel training and disability awareness training for travel providers.

British Red Cross
44 Moorfields, London EC2Y 9AL
☎ 0844 871 1111
    Textphone 020 7562 2050
🌐 www.redcross.org.uk

British Red Cross branches offer a transport service for people who cannot get about easily or use public transport. It helps people to get to medical appointments, go shopping or just to get out of the house. Call or visit the website for details of local Red Cross Branches.

Travelling by sea

Information on ferry operators between the British mainland and the Isle of Wight, the Scottish islands, the Channel Islands, Isle of Man and Ireland is given in the appropriate Regional sections of this Guide. If you require any assistance you should tell the ferry company in advance.

Price concessions on car ferries are often available to disabled people, and to members of one of the organisations for disabled motorists.

FERRY TRAVEL

Large, modern ships used on international journeys may be accessible with lifts between decks, toilets designed for disabled people and adapted cabins. Simpler vessels on estuary crossings with open car decks may not be as accessible.

If you are planning to travel by ferry, you need to remember that in tidal waters, the gradient of any boarding ramp will vary according to the tide. This is the case even in places like the river Thames in London, even though it's quite a long way from the sea. At low tide, ramps may be very steep.

If you need assistance or information, get in touch with the ferry operator in advance. Contact details and other information can be obtained from the public transport information points or motoring organisations.

Travelling by sea
Services on ferries and ships vary considerably, even across the UK, so it is important to plan ahead and ensure all sections of your journey are accessible to you. Port facilities and services (including booking facilities) in the UK should be accessible to disabled people. However, there is currently no legislation requiring operators of passenger vessels to do

HOLIDAYS IN THE BRITISH ISLES

ADVICE & GUIDANCE

the same. Despite this, many ferry and cruise operators provide access to their services for disabled people.

Access to sea travel
The Disabled Persons Transport Advisory Committee (DPTAC) has published Access to Sea Travel – Information for Disabled People and Persons with Reduced Mobility. This document can be downloaded from the DPTAC website:
- dptac.independent.gov.uk/pubs/seatravel/index.htm
- 0207 944 8011

Or you can get a printed copy by calling DPTAC.

Making a complaint about sea services
For information on how to make a complaint about a port or ship service, see the DPTAC document Access to Sea Travel (for details, see above).

Rail travel

Since 1998, all new trains have had to incorporate access features for disabled people, including spaces for passengers using manual wheelchairs, appropriate toilets and signage. Many trains introduced before that date also have spaces for passengers using wheelchairs. Very few trains can accommodate the larger makes of scooters.

The number of spaces available to wheelchair users on each train is usually limited, so it is important that you book your space in advance. Most trains can accommodate wheelchairs that are up to 70cm wide and 120cm long. There are a small number of older trains that can only currently carry wheelchairs that have a maximum width of 67cm. Older trains are gradually being phased out but some are still in service. The maximum combined weight of a person and their wheelchair that can be carried varies from 230kg to 300kg.

Accessibility for disabled passengers at train stations is variable. There has been an active process of adapting premises, but effort has been concentrated on larger stations and those where modernisation was already planned. Many smaller stations still have steps to one or more platforms.

PLANNING YOUR JOURNEY
It is worth looking at options to take through-services across major population centres rather than changing trains. Information on services and disruptions can be obtained from:

National Train Enquiries
- 08457 484950
  Textphone 0845 605 0600
- www.nationalrail.co.uk

The National Rail website also has 'Stations Made Easy' pages showing the layout of stations. This can be useful in planning a journey through a station you are not familiar with.

GETTING THERE & TRAVELLING AROUND

Despite continuing improvements, many disabled passengers may still need help at some points of their rail journey. If you think you may need assistance, it helps to give as much advance notice as possible.

If you will be travelling on more than one train line, you should address any requests for information and assistance to the Train Operating company responsible for the first leg of your journey, the numbers you might need are:

Arriva Trains Wales
- 0845 300 3005
  Textphone 0845 605 0600

C2C
- 01702 357640 (also textphone)

Chiltern Railways
- 0845 600 5165
  Textphone 0845 707 8051

Cross Country
- 0844 811 0124
  Textphone 0844 811 0125

East Coast
- 0845 722 5225
  Textphone 18001 08457 225225

East Midlands Trains
- 0845 712 5678
  Textphone 18001 0845 712 5678

First Capital Connect
- 0800 058 2844
  Textphone 0800 975 1052

First Great Western
- 0800 197 1329
  Textphone 18001 0800 197 1329

First Hull Trains
- 0845 071 0222
  Textphone 0845 678 6867

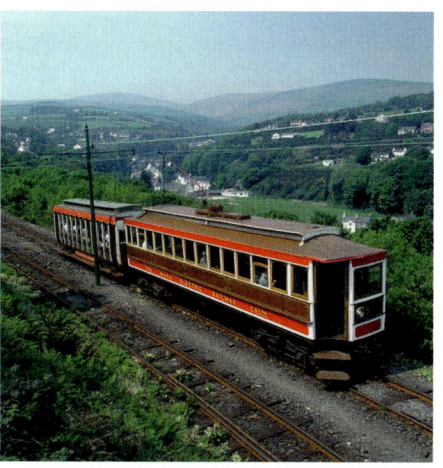

The **Disabled Persons Railcard** gives a third off many rail fares for the cardholder and an adult travelling companion. A list of qualifying criteria and an application form are in the *Rail travel made easy* leaflet, available from Travel Centres and staffed stations. It takes up to two weeks to obtain a new or renewed railcard, so applications should be made ahead of any planned journeys. A one-year railcard currently costs £20 and a three-year card is available for £54. A Disabled Persons Railcard application helpline is available on: Telephone 0845 605 0525 (7am to 10pm, Monday to Sunday); Textphone 0845 601 0132; email disability@atoc.org or see www.disabledpersons-railcard.co.uk. Application forms should be sent to: Disabled Persons Railcard Office, PO Box 11631, Laurencekirk AB30 9AA.

ADVICE & GUIDANCE

First ScotRail
- 0800 912 2901
  Textphone 18001 0800 912 2901

First TransPennine
- 0800 107 2149
  Textphone 0800 107 2061

Grand Central Railway
- 0844 811 007
  Textphone 0845 305 6815

Heathrow Express
- 0845 600 1515

London Midland
- 0800 092 4260
  Textphone 0844 811 0134

London Overground
- 0843 222 1234
  Textphone 0207 918 3015

Merseyrail
- 0800 027 7347 (also textphone)

National Express East Anglia
- 0800 028 2878
  Textphone 0845 606 7245

Northern Rail
- 0808 156 1606
  Textphone 0845 604 5608

SouthEastern
- 0800 783 4524
  Textphone 0800 783 4548

South West Trains
- 0800 528 2100
  Textphone 0800 692 0792

Southern
- 0800 138 1016
  Textphone 0800 138 1018

Virgin Trains
- 0845 744 3366
  Textphone 0845 744 3367

Passenger Focus
Freepost (RRRE-ETTC-LEET), PO Box 4257, Manchester M60 3AR
- 0300 123 2350
- info@passengerfocus.org.uk
- www.passengerfocus.org.uk

Passenger Focus is the national watchdog for train passengers. It can assist with complaints about rail travel where a response from an initial approach to the train operator has been unsatisfactory.

Mainline trains
On mainline (intercity, suburban and cross-country) trains there is a space designed for wheelchair users to travel in safety and comfort. You must always use this space and should apply your brakes when the train is moving. If you use a powered wheelchair, you should make sure that the power is switched off when travelling.

All intercity train services and most other mainline services are wheelchair accessible. Access to the train is provided by a ramp kept either at the station or on the train. Wheelchair accessible sleeper cabins are available on overnight trains between London and Scotland but not on those between London and the West of England.

Local and regional services
Most trains can accommodate wheelchair users and new trains also have facilities to assist sensory

GETTING THERE & TRAVELLING AROUND

impaired people. For example, public information systems that are both visual and audible. To arrange a train journey in the UK, contact National Rail Enquiries:
- ☎ 0845 7484 950
  Textphone 0845 6050 600

National rail and the Disabled People's Protection Policy
Rail companies must produce a Disabled People's Protection Policy (DPPP). The DPPP explains how the company helps disabled passengers to use their stations and trains. You can get copies of a company's DPPP direct from the company.

Traintaxi
You can use Traintaxi to find out if accessible taxis are available at a station. Traintaxi lists up to three local taxi or cab firms serving each station. You can find out more about taxis later in this section.
- 🌐 www.traintaxi.co.uk

Cross-channel services

THE CHANNEL TUNNEL
As an alternative to ferries or planes, the Channel Tunnel offers a useful route to continental Europe. Two services exist:

Eurostar
Eurostar operates train services from London St Pancras, Ebbsfleet and Ashford International to Brussels, Lille and Paris. They offer a limited number of reduced rate tickets for passengers using wheelchairs and their companion. Spaces are limited, so it is worth booking well in advance. Assistance is available on request at check-in but arrive as early as possible.
- ☎ 0870 518 6186
- 🌐 www.eurostar.com

Eurotunnel
Eurotunnel operates vehicle-carrying shuttle trains between Folkestone and Calais. Disabled drivers or passengers should notify staff at check-in so that they can park at the front of the shuttle. A maximum of five vehicles carrying disabled drivers or passengers (who may need assistance in an emergency evacuation) can be carried in any shuttle. Terminals are accessible and have accessible toilets. There is no need for people to get out of their vehicles if they do not wish to.
- ☎ 0800 0969 992
- 🌐 www.eurotunnel.co.uk

Taxis

In London, all licensed taxis must be able to carry a passenger using a standard wheelchair. So all London black cabs manufactured since 1989 have to have space to carry a passenger using a manual wheelchair and either carry or be equipped with a ramp.

ADVICE & GUIDANCE

Black cabs also feature a hidden step up to the cab which the driver can simply swing out from the chassis. In addition, black cabs are fitted with swivel seats that can be rotated through 90 degrees, enabling the passenger to take their seat outside of the taxi and then swivel into the vehicle.

> www.traintaxi.co.uk is a database giving information on the availability of taxis at stations throughout Britain. It includes telephone numbers for up to three taxi companies for advanced bookings and indicates which ones say they have accessible vehicles. You should still check whether the company can meet your requirements when you book.

Similar rules have been introduced by local authorities responsible for regulating taxis in other areas. In some areas price concession systems are available to disabled people for journeys by taxi and/or private hire cars. This may be as part of a more general concession scheme or a separate system. On a local basis, other specialist taxi services may exist for disabled people.

A wide range of other cars are used as private hire vehicles and when you make a booking you should check with the operator whether their vehicles meet your accessibility requirements. Private hire vehicles should carry assistance dogs at no extra charge.

The Government is committed to an accessible public transport system in which disabled people have the same opportunities to travel as other members of society. Taxis and private hire vehicles (PHVs) are a vital link in the accessible transport chain and, although disabled people are reported to travel a third less often than the public in general, they use taxis and PHVs on average 67% more often.

You can find out more about accessible taxi and private hire vehicles from local authorities. Or visit:
 www.transportdirect.info

Stay Safe with Cabwise Transport for London's Text Service

Text CAB to 60835, and you'll receive two minicab numbers and one taxi (black cab) number straight back to your mobile phone by text. You don't even need to say where you are as your location is plotted using GPS. So save 60835 to your mobile now and it'll be there whenever you need it. Text charged at 35p per enquiry plus standard text message rate. Roaming rates apply to overseas networks.

Customers on the 3 network need to enter different information. See www.tfl.gov.uk/cabwise for further details.

GETTING THERE & TRAVELLING AROUND

'Stay Safe in London'
Unbooked minicabs are illegal. You may be approached by minicab drivers seeking passengers or offering a service. Avoid using these as they are unsafe, unlicensed, uninsured and illegal and you put yourself in danger if you use these services.

Booking your minicab with a licensed minicab company guarantees that your trip will be carried out by a licensed driver in a licensed vehicle. It also means that a record is kept of your journey, your driver and the vehicle used. Therefore, in the event of any problems, the driver can be traced.

Only taxis (black cabs) can be stopped by customers and can pick up off the street. Even minicabs lined up outside pubs and clubs are breaking the law if they accept your fare without a booking being made first.

Many clubs have licensed minicab operators inside who can take your booking. Check with staff to see if a minicab service is available.

You can use these two companies to book taxis in London:
Cabwise: text CAB to 60835 (see above for details)
Findaride: find details of licensed private hire and minicab operators in any part of London:
- www.tfl.gov.uk/findaride

To comment or complain about taxi and private hire services contact:
- TfL on 0845 300 7000
- tph.coms@tfl.gov.uk
- www.tfl.gov.uk/contactcabs

Trams and underground systems

Trams and other light rail systems developed over recent years in a number of places, including Croydon, Greater Manchester, Nottingham, Sheffield and the West Midlands, have been designed for use by disabled people.

The Tyne Wear Metro and the Docklands Light Railway in East London are fairly accessible to wheelchair users but you may need to be accompanied. Access for disabled passengers is still limited on the older underground systems in London and Glasgow. In London, new developments, such as the Jubilee Line extension between Westminster and Stratford are designed to be accessible.

Transport for London is running a programme to create step-free routes to the platforms and other access improvements at almost 100 stations. You can find up-to-date information on Underground maps published by Transport for London and available at www.tfl.gov.uk.

ADVICE & GUIDANCE

Chartwell Insurance

Specialist Disabled Travel Insurance

- Single and Multi-trip Policies
- No Age Limit for Single-Trip Policies
- Expertise in Disabled Market
- Affordable Rates

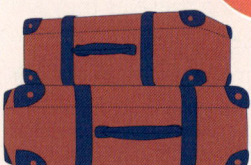

Finding appropriate travel insurance can be stressful if you have any pre-exisiting medical conditions. However Chartwell offer comprehensive travel insurance for most current disabilities.

Our policies can offer:

- Replacement medication cover up to £300
- Stand-in carer flown out to you
- Wheelchair cover up to £2500
- Baggage up to £1500 covered

0800 089 0146 | chartwellinsurance.co.uk

Chartwell Insurance is a trading name of Adrian Flux Insurance Services. Authorised and regulated by the Financial Services Authority.

HOISTS
Starting from £300 for Motability customers

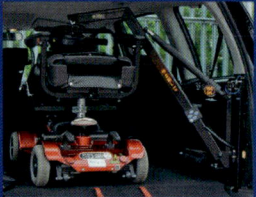

Seven different models to choose from: 40Kg, 75Kg, 80Kg, 100Kg, 120Kg, 150Kg and patented fully automatic Telescopic Hoist.
Enables you to easily lift and load your scooter, wheelchair or powerchair into your hatchback, estate car, MPV or 4x4. Simple and easy to operate.

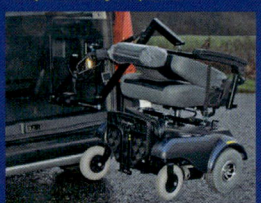

Brig-Ayd Controls Ltd

Brig-Ayd Controls is the UK's largest manufacturer and supplier of lifting and driving aids for disabled drivers and passengers.

From our first day of trading in 1972 our goal has been to create the finest driving adaptations coupled with excellent customer service.

Our products are designed and manufactured by ourselves in our own workshops in Welwyn Garden City, fitted by us or distributed to be fitted by trained installers throughout the UK and Ireland.

Freephone: 0800 0147522
Telephone: 01707 322322
Fax: 01707 394149
sales@brig-aydcontrols.co.uk
www.brig-aydcontrols.co.uk

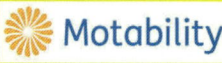

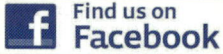

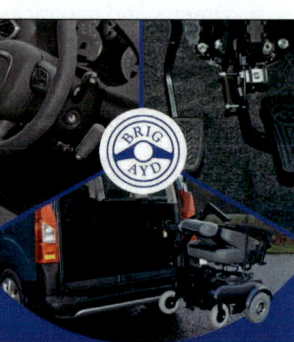

Hand Controls

Single lever hand controls for light and easy operation of throttle and brake. Options for toggle or rotary indicator plus dip switch or horn buttons. We also have an option for an electric trigger throttle and brake.

Left Foot Accelerators

The Twin Flip pedal transfer. Suitable for right or left foot operation.

The Electric Crossover pedal transfer for left or right foot operation at the touch of a button.

The Floor Mounted pedal transfer easily removed when not in use.

GETTING THERE & TRAVELLING AROUND

Motoring

For many disabled people, having a car provides one of the main routes to independent mobility. Developments in technology and vehicle design mean that it is getting easier to find cars that can be adapted to meet the needs of disabled drivers or passengers. Motoring organisations such as the AA and RAC provide particular services for their disabled members and can give help and advice with things like planning routes and insurance. When you are away from home it is also worth finding out in advance about parking facilities.

Parking

THE BLUE BADGE SCHEME

This scheme provides a national system of on-street parking concessions for people with severe mobility problems.

Having a Blue Badge will help you to park closer to your destination, either as the passenger or as the driver. However, the badge is intended for on-street parking only. Off-street car parks, such as those provided in local authority, hospital or supermarket car parks are governed by separate rules. To get a leaflet to tell you more about where you can and cannot park in the on-street environment. To find out more visit
Ⓦ www.gov.uk

Blue Badges are issued by local councils who are responsible for assessing whether you are eligible. In those parts of England where there are County and District Councils, Blue Badges are issued by the County Council.

Blue Badge holders can generally park without charge in areas controlled by parking meters and in pay-and-display bays. They are also exempt from time limits imposed on others and may park for up to three hours on yellow lines, except where loading or other restrictions apply. This time limit does not apply in Scotland.

The scheme does not apply in parts of the centre of London where four local authorities (The Royal Borough of Kensington and Chelsea, City of Westminster, City of London and London Borough of Camden) have set up their own, special disabled badge schemes for people that live, work or study in the central area. You can apply direct to these boroughs for details of their own schemes.

HOLIDAYS IN THE BRITISH ISLES

ADVICE & GUIDANCE

BELFORD TRANSFER LIFT
GIVES YOU FREEDOM TO TRAVEL

Extensively developed, refined and tested by design specialists, the precision-manufactured Belford Transfer Lift makes the touring holiday accessible and affordable for the very first time.

The Lift is an ingenious, neat and unobtrusive invention which allows wheelchair users to access a motor home or caravan without the need for extensive coachwork modification or costly custom build.

It overcomes the uncertainty of travelling to 'accessible' holiday accommodation when you can't be certain that it will be suitable when you arrive.

- Quick and easy to use
- Retro-fitted
- Modular design for compact storage

Contact us to find out more:
Belford Hoist Ltd, Belford, Northumberland, NE70 7DT
Telephone: **07864 17 11 10**
Email: **info@belfordtransferlift.com**

www.belfordtransferlift.com

C&S seating

19 Stirling Road
Castleham Industrial Estate
St Leonard's on Sea
East Sussex TN38 9NP

01424 853331

info@cands-seating.co.uk
www.cands-seating.co.uk

Products designed and developed to aid basic postural management.

T Rolls

T Rolls are used to control position of the body in supine lying.

We also make various other rolls, see our website for more details.

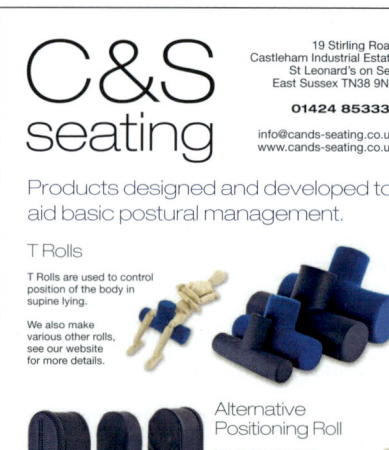

Alternative Positioning Roll

The APR is designed for use where more control of the abducted lower limbs is required.

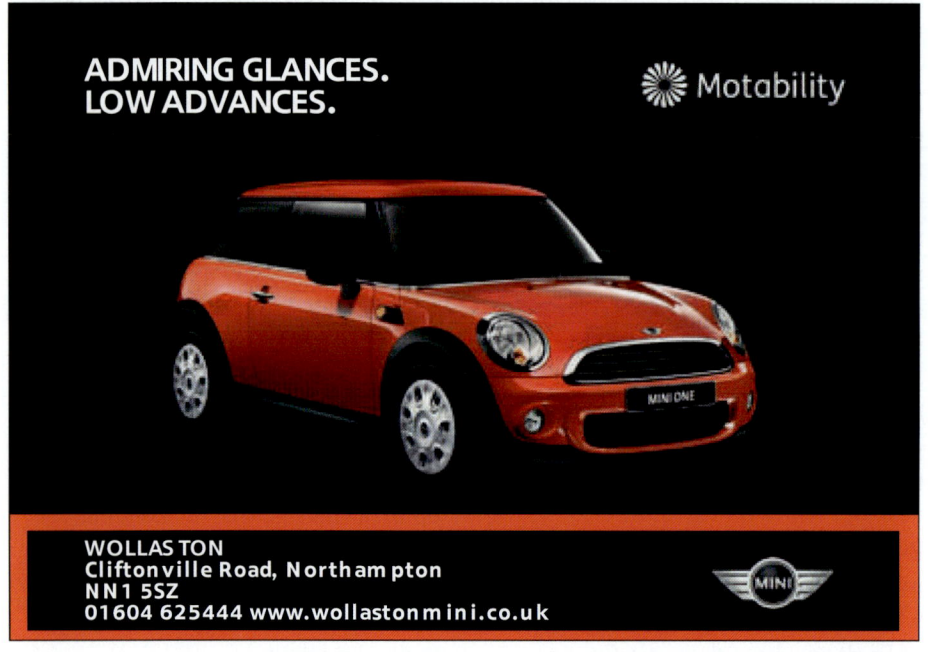

ADMIRING GLANCES. LOW ADVANCES.

Motability

WOLLASTON
Cliftonville Road, Northampton
NN1 5SZ
01604 625444   www.wollastonmini.co.uk

GETTING THERE & TRAVELLING AROUND

Although the Blue Badge Scheme does not apply to off-street parking, it is often used by local authorities as the basis for concessionary use of car parks and to indicate that designated parking bays in privately-owned parking areas are being used correctly. A Blue Badge does not always entitle you to free parking in off-street car parks, even when they are run by the local council. Always check to find out if you need to pay.

> The **Department for Transport** has produced a guide to concessions that are available to disabled people. You can download this list from their website: www.dft.gov.uk

Outside the EU it will be a matter of local policy whether countries will recognise the Blue Badge. Some countries that have high numbers of tourists may award a short-term badge for the duration of your stay. Always check before you use your badge. If you incur a fine that you don't pay you could be refused entry next time you visit the country.

Blue Badge Initial Enquire Support Service
- 0844 463 0213

In Scotland:
- 0844 463 0214

In Wales:
- 0844 463 0215

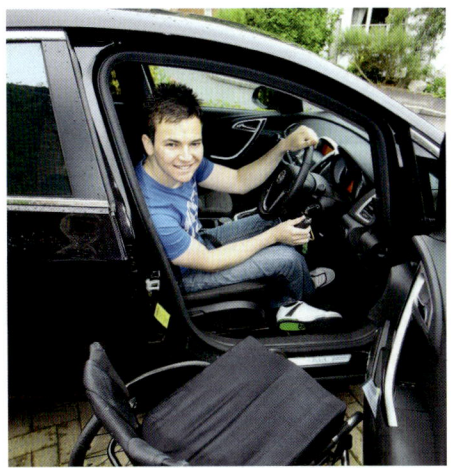

Blue Badge Network
198 Wolverhampton Street, Dudley
DY1 1DZ
- 07964 590060
- headoffice@bluebadgenetwork.org.uk
- www.bluebadgenetwork.org.uk

The Blue Badge Network is a membership organisation aiming to help disabled people, to maintain the integrity of the concessionary parking permit.

Blue Badge Nav (BBNav)
BBNav is a satellite navigation system with all the usual functionality as well as offering full coverage of Blue Badge on-street parking bays, car park access and local council parking rules for over 150 major UK cities and towns. To find out more go to:
- www.bbnav.co.uk

ADVICE & GUIDANCE

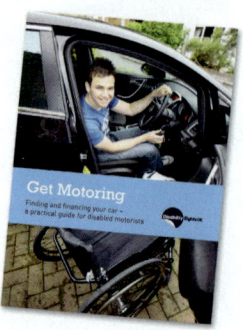

Get Motoring
A practical guide for disabled motorists to help find and finance a car. New 2012 edition.

Available to order from our online shop
www.disabilityrightsuk.org

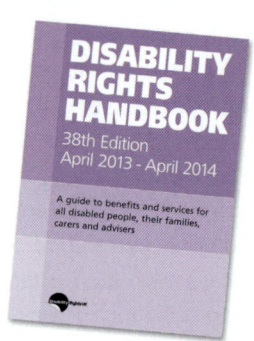

Disability Rights Handbook
Comprehensive information and guidance on benefits and services for all disabled people, their families, carers and advisers.

Available to order from our online shop
www.disabilityrightsuk.org

FREE ATTENDED SERVICE at selected times

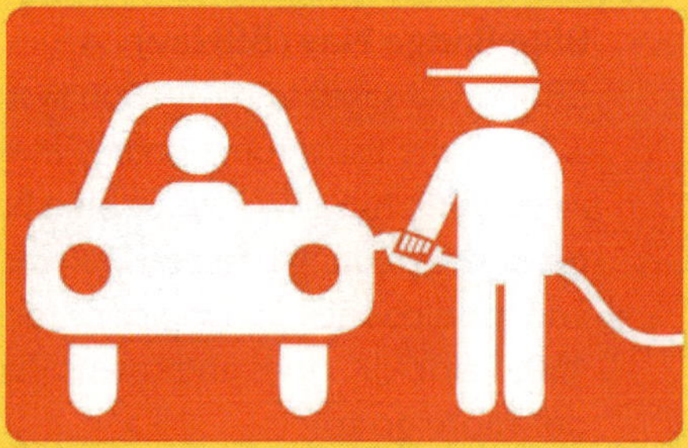

Check in store for the hours when this is available

GETTING THERE & TRAVELLING AROUND

SHELL: AT YOUR SERVICE

Shell reintroduces Attended Service to bring back the golden age of motoring

What is Attended Service?
Attended Service is the reintroduction of Forecourt Attendants at Shell sites across the UK. Attendants are on hand at 300 sites across the country to advise drivers on fuels, fuel efficiency, and safety tips. After an absence of more than 20 years, Shell Forecourt Attendants have returned; harking back to a golden age of customer service for motorists.

How does Attended Service benefit you?
For those with restricted mobility Attended Service has proved to be helpful and convenient.

Attendants can fill your car up, and deploy their Automobile Association (AA) training to offer advice on how your car is running, including checks on oil and screen wash levels, tyre pressures and tread depths.

Attendants can also advise on driving behaviours and how to make the right fuel choices whilst providing tips for driving in British weather.

Find out more about Attended Service:
Find your nearest Shell garage with Attended Service at:
www.shell.co.uk/attendedservice.

We would also love to hear your views on the service – get in touch at:
www.shell.co.uk/tellshell

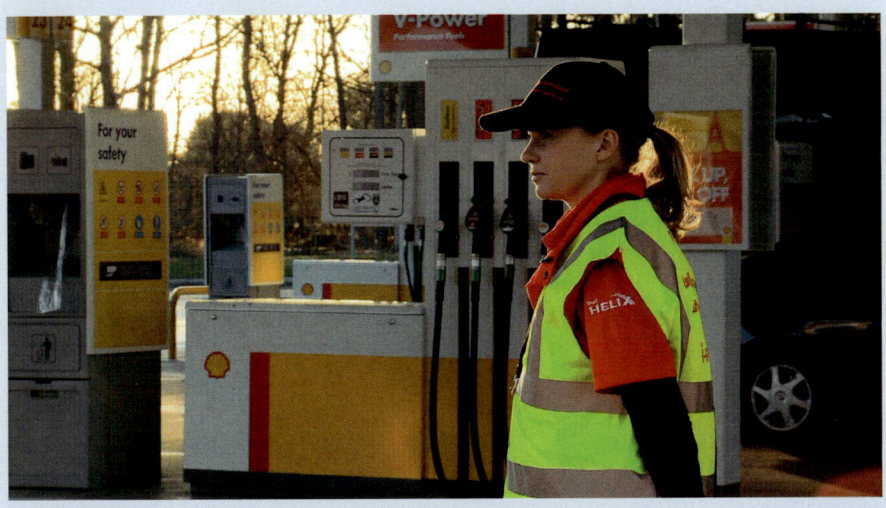

HOLIDAYS IN THE BRITISH ISLES

DISABILITY MOTORING ORGANISATIONS
Disabled Motorists Federation
- 0151 648 3457
- www.dmfed.org.uk

The Disabled Motorists Federation is a national organisation of disabled motorists. It is volunteer-run and can be contacted by phone or via their website.

> Disability Rights UK publish *Get Motoring* – a free, recently updated guide to motoring that includes all the facts you will need: from obtaining a licence, driving lessons, locating and choosing the right vehicle, finding the right finance, price guides and repayment options, adaptations and accessibility ratings, vehicle maintenance and general upkeep, to a list of essential contacts.

Disabled Motoring UK
National Headquarters, Ashwellthorpe, Norwich NR16 1EX
- 01508 489449
- info@disabledmotoring.org
- www.disabledmotoring.org

Disabled Motoring UK is a national charity that campaigns and provides information on all matters related to motoring/mobility and disabled people.

National Association for Bikers with a Disability (NABD)
Unit 20, The Bridgewater Centre, Robson Avenue, Urmston, Manchester M41 7TE
- 0844 415 4849
- office@thenabd.org.uk
- www.nabd.org.uk

NABD caters for disabled people who want to enjoy the freedom of motorcycling. It provides a range of services for its members including advice and help on training, licensing, adaptations and the associated costs and insurance. It has a network of local representatives and produces a quarterly magazine.

Leisure activities

Taking part in leisure activities is one of life's great pleasures. Having a disability or impairment may limit what we do but with the right help, support and equipment we can take part in a wide range of activities. This section of the Guide tells you about some of the things you might like to do while you're away.

Arts

While you are away, you might want to go to a play or a show. The local tourist information service or library should have a list of what is on. You can also get information on taking part in or visiting arts-related activities from a wide range of organisations. Check ahead on the internet before you go or consider an app for your Smartphone, if you have one. These are some of the organisations currently providing information about the arts in the UK:

Arts Council of England
14 Great Peter Street, London SW1P 3NQ
- 0845 300 6200
   Textphone 020 7973 6564
- enquiries@artscouncil.org.uk
- www.artscouncil.org.uk

Responsible for arts funding and development in England. Provides information and advice to artists and arts organisations.

Elsewhere in UK contact:

Arts Council of Northern Ireland
77 Malone Road, Belfast BT9 6AQ
- 028 9038 5200
- www.artscouncil-ni.org

Creative Scotland
Waverley Gate, 2-4 Waterloo Place, Edinburgh EH1 3EG
- 0845 603 6000
- enquiries@creativescotland.com
- www.creativescotland.com

Arts Council of Wales
Bute Place, Cardiff CF10 5AL
- 0845 8734 900
   SMS service 07797 800 504
- www.artswales.org

Artsline
c/o 21 Pine Court, Wood Lodge Gardens, Bromley BR1 2WA
- 020 7388 2227 (also textphone)
- www.artsline.org.uk

Online information for disabled people on arts and leisure events around London. Includes access details at arts and entertainment venues and events.

ADVICE & GUIDANCE

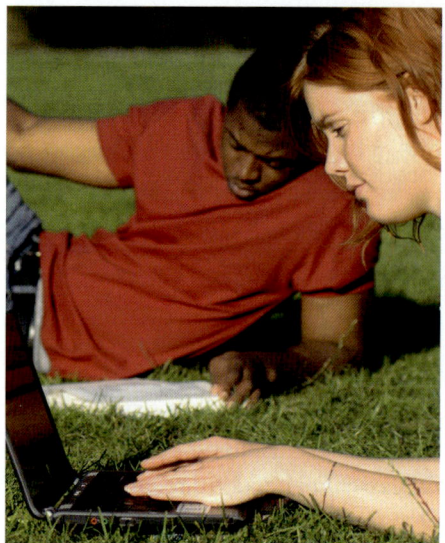

Attitude is Everything
54 Chalton Street, London NW1 1HS
☎ 020 7383 7979
🌐 www.attitudeiseverything.org.uk
Work with audiences, artists and the music industry to improve deaf and disabled people's access to live music. It promotes a 'Charter of Best Practice' to venues and festivals throughout the country.

Disability Cultural Projects (DCP)
🌐 www.disabilityarts.info
DCP Access guide
🌐 www.artsaccessuk.org
DCP produces *EtCetera*, a weekly electronic newsletter of opportunities, an events list and an online arts access guide. The website also contains extensive links to disability arts organisations and archived material from the National Disability Arts Forum that closed in 2008.

MAGIC Deaf Arts is a group of 16 major museums and art galleries in London. Each provides events and facilities for deaf and hard of hearing visitors, including specialist tours and sign language interpreters at public talks and lectures. Visit their website www.magicdeaf.org.uk for a calendar of events.

The Mayflower Theatre
Empire Lane, Southampton SO15 1AP
☎ 02380 711813
🌐 www.mayflower.org.uk
Offers discounts for disabled people and their companions. These discounts are not available for all performances. Other theatres may offer similar discounts but you will have to check with the theatre directly or on the internet before you book your tickets.

Music and the Deaf
The Media Centre, 7 Northumberland Street, Huddersfield HD1 1RL
☎ 01484 483115
   Textphone 01484 483117
🌐 www.matd.org.uk
Help deaf people of all ages access music and the performing arts. It provides talks, signed theatre performances and workshops. In West Yorkshire it runs after-school clubs and a Deaf Youth Orchestra. Music and the Deaf also runs training days and collaborative projects with orchestras, opera, theatre and dance companies and is one of the five lead organisations in Sing-up, a project to promote singing in schools.

National Theatre

South Bank, London SE1 9PX
- 020 7452 3000
- access@nationaltheatre.org.uk
- www.nationaltheatre.org.uk

Aims to be accessible and welcoming to all. Its three auditoriums have allocated wheelchair spaces and assistance dogs are welcome. People with hearing impairments can attend captioned and signed performances. Blind and visually-impaired people can attend audio-described performances and receive synopses notes on CD or cassette. Touch tours and Braille cast lists are also available. Its access mailing list offers free information on CD, in Braille and large print via email.

Nordoff Robbins

2 Lissenden Gardens, London NW5 1PQ
- 020 7267 4496
- admin@nordoff-robbins.org.uk
- www.nordoff-robbins.org.uk

A national organisation that seeks to use the power of music to transform the lives of children and adults living with illness, disability, trauma or in isolation. Their trained practitioners work in a range of settings including music therapy, music and health projects and community music schemes as well as the organisation's own centres.

Official London Theatre (OLT)

- www.officiallondontheatre.co.uk/access

Wants to ensure your trip to the theatre is as fantastic and accessible an experience as possible, and have a variety of resources to help. For extensive venue access information about theatres across London, visit their detailed venue access site made in collaboration with Direct Enquires. You can download the OLT *Access London Theatre* guide, which is updated four times per year and includes detailed access information for more than 70 theatres in London. They also have a selection of Access Enabled maps, detailing step-free journeys to many of London's most popular theatres. Visit their website to find out more.

Zinc Arts (formerly Theatre Resource) aims to advance and promote creativity, culture and heritage of disabled people and other socially excluded groups in Essex and Hertfordshire. It arranges a wide range of programmes and events. Contact Zinc Arts, High Street, Chipping Ongar, Essex CM5 0AD. Telephone 01277 365626; Textphone 01277 365003 or visit www.zincarts.org.uk

ADVICE & GUIDANCE

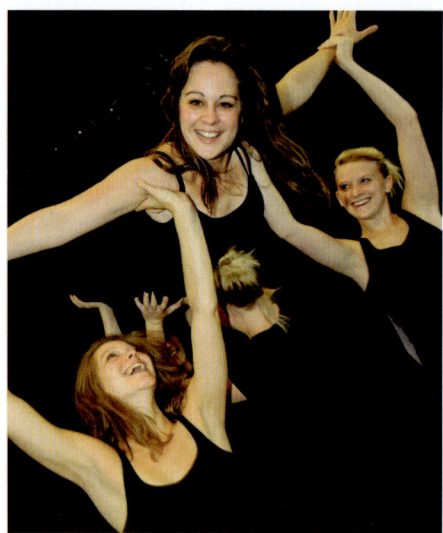

Shape
Deane House Studios, 27 Greenwood Place, London NW5 1LB
- 0845 521 3457
  Textphone 020 7424 7368
- www.shapearts.org.uk

Offers a range of activities to enable disabled people to participate and enjoy arts and cultural activities mainly in the London area. Shape Tickets is a service offering its members tickets, often at reduced prices, at venues throughout London coupled with access assistance and transport if required.

Signed Performances In Theatre (SPIT)
6 Thirlmere Drive, Lymm, Cheshire WA13 9PE
- 01925 754231
- www.spit.org.uk

Promotes British Sign Language interpreted performances in mainstream theatre and provides a link between arts organisations and the Deaf community. Its website includes a directory of signed and captioned performances nationwide.

STAGETEXT
1st Floor, 54 Commercial Street, London E1 6LT
- 020 7377 0540
  Textphone 020 7247 7801
- enquiries@stagetext.org
- www.stagetext.org

Provides access to the theatre for deaf and hard of hearing people through captioning. The full text, together with character names, sound effects and off-stage noises, is shown on LED displays as the words are spoken or sung. Around 200 productions are captioned each year in over 80 venues across the UK. Information on forthcoming performances is given on its website.

VocalEyes
1st Floor, 54 Commercial Street, London E1 6LT
- 020 7375 1043
- enquiries@vocaleyes.co.uk
- www.vocaleyes.co.uk

A national organisation which provides audio description for performances in the theatre and also for museums, galleries and architectural heritage sites. A programme of forthcoming events is published in print, Braille and on tape as well as on their website.

Cinemas

In the past, few cinemas were accessible to people with impaired mobility, hearing or sight. The development of new cinema buildings has meant improvements with respect to physical access, with at least some screens in multiplexes having spaces for wheelchair users.

A programme is now underway to substantially increase both the number of cinemas equipped to show films with digital subtitles and audio description and the number of films that are available. For information on subtitled and audio-described films and where they are being shown, visit:
- www.yourlocalcinema.com

If you are registered blind or receive disability living allowance or attendance allowance, the **Cinema Exhibitors' Association (CEA)** offers a national card verifying entitlement to a free ticket for a person accompanying you to the cinema. There is a £5.50 administration charge and the card has to be renewed each year.

Application forms are available from participating cinemas or from:
- www.ceacard.co.uk

The CEA card is administered and run by: The Card Network, Network House, St Ives Way, Sandycroft CH5 2QS
- 0845 123 1292
  Textphone 0845 123 1296
- email info@ceacard.co.uk

ADVICE & GUIDANCE

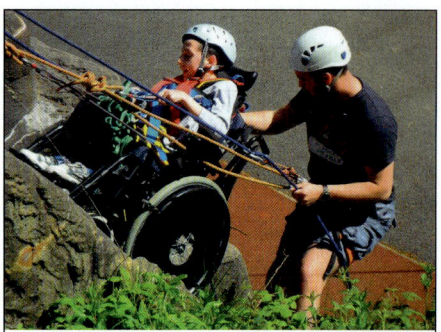

Challenging and enjoyable outdoor activity holidays for all.

Scan here for more info!

At Calvert Trust Exmoor
it's what you CAN do that counts!

01598 763221   exmoor@calvert-trust.org.uk
www.calvert-trust.org.uk/exmoor

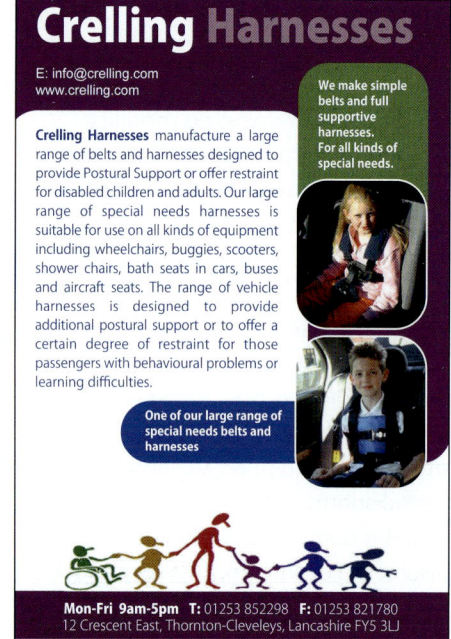

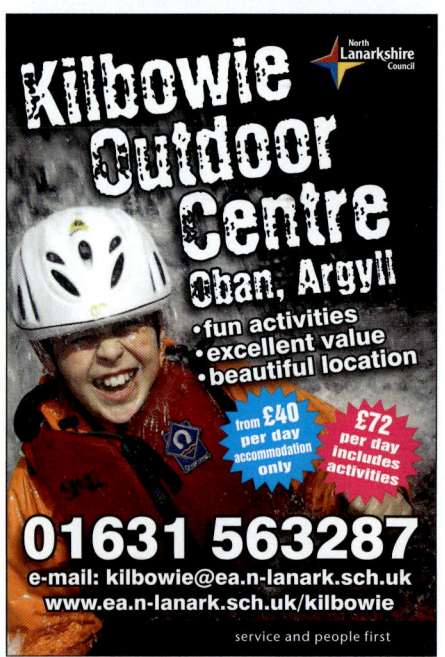

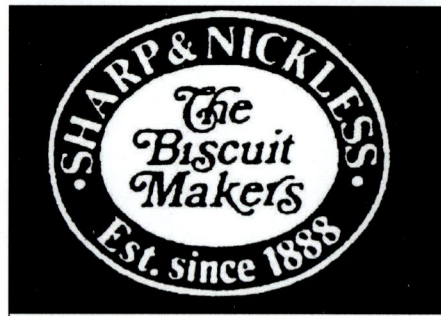

Speciality Brandy Snaps

SHARP & NICKLESS LTD

College Street,
Long Eaton
Nottingham NG10 4NN

Tel & fax 0115 973 2169

WHILE YOU'RE AWAY

Activity holidays

Some people choose their holiday destination based on a particular leisure interest. This section includes a selection of organisations that provide outdoor activity, boating and skiing holidays as well as breaks for people who want to volunteer, take a course or follow a special interest while away.

Outdoor activity holidays

These centres cater for individuals or groups on organised programmes of outdoor and indoor activities including horse riding and rock climbing. Some also offer facilities for self-led groups.

Activenture Holidays
Hindleap Warren, Wych Cross, Forest Row, East Sussex RH18 5JS
- 01342 828215
- activenture@hindleap.com
- www.londonyouth.org

Run week-long activity holidays for young people with disabilities or special needs aged 8-18 during school holidays, and a weekend for over 18s, at Hindleap Warren Outdoor Centre. Owned by London Youth, the Centre has a 300-acre site in Ashdown Forest and can offer 24-hour one-to-one care. Activities available with trained instructors include abseiling, canoeing, archery, and obstacle courses. 30 people are accommodated on each holiday with young and adult staff as companions. Nurse in attendance. Early booking essential.

Avon Tyrrell
Bransgore, Hampshire BH23 8EE
- 01425 672347
- info@ukyouth.org
- www.avontyrrell.org.uk

UK Youth activity centre on a 65-acre site in the New Forest for groups of all ages offering a wide range of activities with qualified instructors including climbing, canoeing, archery, zip wire, high and low rope courses and environmental studies. Accessible accommodation on either full board or self-catering basis is available.

Badaguish Centre
Aviemore, Inverness-shire PH22 1QU
- 01479 861285
- info@badaguish.org
- www.badaguish.org

Provide activity holidays with support predominately for people with learning disabilities. They offer a wide range of activities in an area that includes the Cairngorm Funicular Railway and Morlich Water Sports Centre. Respite care activity holidays with 24-hour care arranged for unaccompanied people with learning disabilities. For groups

HOLIDAYS IN THE BRITISH ISLES

ADVICE & GUIDANCE

there is also accommodation in fully accessible log cabins or under canvas as well as in new, fully accessible self-catering lodges.

Bendrigg Trust
Bendrigg Lodge, Old Hutton, Kendal, Cumbria LA8 0NR
- 01539 722446
- office@bendrigg.org.uk
- www.bendrigg.org.uk

Residential activity centre running courses for people of all ages and abilities and specialising in supporting people with learning disabilities. A wide range of outdoor and indoor activities are available with qualified, experienced staff. Individual programmes are planned for each group. Open weeks are available for individuals and carers. Accommodation for up to 40 people in small dormitories. Lift and ramp to first floor. Adapted showers, washrooms and ceiling and mobile hoists available.

Bowles
Eridge Green, Tunbridge Wells TN3 9LW
- 01892 665665
- admin@bowles.ac
- www.bowles.ac

Offer activity courses for groups of young people and adults including disabled people. Modern accommodation includes twin and single bedrooms with en-suite accommodation plus two twin bedrooms with en-suite shower rooms designed for wheelchair users.

There are also 96 rooms in dormitory accommodation available. Activities include skiing, rope courses, rock climbing, canoeing and archery. Some specialist equipment available.

Calvert Trust Exmoor
Wistlandpound, Kentisbury, Barnstaple, Devon EX31 4SJ
- 01598 763221
- exmoor@calvert-trust.org.uk
- www.calvert-trust.org.uk

Activity centre near the coast and Exmoor, designed for disabled people and their friends and families. All bedrooms have shower rooms accessible to wheelchair users. Indoor swimming pool, jacuzzi and steam room. Activities offered include climbing, bush craft, horse riding, sailing, canoeing, and archery. Self-catering units also available.

The Lake District Calvert Trust
Little Crosthwaite, Keswick, Cumbria CA12 4QD
- 01768 772255
- enquiries@lakedistrict.calvert-trust.org.uk
- www.calvert-trust.org.uk

Outdoor activity holidays and educational or personal development courses designed around individual group requirements. The accommodation has recently been refurbished and is in a converted farmhouse with wheelchair access throughout. All bedrooms all have en-suite shower rooms. Facilities include

HOLIDAYS IN THE BRITISH ISLES

sports hall, climbing wall, indoor pool, games room, TV lounge, and a state of the art hydrotherapy pool. Activities include rock climbing, abseiling, horse riding, water sports, fell walking, orienteering and archery. Adapted equipment available. Qualified staff. Self-catering accommodation also available.

Calvert Trust Kielder
Kielder Water, Hexham,
Northumberland NE48 1BS
- 01434 250232
- enquiries@calvert-kielder.com
- www.calvert-trust.org.uk

Purpose-built holiday centre by Northumberland National Park for disabled people and their families and friends. Activities include water sports, climbing, abseiling, archery and zipwire with king swing and low ropes course. Instruction and equipment available. There is a hydrotherapy pool and recreation hall. All accommodation is fully accessible for wheelchair users with level entry showers throughout. Care packages available.

Castleshaw Centre
Delph, Greater Manchester OL3 5LZ
- 0161 770 8595
- castleshawcentre@oldham.gov.uk
- www.oldham.gov.uk

Outdoor and environmental education centre with activities and wheelchair accessible residential facilities for use by educational or community groups. Ideal for exploring the nearby moors and villages of the South Pennines.

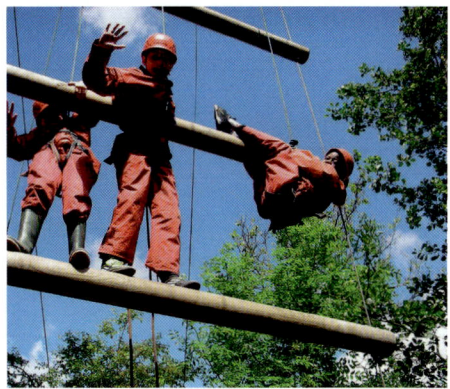

Coldwell Activity Centre
Back Lane, Southfield, Burnley BB10 3RD
- 01282 601819
- bookings@coldwell.org.uk
- www.coldwell.org.uk

Group holiday accommodation in the Pennines by Coldwell Reservoir. Outdoor activity programme available including archery, canoeing and rockclimbing. Reserved parking bays and entrance ramp in place. All public rooms have level access and there's a lift to the first floor. Adapted shower rooms. Accommodation for up to 27 in 12 bedrooms – minimum group size 16.

The Kepplewray Centre
Broughton-in-Furness, Cumbria LA20 6HE
- 01229 716936
- web1@kepplewray.org.uk
- www.kepplewray.org.uk

Fully accessible and inclusive indoor and outdoor activity centre in southern Lake District designed for groups of disabled and non-disabled people.

ADVICE & GUIDANCE

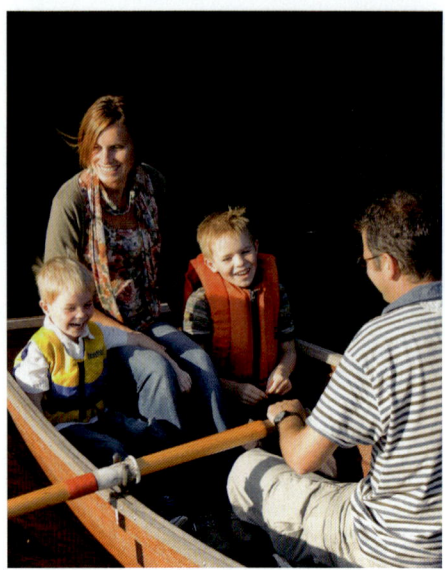

Accommodation for up to 45, ramp to side door and lift available to upper floor. Variety of bedrooms, bathrooms and toilets fitted for a range of disabilities. Equipment includes Clos-o-Mat WC, adjustable height bed, shower chair and electric hoist. A wide variety of outside and indoor activities are available including environmental studies. Programmes offered for families, schools and organisations.

Loch Insh Watersports

Insh Hall, Kincraig, Inverness-shire PH21 1NU
- 01540 651272
- office@lochinsh.com
- www.lochinsh.com

Privately run watersport centre in Cairngorm National Park between Aviemore and Kingussie offering courses for families and groups. The jetty is accessible for wheelchair users from the car park and boathouse/restaurant. Archery and an adapted catamaran are available for wheelchair users. Advance booking required.

Mersea Island Festival

East Mersea Youth Camp, Rewsalls Lane, East Mersea, Colchester CO5 8SX
- 01206 383226
- info@merseyfestival.org.uk
- www.merseafestival.org.uk

Two activity breaks of five and three days are offered in August each year comprising sport, music and art. The programme is designed to be accessible to everyone and includes water-sports, climbing, archery, circus skills and workshops in music, dance, arts and crafts all with qualified instructors. The 70-acre site on the coast has camping accommodation and associated facilities for up to 350 people.

Plas Menai National Watersports Centre

Llanfairisgaer, Caernarfon, Gwynedd LL55 1UE
- 0124 8670 964
- info@plasmenai.co.uk
- www.plasmenai.co.uk

Centre owned by Sports Council for Wales offering watersports courses for groups including disabled people. Accommodation entrance level. 43 bedrooms in separate blocks with level entry and two fully adapted bathrooms with wheelchair accessible shower rooms available and designed for disabled people.

Riding for the Disabled Association
Norfolk House, 1a Tournament Court, Edgehill Drive, Warwick CV34 6LG
- 0845 658 1082
- info@rda.org.uk
- www.rda.org.uk

Has local riding and carriage driving groups for disabled people throughout the country. Organise group, county, regional and national holidays for its members.

> ### TOP THINGS TO SEE OR DO
> **Red Ridge Outdoor Centre**
> Red Ridge at Cefn Coch, near Llanfair Caereinion, Welshpoool, Powys, has been offering accessible activities to people of all ages and abilities since 1978. Providing special breaks for individuals with disabilities, who wish to enjoy an adventure holiday. Guests are of all ages and abilities, and are drawn from a wide range of disabilities including Downs Syndrome, Autism, Epilepsy and Cerebral Palsy.
> - www.redridgecentre.co.uk

Queen Elizabeth II Silver Jubilee Activities Centre
Manor Farm Country Park, Pylands Lane, Bursledon, Hampshire SO31 1BH
- 023 8040 4844
- qe2centre@aol.com
- www.qe2activitycentre.co.uk

Residential activity centre in Country Park by Hamble River near Southampton. Accommodation is in six self-catering cabins each for up to eight people. Adapted cooking facilities, showers and toilets are available for participants with disabilities. Activities offered include canoeing, orienteering and indoor sports. Facilities adapted for disabled people include a motor boat and a climbing wall.

Whitewave – Skye's Outdoor Centre
No. 19 Lincro, Kilmuir, Isle of Skye IV51 9YN
- 01470 542414
- info@whitewave.co.uk
- www.white-wave.co.uk

Family-run centre in north Skye offering activities including canoeing, archery, Gaelic language courses and informal breaks in self-catering accommodation. Apply to Anne Martin and John White.

Woodlarks Camp Site Trust
Tilford Road, Lower Bourne, Farnham GU10 3RN
- 01252 715238
- enquiries@woodlarks.org.uk
- www.woodlarks.org.uk

A woodland site for tented camping with some indoor accommodation including toilets and washing facilities. Tents and beds provided. Fully accessible and equipped for wheelchair users. Heated swimming pool, aerial runway and barbeque sites. Available for group bookings, and for seven weeks are open to individuals as disabled participants and volunteer helpers.

HEADS UP HOLIDAYS

Your journey starts here ...

Let us help your holiday dreams become reality. Heads up Holidays is the first holiday company of its kind in the world and we are proud of it.

With our healthcare background, local knowledge and holiday experience we can offer a safe, supportive and exciting environment for clients who are disabled by brain and spinal cord injury or children and adults with cerebral palsy.

We encourage independence and self-confidence through carefully selected accommodation and activities. We have staff in holiday locations which make our holidays cost effective because you pay for the care at the time you need it.

We have seen and heard our clients after their holiday experience and the results are long lasting.

We know our holidays help in the long-term rehabilitation process which is why we spend so much time ensuring we get each holiday itinerary just right.

Whether you want your holiday to be an action packed experience or simply a relaxing and tranquil getaway, Heads Up Holidays can arrange all aspects of your holiday no matter what your disability may be and needs dictate, turning it from a dream to reality.

Some of our clients have fulfilled life-long ambitions visiting countries they thought were not possible. One of our clients had always wanted to see the Great Wall of China, the Forbidden City and the Terracotta Warriors. We supported this client throughout his holiday and his trip of a lifetime, he had a fabulous time leaving him with some fantastic memories and great photos. He is already arranging his next holiday with Heads Up Holidays, the world is his oyster and we are there to support him every step of the way!

Visit our website for some fabulous holiday ideas – we are here to help you every step of the way and holidays are our passion.

www.headsupholidays.com

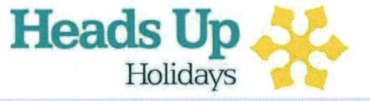

WHILE YOU'RE AWAY

Special interest centres and courses

The following centres and organisations offer residential courses on a variety of non-vocational subjects and areas of special interest from photography and literature to environmental studies and personal development.

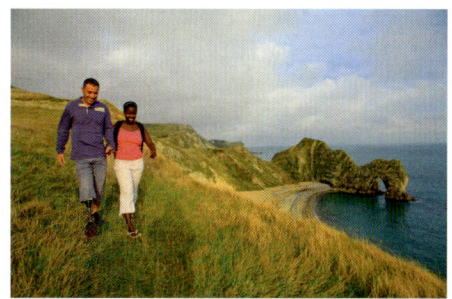

Ammerdown Centre
Ammerdown Park, Radstock, Somerset BA3 56W
- 01761 433709
- centre@ammerdown.org
- www.ammerdown.org

Conference and retreat centre set within a country estate 20 minutes from both Bath and Wells offering a variety of holistic courses suitable for people with disabilities. Specialist break available for people with ME run in September. Entrance level access, public lecture rooms ground floor. Lift to first floor. One twin and two single bedrooms with bathrooms designed for disabled guests. Programme of events and further information is available on request.

Higham Hall
Bassenthwaite Lake, Cockermouth, Cumbria CA13 9SH
- 01768 776276
- admin@highamhall.com
- www.highamhall.com

Residential adult education college in northern Lake District offering a varied programme of short courses all year round. Main public areas and all ground floor rooms are accessible to disabled people and there is a stair lift on the main staircase. Induction loop in the lecture room and also a portable loop for other classes is available. Bungalow in the grounds adapted for wheelchair users and friends and family.

Holton Lee
East Holton, Poole, Dorset BH16 6JN
- 01202 631063
- facilities@holtonlee.co.uk
- www.holtonlee.co.uk

Offer a range of accessible, short-term, self-catering accommodation for individuals and groups of up to 22 people, set within 350 acres of diverse landscape. Ideally situated for the Isle of Purbeck and the Jurassic Coast World Heritage Site. In 2012, introduced Mobility Safaris with Countryside Mobility South West. Guides take groups of disabled people into the countryside and run courses on a variety of subjects including photography and habitat management. From August, four-week long learning breaks will be available covering mixed crafts, wildlife observation and gardening skills.

ADVICE & GUIDANCE

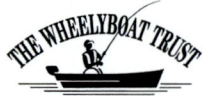

Wheelyboats provide disabled people with hassle-free and independent access to waterborne activities such as nature watching, pleasure boating and angling. More than 150 boats have been supplied by the Trust to venues open to the public all over the UK.

Contact our Director or visit our website to find out about Wheelyboats operating near you.

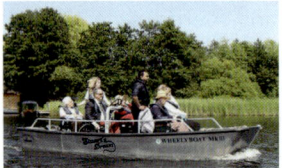

Contact: Andy Beadsley, Director
Tel: 01798 342222 Email: info@wheelyboats.org

www.wheelyboats.org

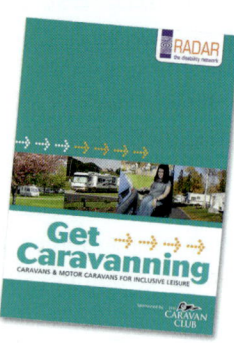

Get Caravanning

A guide to exploring caravanning from a disabled person's point of view. It provides all the information you need to start or resume this popular leisure activity.

Available to order from our online shop
www.disabilityrightsuk.org

 Bruce Wake Charitable Trust
ASSISTING THE PROVISION OF LEISURE FACILITIES FOR THE DISABLED

A Charitable trust assisting the provision of leisure facilities for the disabled

Operate three boats designed for use by disabled people, based at Upton-on-Severn between Tewksbury and Worcester. Two are narrow boats designed for wheelchair users and family with berths for 6-7 people for holidays on the rivers and canals of the south west Midlands. One is wide beamed boat for use on the rivers Severn and Avon and the Gloucester and Sharpness Canal. All three boats have two hydraulic lifts, a hoist over a bed and a specially designed WC/shower.

Hire prices for 2013 are from £650 - £800 per week.

PO Box No. 9335, Oakham, Rutland LE15 0ET
Tel & Fax. 0844 879 3249
e-mail: info@brucewaketrust.co.uk
website: www.brucewaketrust.co.uk

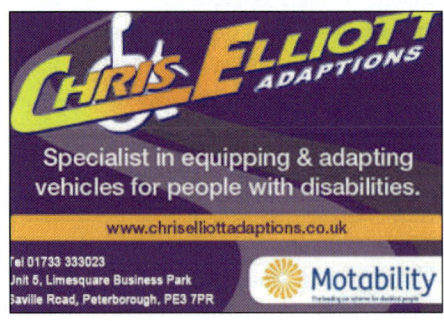

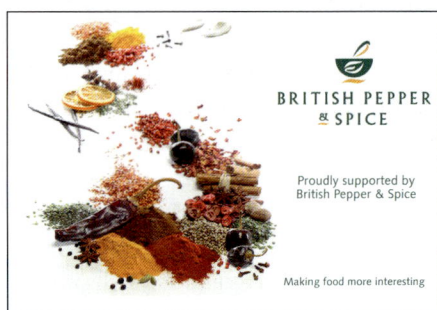

The Kingcombe Centre
Toller Porcorum, Dorchester, Dorset DT2 0EQ
- 01300 320684
- office@kingcombecentre.org.uk
- www.kingcombe.org

Study centre in converted farm buildings surrounded by a nature reserve. A variety of residential and day courses are organised throughout the year, many drawing on the natural history of the surrounding area. Small step to main building, ramp available. Main public rooms on ground floor, level or ramped. Unisex WC. Two bedrooms in annexe, single and twin, designed for disabled people. Roll-in shower room opposite, handrails, transfer space by WC and shower chair available. Accessible paths and boardwalks and all-terrain buggy available.

Knuston Hall Residential College
Irchester, Wellingborough, Northamptonshire NN29 7EU
- 01933 312104
- enquiries@knustonhall.org.uk
- www.knustonhall.org.uk

Offer short residential courses on literature, arts, crafts and music. Reserved parking bays. Entrance level, automatic doors. Main public rooms have level access. Most teaching rooms level and fitted with induction loop. Ramp to six ground floor bedrooms with en-suite bathrooms, one adapted for people with disabilities. Stair lift to first floor bedrooms. Individual requirements should be checked when enquiring about a course.

Sport Wales
Sophia Gardens, Cardiff CF11 9SW
- 0845 0450904
- info@sportwales.org.uk
- www.sportwales.org.uk

Sports centre in central Cardiff offering residential breaks for people of all abilities including specialist residential courses for people with disabilities. Entrance ramp and automatic doors with lift to all floors. Two twin bedrooms designed for guests with disabilities including shower rooms with sliding doors and space for side transfer to WC. Waterproof sheets available. Tactile signs and Braille plan of the premises also available.

Holidays afloat

These organisations and projects run holidays for both self-led and skippered boating holidays ranging from breaks on a canal barge to full ocean sailing.

Accessible Boating
31 Burns Avenue, Church Crookham, Fleet GU52 6BN
- 01252 622520
- bookings@accessibleboating.org.uk
- www.accessibleboating.org.uk

Operate two boats specially designed and equipped with facilities for less-mobile passengers and their companions. 'Madame Butterfly' is a seven-berth cruising canal boat based

ADVICE & GUIDANCE

at Odiham on the Basingstoke Canal. It is equipped with hydraulic lifts at the prow and stern, power assisted steering and hoists for the WC and shower as well as over one bed. 'Dawn', a day boat suitable for six wheelchair users is also available.

The Bruce Trust
Hungerford, Berkshire RG17 9YY
T 01264 356451
E enquiries@brucetrust.org.uk
W www.brucetrust.org.uk

Operate four specially designed boats, two 12, one 10 and one six-berth in the Kennet and Avon Canal. These are based at Great Bedwyn, for cruising between Reading and Devizes Locks from where return cruises to Bath are possible. Each boat is equipped with a hydraulic lift and specially designed toilet. Full training can be given to group leaders.

The Bruce Wake Charitable Trust
Oakam, Rutland LE15 0ET
T 08448 793349
E info@brucewaketrust.co.uk
W www.brucewaketrust.co.uk

Operate two narrow boats; 'Isabella' and 'Lilia' designed for use by disabled people, based at Upton-on-Severn between Tewkesbury and Worcester. Both boats are designed to accommodate one wheelchair user and their family or friends with berths for six-seven people for holidays on the rivers and canals of the south Midlands. They have two hydraulic lifts, a hoist over one bed and a specially designed WC and shower. Also have the 'Charlotte III', a wide beamed boat available for use on the rivers Severn and Avon and on the Gloucester-Sharpness Canal.

The Canal Boat Project
Lock View, Burnt Mill Lane, Essex CM20 2QS
T 01279 424444
E admin@canalboat.org.uk
W www.canalboat.org.uk

Small fleet of purpose built, specially adapted boats for hire to disabled people on the rivers Lee and Stort. Two wide-beamed residential boats sleep 12 or eight people respectively and can only be hired by self-steering parties. Two day boats are also offered with a skipper and crew; one accommodating 12 passengers with the possibility of having six wheelchair users aboard and one for up to 10 passengers that will only accommodate one wheelchair. Each has a lift giving access to most parts of the boats and some have specialist control equipment to enable people with mobility problems to steer.

Docklands Canal Boat Trust
8 Lloyd Villas, Roman Road E6 3SW
T 07511 622747
E bookings@dcbt.org.uk
W www.dcbt.org.uk

'MV Challenge' is a wide-beamed barge based on the Lee and Stort Canal on the Hertfordshire/Essex border. The barge sleeps 10 passengers or 12 people for a day-trip and can take up to five wheelchair users onboard. It has a lift between decks and a wet room for disabled people. A skipper is provided. Bookings are taken from April to October with special Christmas outings available in December.

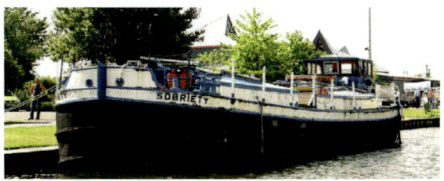

TOP THINGS TO SEE AND DO

Dolphin III Boat, Dolphin Marina

Moored at Poole Quay, Poole, this is a specially designed boat for people of all ages with disabilities, and particularly suitable for those in wheelchairs or with walking difficulties. Free trips are offered for disabled people but early booking is essential. The boat mainly takes groups (up to 12 people in total) but individuals can be catered for.
- www.thefriendsofdolphin.co.uk
- 01258 857806

Jubilee Sailing Trust

12 Hazel Road, Woolston, Southampton SO19 7GA
- 02380 449108
- info@jst.org.uk
- www.jst.org.uk

Offer adventure holidays as crew members of 'Lord Nelson' and 'Tenacious'; purpose built, square-rigged tall sailing ships. Voyages last between four and 10 days and run around the UK, off the Canary Islands and sometimes further afield. Anyone aged over 16 can sail and bursary funding is sometimes available to cover fees. People with disabilities, including wheelchair users, sail alongside an equal number of non-disabled people. Special equipment includes flat wide decks, audio compasses, lifts between decks and an adjustable seat at the helm.

The Lyneal Trust

Lyneal Trust, Shirehall, Abbey Foregate, Shrewsbury SY2 6ND
- 01743 252728
- pushkar.trivedi@shropshire.gov.uk
- www.lynealtrust.org

Provide canal and canal-side holidays on the Llangollen Canal in North Shropshire for people with disabilities and their families and friends from their base at Lyneal Wharf. At the Wharf there is a games room, kitchen and showers and two accessible chalets and a bungalow for up to 16 people. 'Shropshire Lass' is a purpose built, eight berth canal boat that can accommodate up to three wheelchair users and has a specialist WC and shower for people with disabilities. 'Shropshire Lad' is available for day trips and holidays for people staying in the chalets or bungalow. Both boats have a hydraulic lift and hydraulic steering which allows wheelchair users to take part in running the boat. All parts of the boats can be accessed by people in wheelchairs.

ADVICE & GUIDANCE

Peter Le Marchant Trust
Canalside Moorings, Beeches Road, Loughborough LE11 2NS
- 01509 265590
- lynnsmith@peterlemarchanttrust.co.uk
- www.peterlemarchanttrust.org.uk

Have three boats designed for people with disabilities and long term health conditions. 'Serenade' takes up to 10 people on holidays ranging from four days to a fortnight, 'Melody' is available for weekly hire by small groups and 'Symphony' takes up to 26 people on day trips. All boats have hydraulic lifts, toilets and showers designed for wheelchair users.

TOP THINGS TO SEE OR DO

Prince Canal Boat
Fully accessible boat operated by a community and activities centre on Regent's Canal, Camden. The wide beam canal boat is available for residential and day trips. Customised for use by disabled groups. The boat allows disabled crew members to use the steering and throttle controls. It has an open plan indoor space, and an outside deck which can accommodate large groups.
- www.thepiratecastle.org

Reach Out Plus
Suite 3, Citygate, 17 Victoria Street, Hertfordshire AL1 3JJ
- 0845 2160080
- info@reachoutplus.org
- www.reachoutplus.org

Two 12-berth canal boats operate from their boathouse in Hemel Hempstead. All are fully accessible for people with disabilities and ideal for people of all abilities. In summer 2012, a new 35 passenger boat (17 overnight) and an eight-berth family holiday boat joined the fleet. Both new boats include a special complex needs cabin and bed. The Boat Base also includes a 50 seater fully accessible Education and Visitor Centre.

Seagull Trust Cruises
Bantaskine Park, Falkirk FK1 5PT
- 01324 620768
- www.seagulltrust.org.uk

Offer one six-berth boat that can accommodate a family with a wheelchair user for cruises on the Scottish lowland canals. Two toilets on board can be used by a disabled person, one of which can be combined with a shower. There are lifts at the fore and rear and a skipper can be provided. Day cruises for disabled people and their families and friends are also organised from Falkirk, Kirkintilloch and Ratho.

Yorkshire Waterways Museum
Dutch River Side, Goole DN14 5TB
- 01405 768730
- info@waterwaysmuseum.org.uk
- www.waterwaysmuseum.org.uk

The 'Sobriety' is a converted, wheelchair accessible barge used for groups of up to 12 people for residential trips on the waterways of Yorkshire and Lincolnshire. A lift is provided between the cabin and deck level and a skipper can be made available. Week-long, weekend and day bookings can be taken.

Snowsport holidays

If holidays on the water are not for you, you may fancy a holiday on the slopes. These organisations provide holidays that involve skiing activities specially adapted for disabled people.

Disability Snowsport UK
Glenmore Grounds, Aviemore PH22 1QU
- 01479 861272
- admin@disabilitysnowsport.org.uk
- www.disabilitysnowsport.org.uk

Offer ski instruction by fully qualified instructors for disabled people at a purpose built adaptive ski school at Cairngorm. Similar services are based at ski slopes around the country. In addition, activity weeks are held in Europe and USA.

Redpoint Holidays
Trinity Hall, Llangollen Road LL14 3SF
- 0345 6801214
- sales@redpoint.co,uk
- www.redpoint.co.uk

Mainstream winter sports company that also offer adaptive ski programmes for disabled people wanting a skiing holiday with their family or friends. They also offer a 'Buddy Course' for companions.

Working holidays

Whilst on holiday, you may wish to volunteer on a project and meet others who are interested in getting involved in similar activities or causes. The following organisations may be able to provide you with these opportunities:

British Trust for Conservation Volunteers
Sedum House, Mallard Way, Doncaster DN4 8DB
- 01302 388883
- information@btcv.org.uk
- www.btcv.org.uk

Run an extensive programme of conservation holidays all year round in some of the most beautiful landscapes across the UK. Many of the holidays are suitable for disabled people but please call before booking to explain your needs and check suitability. Full details of the holidays offered can be found on their website.

Toc H Projects
PO Box 15824, Birmingham B13 3JU
- 0121 4433552
- info@toch.org.uk
- www.toch-uk.org.uk

Projects of varying lengths are arranged throughout the year bringing together volunteers to work to help local communities.

ADVICE & GUIDANCE

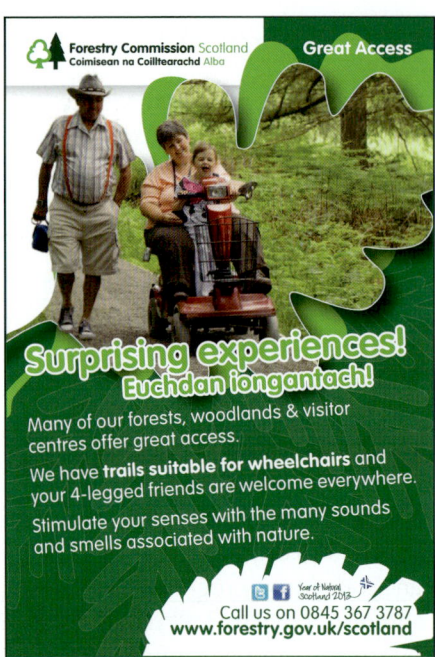

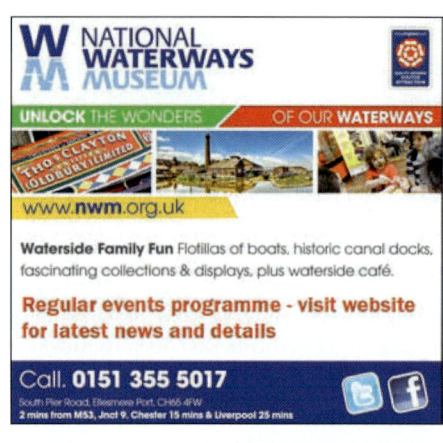

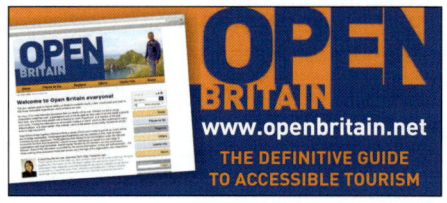

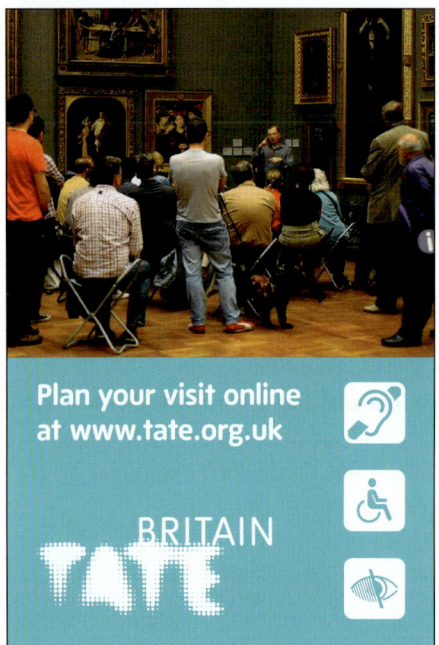

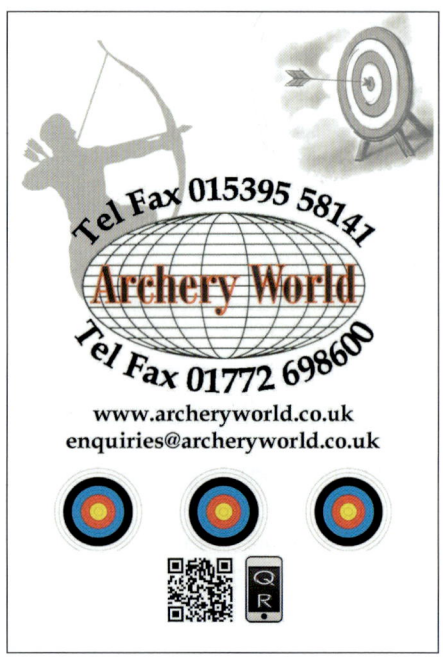

WHILE YOU'RE AWAY

Days out

What you do on your days out – from shopping to visiting stately homes or taking a walk in the forest – will depend on where you are and what you enjoy. Even a day trip can take some planning, so try and find out as much as you can before you head off. Here are some of the things to think about and ideas on where you could go.

Checking accessibility

While most modern tourist attractions should be able to cater for disabled visitors, it is advisable to check in advance if you have any specific requirements, if the attraction is large or for particular events.

Sites with a conservation aim, including historic buildings, nature reserves, forests, industrial heritage displays etc, can have limitations for disabled visitors. Several organisations have improved facilities for their disabled visitors. The following organisations have specialist publications and web pages providing information about their facilities.

Cadw: Welsh Historic Monuments
Plas Carew, Unit 5/7 Cefn Coed, Parck Nantgarw, Cardiff CF15 7QQ
- T 01443 336000
- E cadw@wales.gsi.gov.uk
- W www.cadw.wales.gov.uk

www.disabledgo.info provides online access guides including detailed information gathered by personal inspection around the UK at a wide range of entertainment venues, places to visit, restaurants and shops.

English Heritage
Customer Services Department, Kemble Drive, PO Box 567, Swindon SN2 2YP
- T 0870 333 1181
  Textphone 0800 015 0516
- E customers@english-heritage.org.uk
- W www.english-heritage.org.uk

Historic Scotland
Longmore House, Salisbury Place, Edinburgh EH9 1SH
- T 0131 668 8600
- W www.historic-scotland.gov.uk

The National Trust
PO Box 39, Warrington WA5 7WD
- T 0844 800 1895
  Textphone 0844 800 4410
- E accessforall@nationaltrust.org.uk
- W www.nationaltrust.org.uk

HOLIDAYS IN THE BRITISH ISLES

ADVICE & GUIDANCE

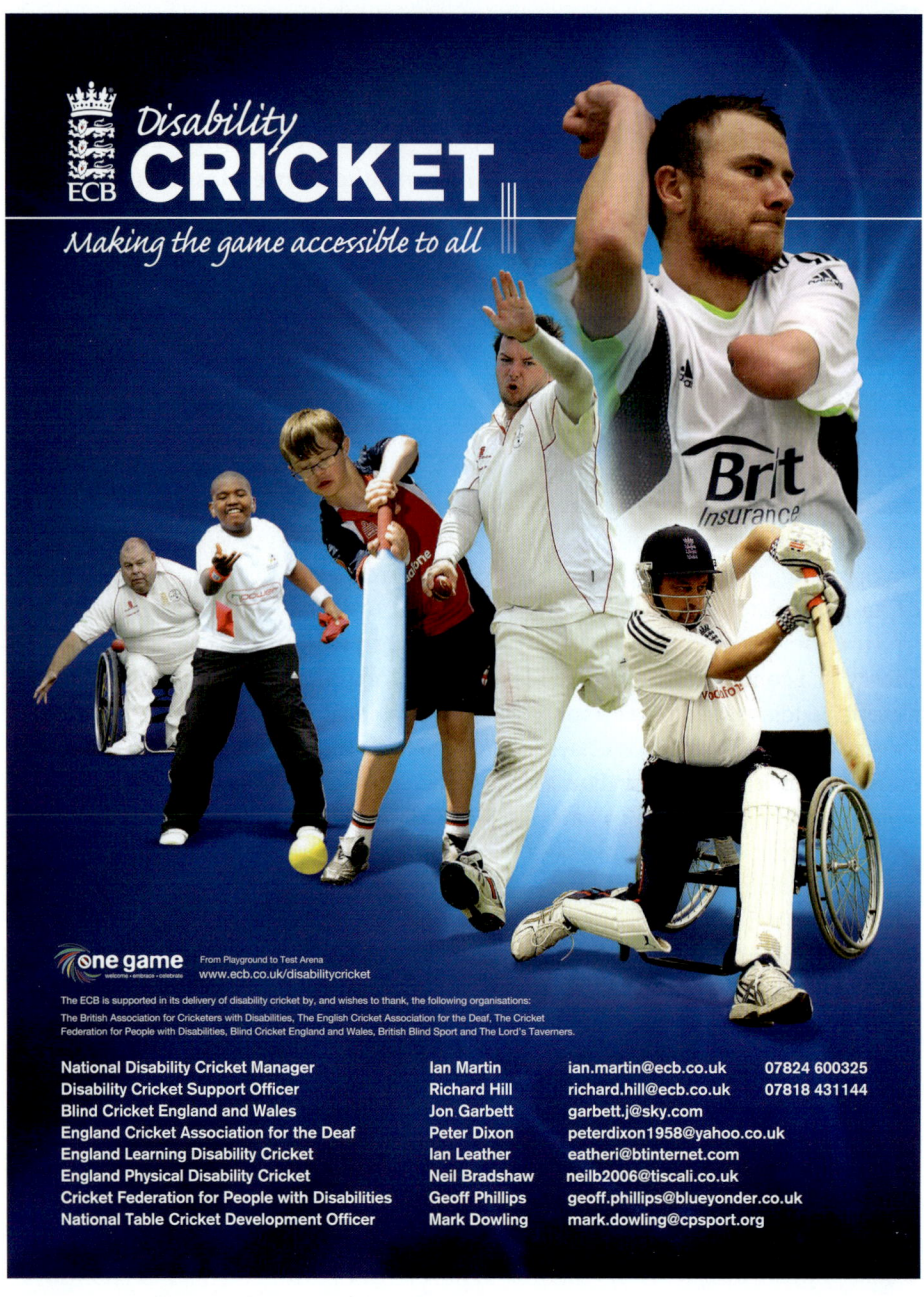

WHILE YOU'RE AWAY

National Trust for Scotland
Hermiston Quay, 5 Cultins Road EH11 4DF
- ☎ 0844 493 2100
- ✉ information@nts.org.uk
- 🌐 www.nts.org.uk

Royal Society for the Protection of Birds
The Lodge, Potton Road, Sandy SG19 2DL
- ☎ 01767 680551
- 🌐 www.rspb.org.uk

> **TOP THINGS TO SEE OR DO**
>
> **Beaumaris Castle, Anglesey**
> World Heritage Site managed by Cadw. The largest of Edward I's fortifications in Wales, it held a strategic position looking across the Menai straits from Anglesey to the mainland. Much of the defences survive and it is surrounded by a partly restored moat. Access into the Castle is via a good pathway, across a wooden drawbridge and in through the 'gate next the sea'. Internal access is mostly over mown grass and compacted surfaces reinforced with matting (there are a few uneven areas). Most of the ground floor can be accessed by wheelchair with the exception of the Chapel and some of the smaller turrets. Disabled car park and toilets on site.
> - 🌐 www.cadw.wales.gov.uk/daysout/beaumaris-castle

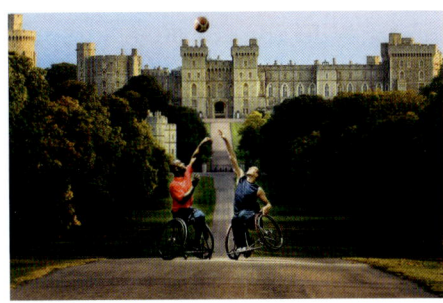

Sport

There are lots of local and national organisations providing and promoting opportunities in sport and facilities for disabled people. In some areas, local organisations have been formed to provide a range of sporting and other recreational activities for disabled people. These groups may use premises owned by the local council or other bodies but a number have their own purpose-built Centres.

Specialist organisations often have an important role in introducing people to sport and for those wishing to be involved in competitions. Taster sessions, which give the opportunity to try a range of activities, are often arranged locally at local sports or leisure centres.

GENERAL INFORMATION

For information on facilities and sporting groups in your local area, contact the local authority Sports Development Officer. The following organisations may also be able to point you in the right direction.

HOLIDAYS IN THE BRITISH ISLES

ADVICE & GUIDANCE

English Federation of Disability Sport (EFDS)
Sport Park, Loughborough University, 3 Oakwood Drive, Loughborough LE11 3QF
- 01509 227 760
- federation@efds.co.uk
- www.efds.co.uk

An umbrella group of disability sports organisations that works with policy makers and mainstream sports governing bodies to develop opportunities for disabled people to become more involved as competitors, recreational participants, administrators, officials and coaches. It seeks to create greater co-operation between disability sports organisations and works with the following national disability sports organisations that are recognised by Sport England: BALASA (British Amputee & Les Autres Sports Association), British Blind Sport, CP Sport, Dwarf Athletics, Mencap Sport, Special Olympics, UK Deaf Sport and WheelPower – British Wheelchair Sport.

The British Paralympics Association (BPA)
60 Charlotte Street, London W1T 2NU
- 020 7842 5789
- info@paralympics.org.uk
- www.paralympics.org.uk

Aside from being the representative organisation for elite paralympians, the BPA also provides, through its website, Parasport, which has been designed to inspire, educate, inform and signpost disabled people, and those interested in disability sport, to high quality opportunities. Parasport aims to help you find your personal best.

For other parts of the UK contact:

Disability Sport Northern Ireland
Adelaide House, Falcon Road, Belfast BT12 6SJ
- 028 9038 7062
- www.dsni.co.uk

Scottish Disability Sport
Caledonia House, South Gyle, Edinburgh EH12 9DQ
- 0131 317 1130
- www.scottishdisabilitysport.com

Disability Sport Wales
Welsh Institute of Sport, Sophia Gardens, Cardiff CF11 9SW
- 0845 846 0021
- www.disabilitysportwales.org

> In 2012, Disability Rights UK published *Doing Sport Differently*, a comprehensive guide to accessing sporting and leisure activities. Generously sponsored by VISA, the guide covers a wide range of sport and fitness activities from rambling to archery. It is available to download for free from the online shop on our website at www.disabilityrightsuk.org

SPECIFIC SPORTING ACTIVITIES

The following are just some of the organisations and projects concerned with helping disabled people to take part in specific sporting activities. More information on this can be found in this section under 'Activity holidays'.

British Disabled Angling Association (BDAA)
9 Yew Tree Road, Delves, Walsall WS5 4NQ
📞 01922 860912
🌐 www.bdaa.co.uk
Represents disabled anglers across the UK, including coarse, sea, specimen and game fishing. Services include: courses, group development, access audits of fishing areas, training people to coach disabled people and disability awareness training.

Inclusive Fitness Initiative (IFI)
Sport Park, Loughborough University, 3 Oakwood Drive, Loughborough LE11 3QF
📞 01509 227 750
✉ info@inclusivefitness.org
🌐 www.inclusivefitness.org
Launched by the English Federation for Disability Sport, IFI promotes the provision and management of integrated facilities for disabled people in general fitness centres. It accredits venues that provide accessible facilities, inclusive fitness equipment, appropriate staff training and inclusive marketing.

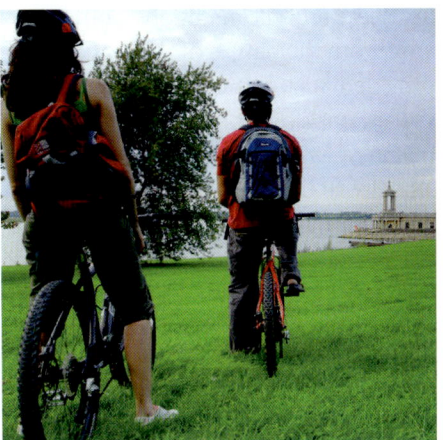

TOP THINGS TO SEE OR DO

Cycle Hire
Based near Buxton, Derbyshire, Hay is part of the 'Wheels for All' network of more than 50 UK centres with bikes for people with limited mobility, including hand-crank cycles, wheelchair cycles, tricycles, electric bikes and an all-terrain mobility scooter. It is one of the few cycle hire providers in the area to have a wide range of equipment for disabled users.
✉ parsleyhay.cyclehire@peakdistrict.gov.uk
📞 01298 84493

SPECTATOR FACILITIES

Facilities for disabled spectators have improved considerably following the creation of new and enlarged stadia, greater awareness of the needs of disabled people and the impact of the Disability Discrimination Act and other regulations.

ADVICE & GUIDANCE

But there are still limitations. Some arise from the nature of the feature provided, such as a commentary for visually impaired spectators at a football match or a raised viewing platform for wheelchair users at a racecourse. Others result from lack of provision, particularly where spectator arrangements are made for a particular event. Contact venues in advance to find out about availability of accessible facilities.

> www.spogo.co.uk is a smart new digital service designed to make it easier for you to find (and in time book) sports and physical activities. Currently only available in England.

Event Mobility Charitable Trust
8 Bayliss Road, Kemerton, Tewkesbury GL20 7JH
- T 01386 725391
- E eventmobility@hotmail.co.uk
- W www.eventmobility.org.uk

Some events can be problematic for disabled people to attend because they extend over a large area or the facilities for spectators are temporary. Event Mobility provides powered scooters and wheelchairs at a range of events including flower shows, agricultural and countryside shows, major golf championships and horse shows. Bookings need to be made in advance. A donation is requested (£18 for scooters and £10 for manual wheelchairs). Visit the website for a list of events that will provide the service or send a stamped addressed envelope to the address above.

Level Playing Field
The Meridian, 4 Copthall House, Station Square, Coventry CV1 2FL
- T 0845 230 6237
- E info@nads.org.uk
- W www.nads.org.uk
  www.levelplayingfield.org.uk

Promotes good facilities for disabled spectators at sports grounds. They have links with Disabled Supporters Associations at many clubs and their website includes information on facilities for disabled fans at grounds around the country.

> **PRESCRIPTION FOOTWEAR**
>
> We offer sophisticated video gait analysis and bio-mechanical assessments, including plantar pressure mapping and electronic in-shoe pressure measurement. This supports the existing footwear and lower limb orthotic service for people with conditions such as arthritis, diabetes, foot deformities and general conditions related to ageing. A full podiatry/chiropody service is also available.
>
> For more information or to book an appointment email us on info@prescriptionfootwear.co.uk or ring 01243 55 4407.
>
> www.prescriptionfootwear.co.uk

Other activities

Here are a few of the organisations devoted to encouraging the participation of disabled people. To find out what's available locally – ask local disability organisations, libraries, or look on the internet.

Disabled Photographers' Society
PO Box 85, Longfield, Kent DA3 9BA
- **T** 01454 317754
- **E** secretary@disabled photographers.co.uk
- **W** www.disabledphotographers.co.uk

Provides information on how you can adapt cameras and other photographic equipment and has access to engineers who can help. It arranges an annual exhibition of members' work and organises occasional photographic holidays and other events. Also has close ties with mainstream photographic bodies.

> *Get Caravanning* is an introductory guide to caravans and motor caravans for leisure use published by Radar with the support of The Caravan Club. The guide is available from Disability Rights UK; Telephone 020 7250 3222 or visit www.disabilityrightsuk.org

Motorsport Endeavour
123 Ealing Village, London W5 2EB
- **T** 020 8991 2358
- **E** info@motorsportendeavour.com
- **W** www.motorsportendeavour.com

Runs events involving disabled people in all forms of motorsport. A wide-ranging programme includes rallies, karting and visits to motorsport venues. The club is open to drivers as well as people wishing to take other roles including as navigators, marshals, timekeepers and spectators. It is also establishing links for disabled people who are seeking employment in the motorsport industry.

TOP THINGS TO SEE OR DO

London Blind Rambling Club
Affiliated to the Ramblers Association, the Club arranges about 24 walks per year, mostly in the Home Counties, with meeting points in Central London. Some walks are located within London, for instance at Hampstead Heath. Each walk is led by the local Ramblers Association group and one-to-one guiding is provided if necessary.
- **W** www.ramblers.org.uk

ADVICE & GUIDANCE

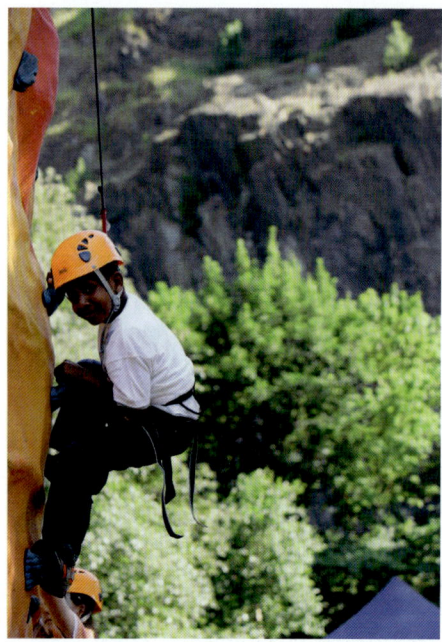

Thrive
The Geoffrey Udall Centre, Beech Hill, Reading RG7 2AT
- 0118 988 5688
- info@thrive.org.uk
- www.thrive.org.uk

Thrive's aim is to improve the lives of elderly and disabled people through gardening and horticulture. It runs demonstration gardens, supports a network of community and therapeutic gardening projects and runs an extensive programme of training courses, many about running community gardening projects. It runs the Blind Gardeners' Club and produces publications and factsheets offering practical advice on a wide variety of gardening topics. Their website www.carryongardening.co.uk provides information about equipment and techniques to make gardening easier. Launched in April 2011, www.accessiblegardens.org.uk has a directory of gardens with accessibility reviews written by people with disabilities. The site also contains information on accessibility, and articles about people, organisations, schools and groups involved with gardens.

The Wheelyboat Trust
- 01798 342222
- info@wheelyboats.org
- www.wheelyboats.org

The principal role of the Trust is to help public waters, groups and organisations acquire Wheelyboats for their disabled visitors, members, beneficiaries, etc., which it does by raising funds to help cover the cost of acquiring Wheelyboats. Wheelyboats have roll-on, roll-off access and can be helmed from a wheelchair. There are four different models – two for multi-purpose use, seating 8 and 12 and two for angling.

Further information

There are further ideas for days out in the 'Useful resources' section of this Guide. You will also find details of a publication called *The Rough Guide to Accessible Britain*. This book contains over 170 ideas and recommendations for days out for disabled people with all suggestions having been reviewed by writers with disabilities.

WHILE YOU'RE AWAY

Public toilets

Accessible toilets can be found in most shopping centres, theatres, theme parks, sports centres and next to public toilet facilities.

Finding accessible toilets

All public toilets in Britain should have an accessible toilet close by. Accessible toilets usually have a level or ramped entrance, a bigger floor space to accommodate a wheelchair or a carer, grab bars and a low-level sink. They may also have a red alarm string that you pull in an emergency.

You might find that many accessible public toilets in Britain are locked – this is to prevent them being vandalised or misused. If you need a key to use an accessible toilet then you can join the National Key Scheme (see below).

TOILET PROVISION

Traditionally, public conveniences or toilets were provided by local authorities. In many areas, accessible features for disabled people have been included for many years, although you may still find inaccessible public conveniences still in use.

Changes in provision
In recent years, there has been an overall reduction in the number of traditional public conveniences, including some unisex units for disabled people operated by local authorities. However, as a result of greater awareness and the impact of Building Regulations and anti-discrimination law, appropriately designed toilets have become more common in privately owned buildings used by the public such as large shops, restaurants and bars and also in public premises including parks and libraries.

There have also been significant changes in the ways that toilets in public places are provided and managed.

In many instances the cleaning and routine maintenance will have been contracted out. Pre-built, self-cleaning toilets (sometimes referred to as 'automatic' or 'superloos') have been installed in an increasing number of locations, and these generally are maintained by the supplier.

In some districts the responsibility for public conveniences has been handed over to other bodies such as Parish Councils or to private companies that are responsible for managing elements of town centre public spaces.

HOLIDAYS IN THE BRITISH ISLES

ADVICE & GUIDANCE

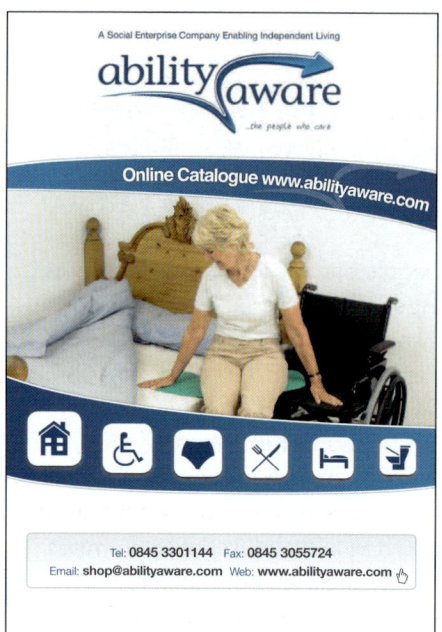

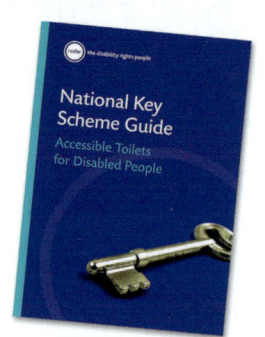

National Key Scheme Guide

Updated every year, this guide lists the location of 9,000 NKS toilets around the UK. It shows opening times, provider name and whether the toilet is unisex.

Available to order from our online shop
www.disabilityrightsuk.org

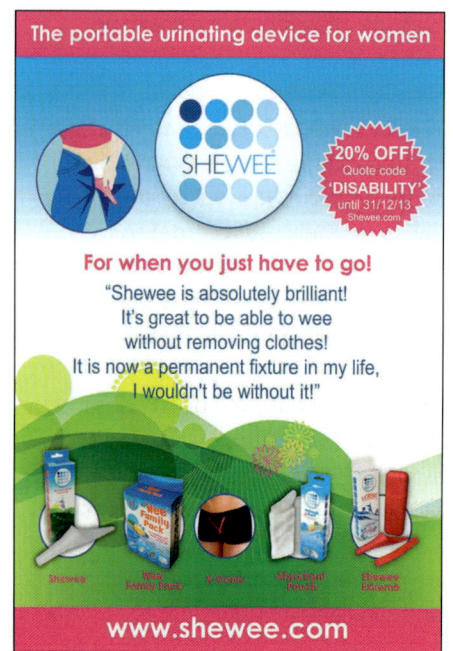

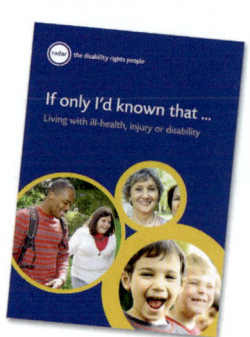

If Only I'd Known That ...

An information-packed guide to services, welfare rights, facilities and support for anyone with a disability or health condition, this guide includes resources for all ages from childhood to later years.

Available to order from our online shop
www.disabilityrightsuk.org

WHILE YOU'RE AWAY

Community toilet schemes have been established in some areas to provide public access to toilets in privately owned places such as pubs and cafes.

Toilets inside the growing number of shopping centres and other semi-public areas are usually the responsibility of the owners or managers of the premises.

B&BF's **Just Can't Wait** card is for people who may need to get to a toilet quickly when a public one is not available. The idea is that the card is shown in a shop or other premises as a request to use a staff or other toilet. Although some high street outlets have signed up to accept it there is no guarantee that the request will be granted, or that those that do accept it will have a toilet available with particular features. The Card, for which a £5 donation is requested, and other information are available from Bladder & Bowel Foundation, SATRA Innovation Park, Rockingham Road, Kettering NN16 9JH. Phone 01536 533255, or visit www.bladderandbowelfoundation.org for more information.

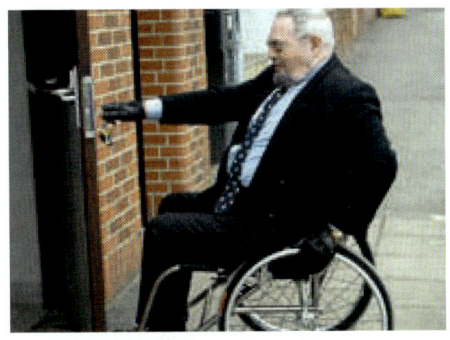

NATIONAL KEY SCHEME FOR TOILETS FOR DISABLED PEOPLE

The National Key Scheme (NKS), sometimes referred to as the Radar key scheme, is widely used throughout the UK. It was introduced over 30 years ago because an increasing number of local authorities and other bodies were finding that they had to lock their toilets for disabled people to prevent them being vandalised, or misused.

How the Scheme works

If toilets have to be locked, providers are asked to fit the standard NKS lock and to make keys available to disabled people in their area. Whenever possible a key should be held somewhere nearby for use by disabled people who have not got one.

The scheme has now been adopted by over 400 local authorities and the NKS lock has also been fitted to over 9000 toilets provided by other organisations including transport undertakings, pub companies, visitor attractions, shops and community bodies.

HOLIDAYS IN THE BRITISH ISLES

ADVICE & GUIDANCE

The National Key Scheme guide
When the scheme was first introduced, Radar (now Disability Rights UK) agreed to keep and maintain a list of all toilets fitted with the NKS lock. This list is regularly updated and published annually in our National Key Scheme Guide.

For news on the latest edition visit:
 www.disabilityrightsuk.org

This information is also available and continually updated as a free Smartphone app available from the Apple App Store, Blackberry World and various e-stores for Android users.

To order a key
Keys can be ordered from our online shop at www.disabilityrightsuk.org or by calling 020 7250 3222.

Changing Places toilets
Some disabled people need facilities that go beyond those found in a 'standard' toilet for disabled people. Changing Places toilets have:
- an adjustable height adult changing table;
- a hoist with tracking, or a mobile one if necessary;
- space both sides of the WC for assistants.

There are around 500 Changing Places toilets around the country. Access may be limited depending on opening times for the premises they are situated in.

For further information about the *Changing Places* campaign or to find details of current and planned Changing Places toilets locations, visit www.changing-places.org

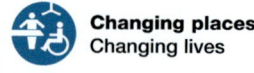
Changing places
Changing lives

Useful resources

This section lists national tourist boards, voluntary and commercial organisations involved in holiday services and tourism for disabled people, leisure providers and equipment and vehicle hire companies. We've also included some specialist organisations offering holidays to destinations outside the UK, in case you're thinking about travelling further afield in the future.

Government resources

GOV.UK
www.gov.uk
The Government's new online information service (formerly DirectGov) providing information on public services with links to government departments and agencies and a wide range of other organisations.

Equality Advisory Support Service
FREEPOST Equality Advisory Support Service FPN4431
0800 444 205
Textphone 0800 444 206
09:00 to 20:00 Monday to Friday
10:00 to 14:00 Saturday

This new service commissioned by the government replaces the helpline run by the Equality and Human Rights Commission. The Helpline is for individuals who think they may have experienced discrimination. The service aims to support individuals referred from local organisations, advisory groups, faith based organisations and other groups working within the community that support people experiencing discrimination and provides advice and information on discrimination and human rights issues.

Tourist boards

The organisations listed below are the key tourist boards in Great Britain and Ireland and include VisitBritain. VisitBritain are primarily sponsored by the Department of Culture, Media and Sport and are responsible for promoting all of the countries within Great Britain & Ireland to visitors from outside these countries.

Each country within Great Britain and Ireland also has its own national tourist board which are also listed below. These board's primary objectives are to provide information for all visitors on public transport, accommodation and tourist attractions within their countries and this will often cover giving information on accessibility.

VisitBritain
1 Palace Street, London SW1E 5HX
0207 578 1000
www.visitbritain.com

ADVICE & GUIDANCE

VisitEngland
1 Palace Street, London SW1E 5HX
- 020 7578 1400
- www.visitengland.com

National tourist board of England. Provide travel and tourism information for all visitors including those with disabilities. There is a huge amount of useful information available free of charge on the VisitEngland website. Most of the listings show the appropriate National Accessible Scheme symbols to indicate those establishments meeting the relevant criteria.

VisitScotland
Ocean Point One, 94 Ocean Drive, Edinburgh EH6 6JH
- 0845 859 1006
- info@visitscotland.com
- www.visitscotland.com

Scotland's national tourism organisation provides information and recommendations to help you plan your visit to Scotland. They provide information on transport, tours, holidays and accommodation. To order a brochure call or email with details of your requirements. Information on accessible accommodation can be found at:
- www.visitscotland.com/accommodation/

VisitWales
- 08708 300 306
- info@visitwales.co.uk
- www.visitwales.co.uk

Welsh Assembly Government's tourism team within the Department of Heritage. First port of call for information on holidays and short breaks in Wales including information on accessible accommodation.

Discover Ireland
- 0800 313 4000
- www.discoverireland.ie

Official Site of Failte Ireland (the Irish Tourist Board). Visit their website for information about accommodation, accessibility, attractions, activities and events in Ireland. An online 'Trip planner' is also available.

Discover Northern Ireland
Northern Ireland Tourist Board, 59 North Street, Belfast BT1 1NB
- 0289 0246609
- info@nitb.com
- www.discovernorthernireland.com

Official Tourist Board for Northern Ireland. Provide tips and guidance on accommodation, activities and things to do and see for all visitors including those with disabilities.

Channel Islands Tourist Board
- www.visitchannelislands.com

Official Tourist Board for the Channel Islands where you can find information about Jersey, Guernsey, Alderny, Herm and Sark. Each Island has its own contact centre, see the main website for relevant contact details.

Isle of Man Department of Tourism & Leisure
Sea Terminal Buildings, Douglas IM1 2RG
- 01624 686766
- tourism@gov.im
- www.visitisleofman.com

The Isle of Man's official tourism organisation. They provide details of accommodation, events and attractions.

USEFUL RESOURCES

Accommodation groups

The hotel groups and other organisations listed below are not specialist providers of accommodation for disabled people but have some properties which may be suitable and include an indication of this in their directories and brochures.

Accor
- 0871 663 0624
- www.accorhotels.com

Accor Hotels is Europe's largest hotel group and includes the chains Sofitel, Pullman, MGallery, Suite Novotel, Mercure, Adagio, All Seasons, Ibis, Etap hotel, Formule 1, hotelF1 and Orbis.

Best Western Hotels GB
Consort House, Amy Johnson Way, Clifton Moor, York YO30 4GP
- Reservations 0845 776 76 76
- www.bestwestern.co.uk

A consortium of independently owned hotels in England, Scotland, Wales and the Channel Islands. Some member hotels have been inspected for accessibility.

Campanile Hotels
Europa House, Church Street, Old Isleworth TW7 6DA
- contactclient@louvre-hotels.com
- www.campanile.com

A chain of purpose-built hotels by main roads and in city centres. Parking is adjacent to the bedrooms and to the building housing reception, bar, restaurant and meeting room. All have rooms designed for disabled guests.

The Camping and Caravanning Club
Greenfields House, Westwood Way, Coventry CV4 8JH
- 0845 130 7633 (also Textphone)
- www.campingandcaravanningclub.co.uk

Operate sites throughout Great Britain, most of which are open to non-members. About 70 have unisex toilet and shower facilities designed for disabled people. This together with information on their sites and membership can be obtained from the above address.

Camping in the Forest
Bath Yard, Moira, Derbyshire DE12 6BD
- 0845 130 8224
- contact@forestholidays.co.uk
- www.campingintheforest.co.uk

The Forestry Commission has 20 caravan and camping sites, most of which have WCs and showers for wheelchair users, and also three self-catering log cabin sites in Cornwall, North Yorkshire and The Trossachs that each have six-person cabins designed for disabled people.

The Caravan Club
East Grinstead House, East Grinstead RH19 1UA
- 01342 326944
- enquiries@caravanclub.co.uk
- www.caravanclub.co.uk

Has about 200 sites throughout the UK. Over 140 have unisex toilet/shower rooms designed for wheelchair users and a further 24 have handrails in amenity blocks. 70 sites have been assessed under the National Accessible Scheme and received the M1 grading. Full details are given in their annual brochure, The Site Collection, which is available free on their website or by calling 0800 521 161.

ADVICE & GUIDANCE

Choice Hotels Europe
Premier House, 112 Station Road, Edgware HA8 7BJ
- 0800 444444
- infouk@choicehotels.com
- www.choicehotelsuk.co.uk

A hotel group including Sleep Inn, Comfort, Quality and Clarion Hotels. Their directory indicates those with facilities for disabled guests.

The Circle
20 Church Road, Horspath, Oxford OX33 1RU
- 01865 875888
- info@circlehotels.co.uk
- www.circlehotels.co.uk

A consortium of individual family run hotels, located throughout the British Isles, with a central reservations office. The Circle Hotel Directory indicates those whose managers say have access to bedrooms for disabled guests.

cottages4you
Spring Mill, Stoney Bank Road, Earby, Lancashire BB94 0AA
- 0845 268 0760
- www.recommended-cottages.co.uk

Company offering self-catering holiday cottages in many parts of Great Britain. Their brochure and website indicate those that have adaptations for wheelchair users and also those with some ground floor accommodation.

Days Inn
- 0800 0280 400
- www.daysinn.co.uk

Accommodation, mainly at Welcome Break Service Areas on motorways and main routes, which have rooms for disabled guests.

Formule 1 Hotels
- www.hotelformule1.com

Budget hotels; each with two rooms for disabled guests with a double and bunk beds. One shared shower room has a roll-in shower, handrails and space for side transfer to the WC. When reception is not open an electronic machine will sell rooms by credit card; an entry code is provided for pre-paid bookings. Reservations may be made through the website or by contacting the hotel.

Haven Holidays
Reservations, 1 Park Lane, Hemel Hempstead HP2 4TU
- 0871 230 2760
- www.havenholidays.com

Operate 35 holiday parks in Great Britain, mainly on the coast. Their brochure, available from travel agents or by calling the above telephone number, indicates that most of these have some units designed for use by disabled people. For detailed information contact a specialist advisor on
- 0871 230 1926

Haven also have some parks with accessible units in France.

Helpful Holidays
Mill Street, Chagford, Devon TQ13 8AW
- 01647 433593
- help@helpfulholidays.com
- www.helpfulholidays.com

Around 600 self-catering properties in Cornwall, Devon, Dorset and Somerset, all of which are regularly inspected. Several have been designed for wheelchair users. These are indicated in their brochure, and can be searched for on the website, as are others that may be suitable for people with mobility difficulties.

USEFUL RESOURCES

Hilton Hotels
Maple Court, Watford WD24 4QQ
- T: 0845 7220055
- W: www.hilton.co.uk

International hotel group with hotels in cities, at airports and in other locations throughout the country. Although mainly used for business travel during the week, special offers for leisure guests are available at weekends.

InterContinental Hotel Group
- T: 0800 405060
- W: www.ichotelsgroup.co.uk

An international hotel group comprising the Express by Holiday Inn brand, middle range Holiday Inn hotels, high class Crowne Plaza hotels and luxury InterContinental hotels. They have a programme of improving their accessibility and services for disabled guests. Information on weekend breaks and other special offers is available by phoning central reservations and on their website.

Ibis Hotels
255 Hammersmith Road, London W6 8SJ
- T: 0871 6630624
- W: www.ibishotel.com

A group of two star hotels, part of the international Accor group, which have rooms designed for disabled guests.

Innkeeper's Lodge
- T: 08451 551 551
- W: www.innkeeperslodge.com

A chain of lodge hotels attached to Mitchells & Butlers pubs and restaurants. The more recent properties have rooms for disabled guests and are indicated in their directory.

National Trust
Holiday Cottage Booking Office, PO Box 536, Melksham SN12 8SX
- T: 0844 800 2072
- E: cottages@nationaltrust.org.uk
- W: www.nationaltrustcottages.co.uk

Have holiday cottages with adaptations for disabled people in a number of parts of England, Wales and Northern Ireland. Further information on these and on other cottages with ground floor accommodation that may be suitable for people with restricted mobility can be obtained from the above address and website.

Novotel Hotels
255 Hammersmith Road, London W6 8SJ
- T: 0871 66 306 26
- W: www.novotel.com

A group of three star hotels, part of the international Accor group, all with rooms designed for disabled guests.

Parkdean Holidays
2nd Floor, 1 Gosforth Park Way, Gosforth Business Park, Newcastle upon Tyne NE12 8ET
- T: 0844 335 3252
- E: enquiries@parkdeanholidays.co.uk
- W: www.parkdeanholidays.co.uk

Operate 20 holiday parks in South West England, East Anglia, Wales and Scotland. Most have some units that have been adapted for disabled guests.

Premier Cottages
- T: 0845 0739421
- W: www.premiercottages.co.uk

Annual brochure of independently owned holiday cottages across Great Britain. Bookings are made direct with the owners who can answer enquiries.

ADVICE & GUIDANCE

Premier Travel Inn
Houghton Hall Business Park, Porz Avenue, Dunstable LU5 5XE
- ☎ 0870 242 8000
- 🌐 www.premierinn.com

A group of over 470 lodge hotels around Great Britain mainly adjoining restaurants or pubs where meals are available, although some have integral restaurants. Almost all have rooms designed for disabled guests and the number of these is indicated in their directory. Bookings can be made online, or by telephone to the central reservations number or to the individual hotels which are listed on their website.

Travelodge
- 🌐 www.travelodge.co.uk

Located beside main roads and in city centres in over 300 locations. Most have rooms designed for disabled guests and guests with limited mobility. These can be specified when booking. Directory available.

Venuemasters
The Workstation, Paternoster Row, Sheffield S1 2BX
- ☎ 0114 249 3090
- ✉ info@venuemasters.co.uk
- 🌐 www.venuemasters.co.uk

Offer holiday accommodation at Universities and Colleges throughout Britain during vacations on self-catering, bed & breakfast and fully serviced terms.

Youth Hostels
Youth Hostels offer inexpensive accommodation with meals or self-catering. A small but growing number of hostels have some adaptations for disabled people. Other hostels vary considerably in the extent of their accessibility. Especially for groups it is recommended that an advance visit is made before booking. Some hostels can be block-booked by groups or offer special activity programmes. For information on membership, hostels and other matters contact the Associations at the addresses below:

Youth Hostels Association (England & Wales)
Trevelyan House, Dimple Road, Matlock DE4 3YH
- ☎ 0800 0191 700
- ✉ customerservices@yha.org.uk
- 🌐 www.yha.org.uk

Scottish Youth Hostels Association
7 Glebe Crescent, Stirling FK8 2JA
- ☎ 0845 293 7373
- ✉ reservations@syha.org.uk
- 🌐 www.syha.org.uk

Hostelling International Northern Ireland
22-32 Donegal Road, Belfast BT12 5JN
- ☎ 028 9032 4733
- ✉ office@hini.org.uk
- 🌐 www.hini.org.uk

An Óige, Irish Youth Hostel Association
61 Mountjoy Street, Dublin 7
- ☎ +353 (0)1 830 4555
- ✉ info@anoige.ie
- 🌐 www.irelandyha.org

USEFUL RESOURCES

Voluntary organisations

The following voluntary organisations are involved in holiday provision for disabled people. Other organisations with a more localised remit are listed in the regional sections of this Guide.

Tourism for All
- 0845 124 9971
  Textphone 0845 124 9976
- info@tourismforall.org.uk
- www.tourismforall.org.uk

Registered charity and the UK's central source of holiday and travel information and support for disabled and older people and carers. Provide information on accessible accommodation, visitor attractions and transport, in the UK and at selected overseas destinations. Identify sources of funding for disabled people on low incomes. Reservations service for inspected accessible accommodation is also offered. Work with all sectors of the tourism industry to improve accessibility and carry out inspections under the National Accessible Scheme. They aim to become a one-stop shop on UK tourism and holidays for anyone needing accessibility information and assistance. Tourism for All have developed the Open Britain brand and launched the new Open Britain website in March 2013. This new information resource aims to help make Britain the most accessible destination in the Europe.

3H Fund
Unit 2B, Speldhurst Business Park, Langdon Road, Tunbridge Wells, Kent TN1 2RA
- 01892 860207
- info@3hfund.org.uk
- www.3hfund.org.uk

Organise subsidised group holidays for physically disabled people accompanied by volunteer carers.

Action Against Allergy
PO Box 278, Twickenham TW1 4QQ
- 020 8892 2711
- aaa@actionagainstallergy.freeserve.co.uk
- www.actionagainstallergy.co.uk

Publish a large number of information leaflets for people with allergies including the leaflet Holiday Accommodation – a useful list of places to stay for people with allergies, price £2.

Action for Blind People
55 Sandgate Street, London SE15 1LE
- 030 3123 9999
- helpline@rnib.org.uk
- www.actionforblindpeople.org.uk
  www.visionhotels.co.uk

Operates four 'Vision Hotels' for blind and partially sighted people in South Devon, West Sussex, Somerset and Windermere. Self-catering units also available at Teignmouth (South Devon) and Windermere. The hotels aim to be accessible for all and welcome visually impaired guests. Brochures are available in large print, braille and cassette format.

HOLIDAYS IN THE BRITISH ISLES

radar the disability rights people
If only I'd known that ...
Living with ill-health, injury or disability

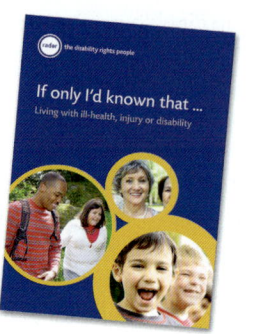

If Only I'd Known That ...

An information-packed guide to services, welfare rights, facilities and support for anyone with a disability or health condition, this guide includes resources for all ages from childhood to later years.

Available to order from our online shop
www.disabilityrightsuk.org

radar the disability rights people
National Key Scheme Guide
Accessible Toilets for Disabled People

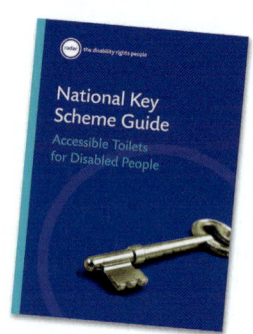

National Key Scheme Guide

Updated every year, this guide lists the location of 9,000 NKS toilets around the UK. It shows opening times, provider name and whether the toilet is unisex.

Available to order from our online shop
www.disabilityrightsuk.org

No more working for a week or two?
Livability provides holidays for more than 4,000 people a year. Our fully-accessible catered accommodation and self-catering holiday homes offer great breaks. We specialise in providing affordable holidays for disabled people as well as their families and friends.
Let us book you in.
08456 584478
www.livability.org.uk
livability
Holidays
Quality Access Choice

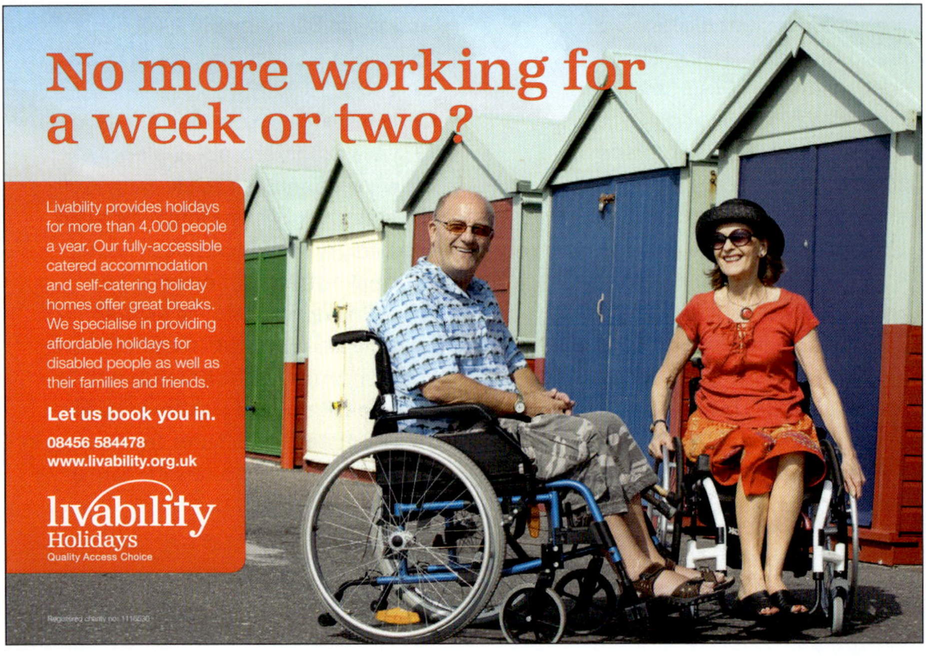

USEFUL RESOURCES

Arthritis Care
18 Stephenson Way, London NW1 2HD
- 📞 020 7380 6500
  Advice Line 0808 8004050
- ✉ info@arthiritiscare.org.uk
- 🌐 www.arthritiscare.org.uk

Campaign and provide a range of services and information for people with arthritis and their families. Free and confidential helpline offers specific advice on arthritis and holidays.

Elsewhere in the UK:
Arthritis Care Northern Ireland, The McCune Building, 1 Shore Road, Belfast BT15 3PG
- 📞 028 9078 2940
  Helpline 0808 800 4050
- ✉ Nireland@arthritiscare.org.uk
- 🌐 www.arthritiscare.org.uk/InyourArea/NorthernIreland

Arthritis Care Scotland, Unit 25A, Anniesland Business Park, Glasgow G13 1EU
- 📞 0141 954 7776
  Helpline 0808 800 4050
- ✉ Scotland@arthritiscare.org.uk
- 🌐 www.arthritiscare.org.uk/InyourArea/Scotland

Arthritis Care Wales, One Caspian Point, Pierhead Street, Cardiff Bay CF10 4DQ
- 📞 02920 444 155
  Helpline 0808 800 4050
- ✉ Wales@arthritiscare.org.uk
- 🌐 www.arthritiscare.org.uk/InyourArea/Wales

Asthma UK
Summit House, 70 Wilson Street, London EC2A 2DB
- 📞 020 7786 4900
- ✉ info@asthma.org.uk
- 🌐 www.asthma.org.uk

Run 'Kick Asthma' adventure holidays for young people with asthma and related conditions. Adventure activities are combined with educational sessions on managing asthma. Holidays held at a variety of locations in the UK divided into 6-11 and 12-17 age groups. For more information:
- 📞 0800 121 62 55
- ✉ holidays@asthma.org.uk

Around the UK:
Asthma UK Cymru, 3rd Floor, Eastgate House, 354-43 Newport Road, Cardiff CF24 0AB
- 📞 029 2043 5400
  Helpline 0800 121 6244
- ✉ wales@asthma.org.uk
- 🌐 www.asthma.org.uk

Asthma UK Northern Ireland, Ground Floor, Unit 2, College house, City Link Business Park, Durham Street, Belfast BT12 4HQ
- 📞 0800 151 3035
  Helpline 0800 121 6244
- ✉ ni@asthma.org.uk
- 🌐 www.asthma.org.uk

Asthma UK Scotland, 4 Queen Street, Edinburgh EH2 1JE
- 📞 0131 226 2544
  Helpline 0800 121 6244
- ✉ scotland@asthma.org.uk
- 🌐 www.asthma.org.uk

ADVICE & GUIDANCE

BREAK
Davison House, 1 Montague Road, Sheringham NR26 8WN
- 01263 822161
- office@break-charity.org
- www.break-charity.org

Charity that supports children, adults and families with care needs at a centre in Norfolk. Offer supported holidays, short breaks, respite care and day care support. Provide special care services for children and adults with learning or physical disabilities and their families. Other services include children's homes, adult day care and residential assessments for families in crisis. Also operate a mentoring scheme where volunteers support young people who have recently left local authority care. Have two holiday chalets in Westward Ho!, Devon.

British Kidney Patient Association
3 The Windmills, St Mary's Close, Turk Street, Alton GU34 1EF
- 01420 54 1424
- info@britishkidney-pa.co.uk
- www.britishkidney-pa.co.uk

Offer financial assistance to kidney patients for holidays. Any requests should be made on your behalf by your renal social worker. Group holidays arranged for young kidney patients at three activity centres and arrangements can be made for adults at some Mediterranean resorts. For information contact the Holiday Secretary.

British Limbless Ex-Service Men's Association (BLESMA)
Frankland Moore House, 185/187 High Road, Chadwell Heath RM6 6NA
- 020 8590 1124
- headquarters@blesma.org
- www.blesma.org

Holiday accommodation available at BLESMA residential and nursing homes in Blackpool for limbless ex-service men and their wives and to widows of former members. Convalescent and holiday accommodation may also be available to other ex-service men.

British Lung Foundation (BLF)
73-75 Goswell Road, London EC1V 7ER
- 020 7688 5555
  Helpline 030 0003 0555
- adminassistant@blf-uk.org
- www.lunguk.org

Among a range of free information sheets and booklets on lung diseases and related issues is *Going on Holiday with a Lung Condition*.

Around the UK:

BLF Scotland and Northern Ireland, Suite 104 Baltic Chambers, 50 Wellington Street, Glasgow G2 6HJ
- 0141 248 0050 or 079 0204 4363
- scotland@blf.org.uk
- northernireland@blf.org.uk

BLF Wales, 6a Prospect Place, Swansea SA1 1QP
- 01792 45 5764
- wales@blf.org.uk

British Polio Fellowship
Eagle Office Centre, The Runway, South Ruislip, Middlesex HA4 6SE
- 0800 018 0586
- info@britishpolio.org.uk
- www.britishpolio.org.uk

Run a self-catering bungalow equipped for wheelchair users at Burnham-on-Sea. Holiday information and grants available to their members.

USEFUL RESOURCES

Calvert Trust
- www.calvert-trust.org.uk

Have three outdoor activity centres equipped for disabled people in the Lake District, Northumbria and Exmoor. At each there is also accessible self-catering for families and similar sized groups. For information on each centre please see the section in this Guide on 'Activity holidays'.

Contact a Family
209-211 City Road, London EC1V 1JN
- 0808 808 3555
  Textphone 0808 808 3556
- helpline@cafamily.org.uk
- www.cafamily.org.uk

Among a range of publications offering information to families with disabled children is a free factsheet – *Holidays, Play and Leisure*.

Cystic Fibrosis Trust
11 London Road, Bromley, Kent BR1 1BY
- Helpline 030 0373 1000
- enquiries@cftrust.org.uk
- www.cftrust.org.uk

Can give information to people with cystic fibrosis and their families on holidays, travel and travel insurance.

Diabetes UK
Macleod House, 10 Parkway, London NW1 7AA
- 020 7424 1000
  Careline 0845 120 2960
  (9am-5pm weekdays)
  Textphone 020 7424 1031
- info@diabetes.org.uk
- www.diabetes.org.uk

Offer advice to people with diabetes on travel planning and have a Travel Guide (price £2). Activity holidays are arranged at a number of locations during the summer for children and young people with diabetes. Contact Careline for details.

DIAL UK
PO Box 833, Milton Keynes, Buckinghamshire MK12 5NY
- 01302 31 0123
- informationenquiries@dialuk.org.uk
- www.scope.org.uk/dial

National network of local disability advice centres run by and for disabled people. Provide independent advice on all aspects of disability, mainly by phone but also in person. DIAL merged with Scope in 2008. Some local DIAL groups are listed in the regional sections of this Guide.

Disabled Christians Fellowship/Through the Roof
PO Box 353, Epsom KT18 5WS
- 01372 749955
- info@throughtheroof.org
- www.throughtheroof.org

Organise holidays for disabled people of all ages both in the UK and overseas. Personal help may be available as required.

Disabled Ramblers
c/o 14 Belmont Park Road, Maidenhead SL6 6HT
- www.disabledramblers.co.uk

Organisation of disabled people promoting improved access in the countryside. Run an annual programme of one and two day supported rambles in a variety of settings mainly for users of mobility vehicles including wheelchairs, scooters and buggies. Advice on accommodation can be given to participants if required.

ADVICE & GUIDANCE

Disaway Trust
55 Tolworth Park Road, Surbiton, Surrey KT6 7RJ
- ☎ 020 8390 2576
- ✉ lynnesimpkins@hotmail.com
- 🌐 www.disaway.co.uk

Organise group holidays for physically disabled people, putting holiday packages together including visiting the venues to ensure suitability and accessibility throughout the holiday. Volunteer helpers are paired with disabled holidaymakers to provide assistance during the holiday.

Epilepsy Society
Chesham Lane, Chalfont St Peter, Bucks SL9 0RJ
- ☎ 01494 60 1300
  Helpline 01494 60 1400
- 🌐 www.epilepsynse.org.uk

Provide respite and residential care and medical services including assessments for people living with epilepsy.

Fieldfare Trust
69 Crossgate, Cupar, Fife KY15 5AS
- ☎ 01334 657708
- ✉ info@fieldfare.org.uk
- 🌐 www.fieldfare.org.uk

Work with people with disabilities and countryside managers to improve access to the countryside for everyone. Run projects which can enable people to take action locally, provide information on accessible places to visit and run events.

Handicapped Aid Trust
Northchapel House, North Street, Horsham, RH12 1RD
- ☎ 0800 028 0647
- ✉ secretary@handicappedaidtrust.org.uk
- 🌐 www.handicappedaidtrust.org.uk

Give grants towards the cost of helpers to assist disabled people on holiday, and towards the cost of holidays and helpers to give carers a break.

Holidays for All
- ☎ 08451 249973
- 🌐 www.holidaysforall.org

Group of UK disability charities and specialist tour companies. Work together to promote quality, accessible holiday breaks providing improved choice and flexibility for holidaymakers. Offer leisure activities and accommodation throughout the UK and abroad for people with sensory and physical impairments, their friends and families.

Holidays for Disabled People
Holidaymaker Liaison Team, PO Box 164, Totton, Southampton SO40 9WZ
- ✉ disholspw@aol.com
- 🌐 www.holidaysfordisabled.com

Organise an annual group holiday for people with physical disabilities at a holiday centre in the UK. Assistance provided by volunteers as required with medical and nursing cover. Participants can take their own companions.

Holidays with Help
4 Pebblecombe, Adelaide Road, Surbiton, Surrey KT4 6LL
- ☎ 020 8390 9752
- ✉ hwhholidays@btinternet.com
- 🌐 www.holidayswithhelp.org.uk

Run group holidays for disabled people at holiday centres in England. Activities and outings arranged. Applications accepted from groups, families and individuals. Experienced helpers and medical and nursing personnel are available. Apply to Rosemary McIntyre at the above address.

USEFUL RESOURCES

Incontact
SATRA Innovation Park, Rockingham Road, Kettering NN16 9JH
- 01536 533255
- info@bladderandbowelfoundation.org
- www.incontact.org

Provide advice and information for people with bowel and bladder control problems, including guidance on taking a holiday.

Livability Holidays
50 Scrutton Street, London EC2A 4XQ
- 0845 658 4478
- holidays@livability.org.uk
- www.livability.org.uk

Offer a range of holiday accommodation including hotels at Minehead and Llandudno and self-catering units, houses and flats around England and Wales including units at holiday parks and self-contained houses and flats equipped for disabled holidaymakers.

Mencap
123 Golden Lane, London EC1Y 0RT
- 020 7454 0454
- help@mencap.org.uk
- www.mencap.org.uk

Charity providing children and adults with learning disabilities support and advice in the areas of benefits, independent living, housing, education, employment and leisure activities through its 500 affiliated local societies. To find services in your local area call 0808 808 111.

Around the UK:
Mencap Cymru, 31 Lambourne Crescent, Cardiff Business Park, Llanishen, Cardiff CF14 5GF
- 029 2074 7588
  Helpline 0808 808 1111
- helpline.wales@mencap.org.uk
- www.mencap.org.uk/wales

Mencap Northern Ireland, Segal House, 4 Annadale Avenue, Belfast BT7 3JH
- 028 9069 135; helpline 0808 808 1111
- helpline.ni@mencap.org.uk
- www.mencap.org.uk/northern-ireland

Mind
15-19 Broadway, Stratford, London E15 4BQ; Mind infoline, PO Box 277, Manchester M60 3XN
- 020 8519 2122
  Mindinfoline 030 0123 3393
- info@mind.org.uk
- www.mind.org.uk

The leading mental health charity in England and Wales, it provides support through over 180 local associations; provides training for health professionals and the public; and campaigns for improved services and better legislation.

Mind Cymru
3rd Floor, Quebec House, Castlebridge, 5-19 Cowbridge Road East, Cardiff CF11 9AB
- 029 2039 5123
  Mindinfoline 0300 123 3393
- contactwales@mind.org.uk
- www.mind.org.uk/mind_cymru

Multiple Sclerosis Society
MS National Centre (MSNC), 372 Edgware Road, London NW2 6ND
- Helpline 0808 800 8000
  Switchboard 0208 4380700
  Information team 0208 4380799
- helpline@mssociety.org.uk
- www.mssociety.org.uk

Provide financial support for people with MS and their families and carers to access short breaks, holidays and respite care. Also provide information about planning and

ADVICE & GUIDANCE

taking a break through their *Guide to Short Breaks*, information team, website and support volunteers in local branches across the UK. Work with partners to introduce special offers, discounts and opportunities for people with MS to take a variety of accessible breaks.

Elsewhere in the UK:
Multiple Sclerosis Society Northern Ireland
The Resource Centre, 34 Annadale Avenue, Belfast BT7 3JJ
- 028 9080 2802

Multiple Sclerosis Society Scotland
Ratho Park, 88 Glasgow Road, Ratho Station, Newbridge EH28 8PP
- 0131 335 4050

Multiple Sclerosis Society Wales/Cymru
Temple Court, Cathedral Road, Cardiff CF11 9HA
- 029 2078 6676

The National Autistic Society
393 City Road, London EC1V 1NG
- 020 7833 2299
  Helpline 0808 800 4104
- nas@nas.org.uk
- www.autism.org.uk

Issue Holiday Help: a guide giving information on places that may be appropriate for children and adults with autism and Asperger syndrome.

Around the UK:
NAS Cymru, 6/7 Village Way, Greenmeadow Springs Business Park, Tongwynlais, Cardiff CF15 7NE
- 029 2062 9312
- wales@nas.org.uk

NAS Northern Ireland, 59 Malone Road, Belfast BT9 6SA
- 028 9068 7066
- northern.ireland@nas.org.uk

NAS Scotland, Central Chambers, 1st Floor, 109 Hope Street, Glasgow G2 6LL
- 0141 221 8090
- scotland@nas.org.uk

National Blind Children's Society
Bradbury House, Market Street, Highbridge, Somerset TA9 3BW
- 01278 764764
- enquiries@nbcs.org.uk
- www.nbcs.org.uk

Provide and organise activity holidays for children with a visual impairment and family weekends among other services. They have a specially adapted mobile home at Burnham-on-Sea.

National Deaf Children's Society
15 Dufferin Street, London EC1Y 8UR
- 020 7490 8656
  Helpline 0808 800 8880
- ndcs@ndcs.org.uk
- www.ndcs.org.uk

Organise activities for deaf children and their families, including a series of residential and day adventure and activity events. Volunteer interpreters and lip speakers provide communication support.

USEFUL RESOURCES

Around the UK:
NDCS Northern Ireland, 38-42 Hill Street, Belfast BT1 2LB
- T 028 9031 3170
  Textphone 028 9027 8177
- E nioffice@ndcsni.co.uk

NDCS Scotland, 2nd Floor, Empire House, 131 West Nile Street, Glasgow G1 2RX
- T 0141 354 7850
- E ndcs.scotland@ndcs.org.uk

NDCS Wales/Cymru, 4 Cathedral Road, Cardiff CF11 9LJ
- T 029 2037 3474
  Textphone 029 2023 2739
- E ndcswales@ndcs.org.uk

National Kidney Federation
The Point, Coach Road, Shireoaks, Worksop, Notts S81 8BW
- T 01909 54 4999
  Helpline 0845 601 0209
- E nkf@kidney.org.uk
- W www.kidney.org.uk

The holiday pages on the website give general advice for kidney patients travelling away from home and contact details for dialysis units in the UK that are particularly geared up for people on holiday.

Papillon Holidays
1 Exeter Drive, Ashton-under-Lyne OL6 8BZ
- T 0774 959 8423
- E papillonholidays@aol.com
- W www.papillonholidays.co.uk

Offer a range of holidays with support in Britain particularly for people with learning and physical disabilities. The programme, which runs through the year, includes a variety of activity and themed breaks as well as less structured seaside holidays.

Parkinson's Disease Society
215 Vauxhall Bridge Road, London SW1V 1EJ
- T 0808 800 0303
  Text relay 18001 0808 800 0303
- E hello@parkinsons.org.uk
- W www.parkinsons.org.uk

Provide support and information to people with Parkinson's, their relatives and carers through a team of information and support workers, local groups, publications and education and training. Publish an information sheet on International Travel & Parkinson's.

Phab England
Summit House, 50 Wandle Road, Croydon CR0 1DF
- T 020 8667 9443
- E info@phab.org.uk
- W www.phab.org.uk

Their Phab Kids Integrated Living Experience offer one week breaks at activity centres for disabled young people aged 9-18. Details on these and information on the network of Phab clubs throughout the country are available from the above address.

PINNT – Patients on Intravenous and Nasogastric Nutrition Therapy
PO Box 3126, Christchurch, Dorset BH23 2XS
- W www.pinnt.com

A self-help organisation for people requiring intravenous, naso-gastric and other artificial nutrition therapy. Produce holiday guidelines giving information on planning a holiday, transporting and obtaining equipment and supplies and other matters. Half PINNT has been established for younger members and their parents.

HOLIDAYS IN THE BRITISH ISLES

ADVICE & GUIDANCE

The Ramblers
2nd Floor, Camelford House, 87-90 Victoria Embankment SE1 7TW
- 0207 3398500
- ramblers@ramblers.org.uk
- www.ramblers.org.uk

Britain's only walking charity, working to safeguard footpaths, countryside and other places and to encourage more people to take up walking. Many local groups and are a good source of local information and some cater for people with disabilities or mobility impairments. You can find your local group by visiting their website.

Rethink
89 Albert Embankment, London SE1 7TP
- 0300 500 0927
- info@rethink.org; advice@rethink.org
- www.rethink.org

Provide services and advice to people affected by severe mental illness including information on holidays and respite care. A factsheet on respite care is available on their website.

In Northern Ireland contact:
Mindwise, Wyndhurst, Knockbracken Healthcare Park, Saintfield Road, Belfast BT8 8BH
- 028 9040 2323
- info@mindwisenv.org
- www.mindwisenv.org

In Scotland contact:
Support in Mind Scotland, 6 Newington Business Centre, Dalkeith Road Mews, Edinburgh EH16 5GA
- 0131 662 4359
- info@supportmindscotland.org.uk
- www.supportinmindscotland.org.uk

In Wales contact:
Hafal, Suite C2, William Knox House, Britannic Way, Llandarcy, Neath SA10 6EL
- 01792 81 6600
- hafal@hafal.org
- www.hafal.org

The Royal Blind Society
- 01827 722574
- Peterhards@royalblindsociety.org
- www.royalsociety.org.uk

Charity who offer self-catering holidays at 37 UK seaside holiday parks for people with a visual impairment.

Royal British Legion
48 Pall Mall, London SW1Y 5JY
- 0845 772 5725
- www.britishlegion.org.uk

Has four Poppy Break Centres for service and ex-service people, their dependants and carers recovering from an illness or bereavement. Centres are in Bridlington, Portrush, Southport and Weston-super-Mare. Personal and nursing care is not provided.

Royal National Institute of Blind People
Leisure Services, 105 Judd Street, London WC1H 9NE
- 0303 123 9999
- helpline@rnib.org.uk
- www.rnib.org.uk

The country's largest charity promoting the rights and interests of, and providing services for anyone with a sight problem. Provide holiday and leisure information for people with sight loss and run vacation schemes together with Action for Blind People for blind and partially sighted children. They also work with the leisure industry to improve access to leisure.

USEFUL RESOURCES

Around the UK:
RNIB Cymru, Trident Court, East Moors Road, Cardiff CF24 5TD
- 029 2045 0440
- cymruevents@rnib.org.uk

RNIB Northern Ireland and Isle of Man,
40 Linenhall Street, Belfast BT2 8BA
- 028 9032 9373
- rnibni@rnib.org.uk

RNIB Scotland, 12-14 Hillside Crescent, Edinburgh EH7 5EA
- 0131 652 3140
- rnibscotland@rnib.org.uk

Sailability
RYA House, Ensign Way, Hamble, Southampton SO31 4YA
- 0845 345 0403
  Textphone 023 8060 4248
- sailability@rya.org.uk
- www.rya.org.uk/sailability

An initiative of the Royal Yachting Association with the aim of promoting and co-ordinating participation by disabled people in the sailing community. It provides information to the public on where they can sail and supports sailing centres and clubs in improving opportunities open to people with disabilities.

Scope
6 Market Road, London N7 9PW
- 020 7619 7100
  Helpline 0808 800 3333
- response@scope.org.uk
- www.scope.org.uk

Provide a range of services including information on schooling, employment and training, care and respite, leisure activities, and communication technologies for people with disabilities.

Scout Holiday Homes Trust
Gilwell Park, Bury Road, Chingford, London E4 7QW
- 020 8433 7290
- scout.holiday.homes@scouts.org.uk
- www.holidayhomestrust.org

Offer low cost self-catering holidays in six-berth chalets and caravans at a number of holiday parks. Any family with a disabled member welcomed – not only those in Scouting. The season is generally from Easter-October and bookings are taken from the previous October.

Scripture Union Holidays
207-209 Queensway, Bletchley, Milton Keynes MK2 2EB
- holidays@scriptureunion.org.uk
- www.scriptureunion.org.uk

Organise holidays for young people. One holiday each year caters for disabled youngsters alongside non-disabled children aged 15-19 and another for 13-19 year-olds with learning difficulties. Applications via the Holidays Administrator.

HOLIDAYS IN THE BRITISH ISLES

ADVICE & GUIDANCE

Sense
101 Pentonville Road, London, N1 9LG
☎ 0845 127 0060 or
   020 7520 0972 (also textphone)
✉ holidays@sense.org.uk
🌐 www.sense.org.uk
Organise over 25 holidays each year for 120 deafblind children and adults. Each holiday has one or more paid leader supported by a team of volunteers to ensure that it is centred on individual needs and choices of holidaymakers. Sense holidays enable participants to have fun in a supportive environment, gain new experiences and meet new people. For further information contact the Holidays Co-ordinator.

Around the UK:
Sense Cymru, Ty Penderyn, 26 High Street, Merthyr Tydfil CF47 8DP
☎ 0845 127 0090
   Textphone 0845 127 0092
✉ cymruenquiries@sense.org.uk

Sense Northern Ireland, Sense Family Centre, The Manor House, 51 Mallusk Road, Mallusk, County Antrim BT36 4RU
☎ 028 9083 3430 (also textphone)
✉ nienquiries@sense.org.uk

Sense Scotland, 43 Middlesex Street, Kinning Park, Glasgow G41 1EE
☎ 0141 429 0294
   Textphone 0141 418 7170
✉ info@sensescotland.org.uk

Spinal Injuries Association (SIA)
SIA House, 2 Trueman Place, Oldbrook, Milton Keynes MK6 2HH
☎ 0845 678 6633
   Helpline 0800 980 0501
✉ sia@spinal.co.uk
🌐 www.spinal.co.uk
Website includes information on holiday opportunities taken from information provided by members and articles and advertisements placed in the Association's magazine.

In Scotland similar services are provided by:
Spinal Injuries Scotland
Festival Business Centre, 150 Brand Street, Govan, Glasgow G51 1DH
☎ 0141 427 7686 or 0800 013 2305
✉ info@sisonline.org
🌐 www.sisonline.org

Vitalise
212 Business Design Centre, 52 Upper Street N1 0QH
☎ 0303 3030147
✉ info@vitalise.org.uk
🌐 www.vitalise.org.uk
Provide breaks for disabled people and carers in three accessible centres in Southampton, Chigwell and Southport. Each centre offers a programme of short breaks with care on-call and personal support. Many activities are offered throughout the year with several special interest weeks, including special Alzheimer's weeks, sightseeing, theatre and music.

Commercial organisations

The following companies and organisations offer holidays or other tourist services specifically geared to meet the needs of disabled people.

AA Disability Helpline
☎ 0800 26 20 50
🌐 www.theaa.com

This Helpline provides information on a range of disability-related subjects, such as motoring in the UK and overseas, route requests, car adaptations and wheelchair maintenance. This service is free to AA Members.

Access at Last Ltd
18 Hazel Grove, Tarleton, Preston PR4 6XL
☎ 01772 814555
🌐 www.accessatlast.com

Travel company formed by a wheelchair user. The website details accessible hotels, adapted vehicles, equipment and holiday packages, and users can post comments. All of these inspected hotels have at least one room with a wheel-in shower.

Accessible Travel & Leisure
Avionics House, Naas Lane, Quedgeley, Gloucester GL2 2SN
☎ 01452 729739
✉ info@accessibletravel.co.uk
🌐 www.accessibletravel.co.uk

Offer a wide range of holidays and related services for disabled people including Mediterranean holidays, cruises and tours in South Africa and Egypt. Accessible villas, apartments and hotels are offered together with accessible transfers or car hire, local representatives and insurance.

Can Be Done Ltd
11 Woodcock Hill, Harrow HA3 0XP
☎ 020 8907 2400
✉ holidays@canbedone.co.uk
🌐 www.canbedone.co.uk

Tour Operator founded by a wheelchair user, offering holidays for people with access or mobility problems. Their brochures include a wide range of destinations in Europe (including Britain and Ireland), Asia, Australia, Africa and America but tailor made holidays can be arranged anywhere.

Chalfont Line
Chalfont House, 4 Providence Road, West Drayton UB7 8HJ
☎ 01895 459540
✉ holidays@chalfont-line.co.uk
🌐 www.chalfont-line.co.uk

Long-established adapted coach hire company with a programme of leisurely paced holidays for wheelchair users and others with impaired mobility mainly to destinations in Britain and Europe. Their own wheelchair accessible coaches are used for these. Also run worldwide cruise holidays. A door-to-door service can be provided at an extra cost. Assistance with planning can be given to groups hiring coaches for their own programmes.

ADVICE & GUIDANCE

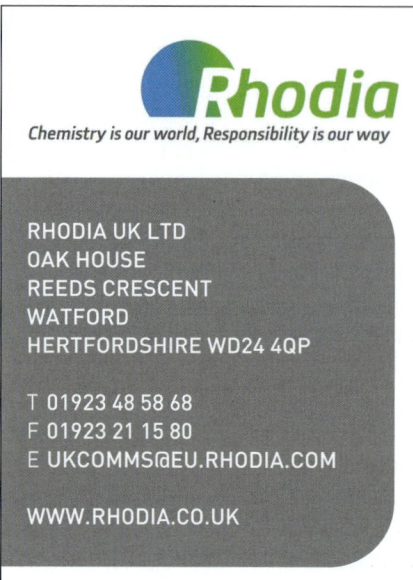

RHODIA UK LTD
OAK HOUSE
REEDS CRESCENT
WATFORD
HERTFORDSHIRE WD24 4QP

T 01923 48 58 68
F 01923 21 15 80
E UKCOMMS@EU.RHODIA.COM

WWW.RHODIA.CO.UK

Best wishes
to Disability Rights UK
in all its work

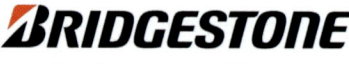

Performance Tyres

Telephone: 01926 488 500
Fax: 01926 488 600

www.bridgestone.co.uk

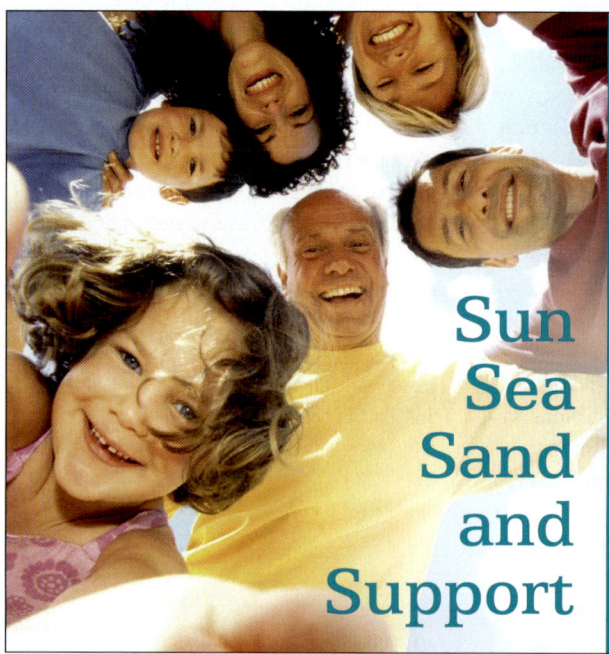

Sun
Sea
Sand
and
Support

We create the holiday designed especially for you, whatever your needs dictate

Whether you want your holiday to be an action packed experience or simply a relaxing and tranquil getaway, Heads Up Holidays can arrange all aspects of your holiday no matter what your needs may be, turning it from a dream to reality.

Let us help you plan your perfect holiday, starting now.

0115 711 7071
www.headsupholidays.com

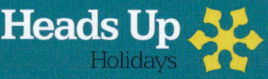

FITTLEWORTH

Is it difficult or just a plain nuisance to organise the medical appliances you need? Yes? Then Fittleworth has the simplest solution to make your life easier.

Fittleworth has been providing free, discreet and reliable home delivery of prescription medical devices since 1984. Specialising in stoma, continence and wound care, we are now one of the UKs leading appliances dispensers. Whether you use our Free Phone number, send your prescription to us in the postage-paid envelope or order on-line; that is all you need to do to use our service.

Having a local supplier is important. We have 32 care centres across the UK dispensing products into their local community. Anyone living in England is no more than 31 miles from Fittleworth. We are a national service, locally based.

We know that absolute discretion is essential to you, just as reliability is. So, your package will arrive on your doorstep in plain wrapping delivered by drivers wearing no Company logos, in vans with no branding and within 24-48 hours. Only you will know what's in the parcel.

If there are times when you wish you had someone to talk to about new products or issues you may have; Fittleworth Customer Service is open 6 days a week and ready to help. We have in-depth knowledge of products available and offer a sampling service if you want to try something new or your needs change. We also have a range of complimentary accessories.

You can rest assured that whatever type or brand of appliance your nurse or doctor prescribes, Fittleworth can provide for you – because we are not tied to any manufacturers.

To work with and support your doctor or nurse, our team of nurses is also on hand for telephone advice and, in some cases, home visits. If needed, expert hand cutters will ensure that your stoma bags are custom cut before delivery.

Do you worry about travelling because of your appliance needs? As the only UK member of World Assist Alliance, clients who need emergency products when abroad can still call us for assistance. This has proved invaluable when luggage is lost or a trip is unexpectedly extended. Knowing that should you have a problem, we are still just a phone call away, means you can relax and enjoy your trip.

So, if you want hassle-free and convenient home delivery of your appliances all you have to do is call us – we'll do the rest. What could be easier?

Fittleworth
0800 378 846
Hawthorn Road, Littlehampton, West Sussex BN17 7LT
Fittleworth Scotland
0800 783 7148
Unit 1, Riverside Business Park, 45 Moffat Street, Glasgow G5 0PD

email: caring@fittleworth.com
www.fittleworth.com

ADVICE & GUIDANCE

Diana's Supported Holidays
18 Parish Close, St Peters, Broadstairs, Kent CT10 2UU
- 0844 800 9373
- enquiries@dsh.org.uk
- www.dsh.org.uk

A range of holidays are offered with support for people with learning disabilities at seaside resorts and countryside areas in Britain and a number of destinations abroad. Groups are of at least six with a qualified leader and support staff, with one-to-one support if required although a lower ratio is normally provided. In addition to the programmed holidays, other destinations can be arranged for groups.

Mosaic Community Care Ltd
Unit 2 Cottam Business Centre, Cottam Lane, Ashton, Preston, Lancashire, PR2 1JR
- 01772 325350
- info@mosaiccommunitycare.co.uk
- www.mosaiccommunitycare.co.uk

Specialise in the provision of supported luxury holidays and respite breaks for disabled people who require support and care with daily living tasks. Their programme includes cruises and destinations in Florida and the UK.

William Forrester
1 Belvedere Close, off Manor Road, Guildford GU2 9NP
- 01483 575401

A wheelchair user who is a registered Blue Badge tour guide. Can help plan an itinerary in London or throughout the country, give lectures and assist visiting study groups. A telephone advice service is offered for wheelchair users visiting the country.

Matching Houses
- www.matchinghouses.com

A website for disabled people who wish to house-swap for their holidays based on the principle that if an exchange can be arranged between people with similar access needs they should both be able to travel with greater confidence within this country or further afield. They have over 600 members worldwide.

Countryside information

Areas of Outstanding Natural Beauty (AONB)
- www.landscapesforlife.org.uk

This website has details and links to all 46 AONB across the UK. Many have information about accessibility and have published easy access walks.

Keep Britain Tidy (Green Flag)
- greenflag.keepbritaintidy.org

The Green Flag Award® Scheme recognises and rewards the best green spaces in the country. For 2012, a record number of awards were made with 1424 parks and green spaces flying a Green Flag or Green Flag Community Award. These areas generally have good disabled access and facilities.

National Parks
- www.nationalparks.gov.uk

15 parks are members of the National Parks scheme. They are areas of protected mountains, meadows, moorlands, woods and wetlands and each one has an organisation that looks after the landscape and wildlife and helps people enjoy and learn about the area. Each park has its own website which can be reached via the website above and publish details of accessibility and facilties.

USEFUL RESOURCES

National Trails
🌐 www.nationaltrail.co.uk

Long distance routes for walking, cycling and horse riding through the finest landscapes in England and Wales. Most National Trails have their own website which can be reached through the central address above and some have information on sections of trails suitable for wheelchair users and buggies.

The Wildlife Trusts
🌐 www.wildlifetrusts.org

The largest UK voluntary organisation dedicated to protecting wildlife and wild places. There are 47 local Trusts across the UK, the Isle of Man and Alderney. Many local trusts publish accessibility information and you can find your local trust through their main website above.

Shopping

The following organisations, shopping areas and shopping centres offer specially adapted facilities and support to disabled people so that you can enjoy getting out and around the shops.

National Federation of Shopmobilty
PO Box 6641, Christchurch, BH23 9DQ
📞 0844 41 41 850
✉ info@shopmobility.org
🌐 www.shopmobilityuk.org

Provide wheelchairs and scooters for use in around 300 shopping centres and other shopping areas throughout UK. Services can provide a great deal of support and independence when you are shopping. Some schemes provide children's wheelchairs, escorts or special services for people visiting their area. The locations of regional branches and the services offered change all the time so although you will find some details in our regional listings, you must call the number above or visit the online directory on their website to double check the costs and what's available.

Capital Shopping Centres Group PLC
📞 020 7887 4220
✉ feedback@capshop.co.uk

Own some of the biggest shopping centres in the country including five of the UK's top six – The Trafford Centre, Manchester; Lakeside, Thurrock; Metrocentre, Gateshead; Braehead, Glasgow and The Mall at Cribbs Causeway, Bristol plus nine 'in-town centres' including Cardiff, Manchester, Newcastle, Norwich and Nottingham. They have made efforts to make their shopping experience fully accessible for disabled shoppers.

The Glades, Bromley, Kent
📞 0208 313 9292
🌐 www.theglades.uk.com

Shopping centre that is completely step-free. There are lifts to the second floor and disabled toilets on the ground level. Good selection of popular stores and leads out on to the High Street, where you will find more accessible shops. Surrounded by a number of car parks with free disabled parking and wheelchair/scooter hire.

The Whitgift Centre & Centrale Centres, Croydon, Surrey
🌐 www.thewhitgiftcroydon.co.uk

Shopping centres in Croydon divided by the High Street. Both contain large department stores, as well as independent and high street shops. There are lifts and disabled toilets in the malls and in some of the shops. Both the shopping centres have car parks with disabled bays close to the entrances. The Whitgift Centre car park offers wheelchair hire on 0208 688 7336.

Romford, Essex
If you are looking for somewhere to shop but want to avoid the London crowds, Romford offers the Brewery and the Mercury joint shopping centre. The Brewery has a wide range of shops, bars and accessible restaurants and also has 85 disabled pay and display car parking spaces. There is a 16 screen cinema with spaces for wheelchairs and a 24-lane bowling alley. For children, there is Kidspace, Europe's largest play area. The Liberty has over 100 shops, with a mixture of mainstream, and specialist stores. It leads out on to the High Street and Market Place where more shops and banks lie. The shopping streets are step-free with lifts to go upstairs so is accessible for all. The shops are very spacious and the restaurants have disabled toilets.

St David's Dewisant, Cardiff
Ⓦ www.stdavidscardiff.com
Shopping centre in the heart of Cardiff city centre. Home to designer shops, big high street names and a large restaurant quarter housing a variety of restaurants. Car parking spaces for disabled visitors and level access entry to most entrances. A lift gives access to all floors and accessible toilets and one Changing Places toilet is also available.

Trafford Centre, Manchester
Ⓦ www.traffordcentre.co.uk
Large indoor shopping and leisure facility situated five miles from the centre of Manchester and the largest shopping centre in the UK by actual size. Every toilet block in the centre contains an accessible toilet which can be opened by a National Key Scheme (Radar) key that can be collected from a member of the centre's staff. Further facilities for disabled visitors include an assisted changing facility with a Clos o Mat WC and an electric hoist. There are 260 designated parking spaces for disabled visitors situated near various entrances to the centre and there are ramps, or dropped kerbs at every entrance and a talking lift to all floors.

Westfield, London
Ⓦ uk.westfield.com/london
Shopping centres based in Stratford, East London and Shepherds Bush in the West with 300 designer and high street shops, a variety of restaurants and a large cinema. The centres are step-free with disabled toilets, wheelchair-friendly malls and lifts. Over 5% of the parking bays are dedicated to disabled parking and customers can book a free wheelchair or motorised scooter. Parking is free Monday – Friday for Blue Badge holders.

Theme parks & attractions

This section includes details of some of the UK's most popular theme parks and attractions. Most major theme parks and attractions have concessions for disabled children and adults. Ask in advance what evidence you will need to bring with you to get a concession. It is normally a Disability Living Allowance (DLA) or Attendance Allowance (AA) award letter but it's worth confirming this before you go to avoid any disappointments or difficulties. Parks may allow a limited number of friends, carers or support workers to go on rides with you or into the park at a discount.

USEFUL RESOURCES

Alton Towers
Alton Towers Resort, Alton, Staffordshire, ST10 4DB
- 📞 0871 222 3330
- 🌐 www.altontowers.com

Charge full entry fee for disabled visitors but offer concessions for up to three helpers. A guide for visitors with disabilities can be downloaded from their website.

Chessington World of Adventures
Chessington World of Adventures Resort, Leatherhead Road, Chessington, Surrey KT9 2NE
- 📞 01372 731582
- 🌐 www.chessington.com

Offer discounted rates for disabled guests and up to two carers. They publish a guide for guests with disabilities available at www.chessington.com/plan-your-trip/disabled-guide.aspx.

Drayton Manor Park and Zoo
Drayton Manor Park, Tamworth B78 3TW
- 📞 0844 472 1950
- ✉ info@draytonmanor.co.uk
- 🌐 www.draytonmanor.co.uk

Offer discounts for disabled people and a carer on the day.

The Eden Project
Bodelva, Cornwall PL24 2SG
- 📞 01726 811911
- 🌐 www.edenproject.com

Offers one free entry for a carer when accompanied by the disabled person.

Hatton Country World
Hatton Farm Village, Dark Lane, Hatton, Warwick, Warwickshire CV35 8XA
- 📞 01926 843 411
- ✉ hatton@hattonworld.com
- 🌐 www.hattonworld.com/farmvillage/contact

Offer discounted rates for disabled people and free entry for a carer.

Howletts Wild Animal Park
Bekesbourne, Nr Canterbury, Kent CT4 5EL
- 📞 0844 842 4647
- 🌐 www.aspinallfoundation.org/howletts

Offer discounted rates for disabled children.

Legoland Windsor
Winkfield Road, Windsor, Berkshire, SL4 4AY
- 📞 01753 626182
  Textphone 18001 0871 2222 001
- ✉ customer.services@legoland.co.uk
- 🌐 www.legoland.co.uk

Offer free entry for a carer who is looking after a disabled child for the day, documentary evidence will be required. Offer free admission for registered personal assistants with documented proof of disability. Publish a guide for disabled guests, available at:
- 🌐 www.legoland.co.uk/Plan/Guests-With-Disabilities

Lightwater Valley
Lightwater Valley Attractions Ltd, North Stainley, Ripon, North Yorkshire HG4 3HT
- 📞 0871 720 0011
- 🌐 www.lightwatervalley.co.uk

Offer discounted rates for disabled people and up to two helpers on proof of disability.

HOLIDAYS IN THE BRITISH ISLES

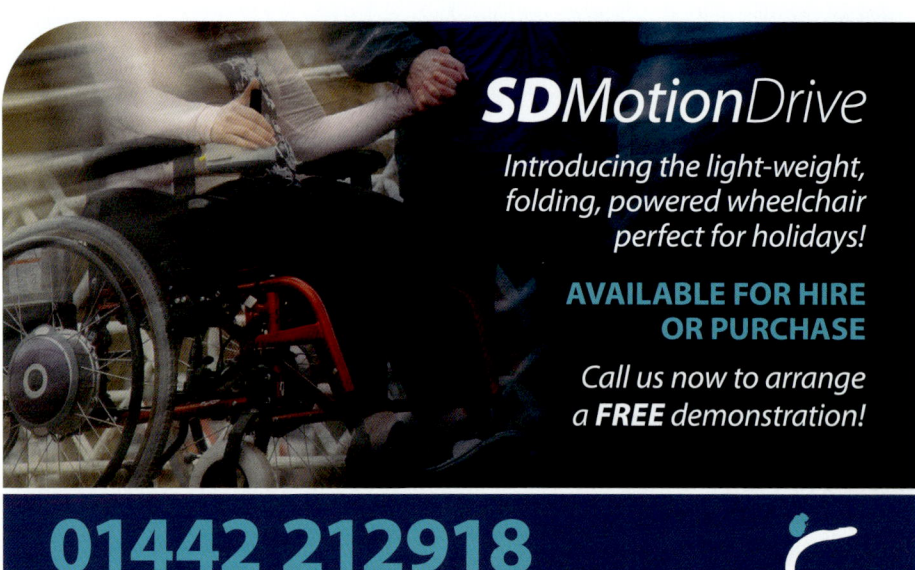

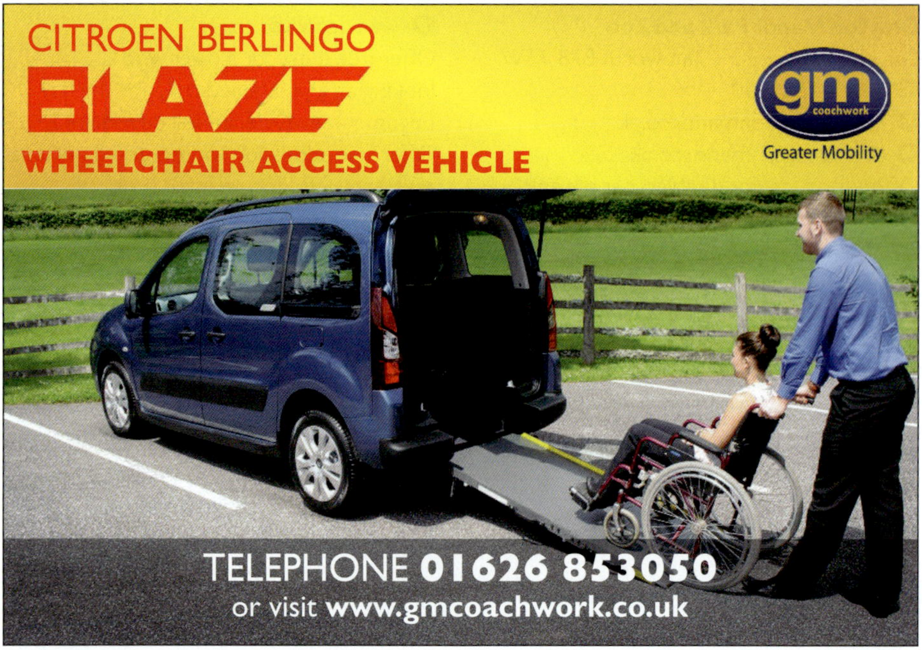

USEFUL RESOURCES

Madame Tussauds
London: Marylebone Road, London NW1 5LR
☎ 0871 894 3000
✉ guest.enquiries@madame-tussauds.com
🌐 www.madametussauds.com/London

Blackpool: 89 Promenade, Blackpool FY1 5AA
☎ 0871 282 9200
✉ guest.enquiries@madame-tussauds.com
🌐 www.madametussauds.com/Blackpool
Museum that contains wax models of famous people including the Royal Family, world leaders and sports and music stars, welcomes disabled visitors and one helper, without charge. You will need to provide documentary proof of disability eg. blue badge or similar.

Oakwood Theme Park
Canaston Bridge, Narberth, Pembrokeshire SA67 8DE
☎ 01834 891273 (General enquiries)
 01834 891376 (24-hour info line)
✉ info@oakwoodthemepark.co.uk
🌐 www.oakwoodthemepark.co.uk
Theme Park in Pembrokeshire that offers discounts for disabled visitors and easy entry on to rides. Offer concessions for the disabled person and a carer at their discretion.

Thorpe Park
Thorpe Park, Staines Road, Chertsey, Surrey KT16 8PN
☎ 0871 663 1673 (9am to 5pm)
🌐 www.thorpepark.com
Theme park in Surrey that offer concessions for disabled children and a carer.

Warwick Arts Centre
Warwick Arts Centre, University of Warwick, Coventry CV4 7AL
☎ 024 7652 4524
✉ arts.centre@warwick.ac.uk
🌐 www.warwickartscentre.co.uk
Allow disabled visitors to bring a companion or carer with them free of charge subject to availability.

Vehicles

Adapted Vehicle Hire
Unit 508 Stone Close, West Drayton, Middlesex UB7 8JU
☎ 0845 257 1670
✉ info@adaptedvehiclehire.com
🌐 www.adaptedvehiclehire.com
Rent out adapted cars and wheelchair accessible vehicles and have launched a 'Car and driver' service. They have branches around the UK and offer a delivery & collection service.

Atlas Vehicle Conversions
3 Aysgarth, Road, Waterlooville, Hampshire PO7 7UG
☎ 023 9226 5600
🌐 www.avcltd.co.uk
In addition to selling adapted cars, have a number of wheelchair accessible vehicles for hire including the Renault Kangoo, which can carry one passenger in a wheelchair and a minibus with removable seats that can carry up to two. Daily, weekly and monthly terms are available with special rates for weekends. Drivers must be over 25.

HOLIDAYS IN THE BRITISH ISLES

ADVICE & GUIDANCE

Freephone 0800 092 5092

adapt-ABILITY

www.adapt-ability.co.uk

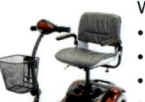

- Buy or hire
- FREE Home Demonstration
- Sales, Service & Repair
- New & Pre-owned
- Home Delivery Service
- Wheelchair & Scooter Service

WHEELCHAIRS, SCOOTERS, BATHLIFTS, WALKING FRAMES, TOILET & BATHROOM AIDS, DINING AIDS, COMMODES, HIGH SEAT & RISER CHAIRS, KITCHEN AIDS, WIDE FITTING SHOES & SLIPPERS, BEDS, STAIRLIFTS and lots more!

Finance Available (Written details on request)

Showroom:
M.Whitfield Ltd,.
Sanderson Street,
Coxhoe,
City of Durham
DH6 4DD
Tel: 0191 377 3705
Email: info@adapt-ability.co.uk

NEBULISERS
Supplied, serviced or repaired. Courtesy Nebuliser while we service yours

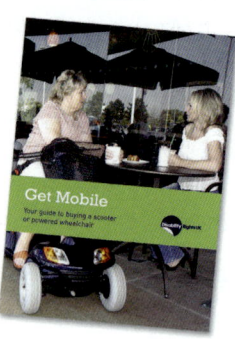

Get Mobile

A guide to buying a mobility scooter or powered wheelchair. New 2012 edition.

Available to order from our online shop
www.disabilityrightsuk.org

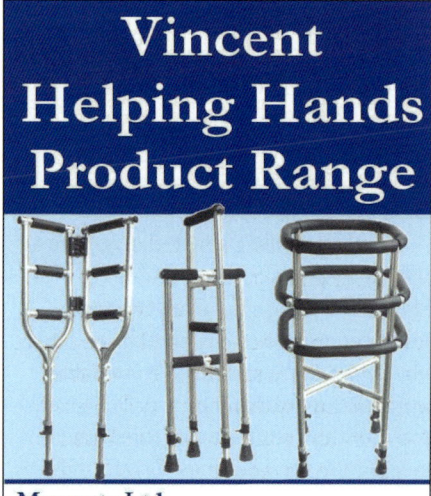

Vincent Helping Hands Product Range

Musmate Ltd
18-19 Mill Road, Radstock BA3 5TX
Tel./ fax (0845 094 4674
email sales@musmate.co.uk
www.musmate.co.uk/vincent

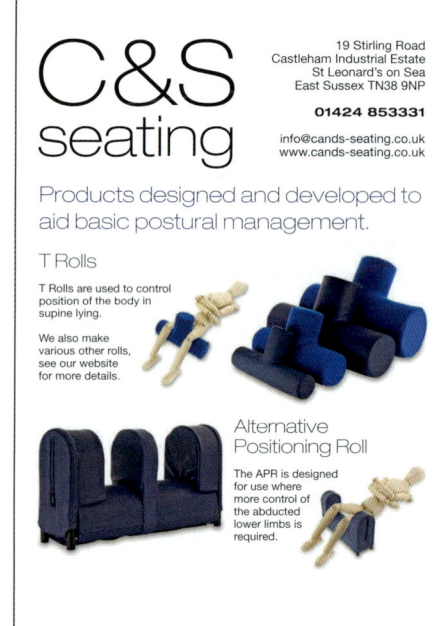

C&S seating

19 Stirling Road
Castleham Industrial Estate
St Leonard's on Sea
East Sussex TN38 9NP

01424 853331

info@cands-seating.co.uk
www.cands-seating.co.uk

Products designed and developed to aid basic postural management.

T Rolls

T Rolls are used to control position of the body in supine lying.

We also make various other rolls, see our website for more details.

Alternative Positioning Roll

The APR is designed for use where more control of the abducted lower limbs is required.

HOLIDAYS IN THE BRITISH ISLES

USEFUL RESOURCES

Autobility
Unit 2, Newburgh Industrial Estate, Cupar Road, Newburgh, Fife KY14 6HA
- 0800 298 9290
- www.autobility.co.uk

Have wheelchair accessible vehicles for hire on weekend, weekly and monthly rates. From their base in central Scotland they can arrange delivery throughout Britain or to airports and railway stations for an additional charge.

Brotherwood Automobility
Lambert House, Pillar Box Lane, Beer Hackett, Sherborne, Dorset DT9 6QP
- 0844 822 7939
- sales@brotherwood.com
- www.brotherwood.com

Convert cars for wheelchair users and have a range of cars available for long or short-term hire from their premises in North Dorset.

Caldew Coaches
6 Caldew Drive, Dalston, Carlisle CA5 7NS
- 01228 711690
- caldewcoachesltd@aol.com
- www.caldewcoaches.co.uk

Company with a range of accessible coaches for hire. These are available for holidays and day trips for groups of eight and above.

GM Coachwork Ltd
Teign Valley, Trusham, Newton Abbot, Devon TQ13 0NX
- 0845 8501860
- sales@gmcoachwork.co.uk
- www.gmcoachwork.co.uk

A Motability Premier Partner supplying wheelchair accessible vehicles including wheelchair access vehicles, drive-from wheelchair vehicles, accessible minibuses, used wheelchair accessible vehicles, wheelchair cars and minibuses. They also offer a full range of mobility conversions and adaptations.

John Flanagan Coach Travel
2 Reddish Hall Cottages, Broad Lane, Grappenhall, Warrington WA4 3HS
- admin@flanagancoaches.org.uk
- www.flaganscoaches.org.uk

Have coaches equipped with lifts that can carry passengers in wheelchairs that are available for hire by groups for day and longer trips. Holidays can be arranged in UK, Ireland and Holland for groups.

Motorvation Hull & East Riding
31a Northfield Close, West End, South Cave, Brough HU15 2EW
- 01430 422809
- mikliz.ten@virgin.net

Have three vehicles adapted to carry a passenger in a wheelchair and three others. Mainly used in East Yorkshire. Available with a voluntary driver on a daily basis. A donation towards running costs based on mileage used is requested.

ADVICE & GUIDANCE

Share more moments like this!

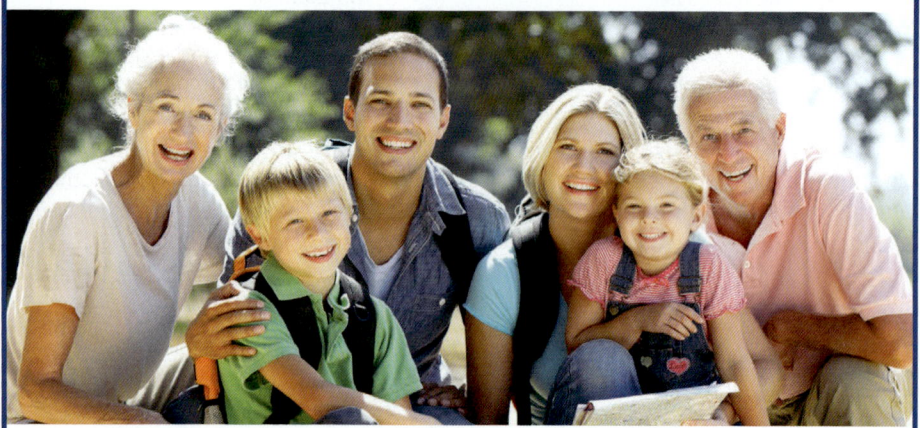

Simply... a secure home delivery service

- A dispensing centre local to you
- Convenient opening hours, six days a week
- Overseas emergency cover - World Assist Alliance

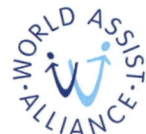

www.fittleworth.com

Opening Hours:
8am - 8pm Monday to Friday
9am to 1pm Saturday

We are Social:

Delivering emergency appliances to our customers abroad on holiday or business

---

We have a range of information sheets available, please tick the relevant boxes and we will post them to you.

I am interested in:
Stoma ❏   Continence ❏   Wound Care ❏

Name:* (Mr/Mrs/Miss) .... Date of Birth:* ....
Address:* ....
.... Postcode:* ....
Telephone No:* .... E-mail:* ....
* All fields must be completed   DISRIGHTSBRITISLEGUIDE-2013

Fittleworth
Hawthorn Road, Littlehampton,
West Sussex, BN17 7LT
www.fittleworth.com

Contact us today on:
Priority FREEPHONE Line
☎ **0800 521 740**

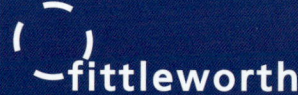

HOLIDAYS IN THE BRITISH ISLES

USEFUL RESOURCES

Nirvana Motorhomes
Court Farm, Pilgrims Road, Upper Halling, Rochester, Kent ME2 1HR
- 0800 328 1475
- info@nirvanarv.com
- www.nirvanarv.com

Hire out a motor home that is purpose-designed to be accessible for a wheelchair user and companions. It is equipped with a lift at the wide entrance, lower level kitchen fitments and a shower room with sliding walls to increase the size. Clamps are available to enable a passenger in a wheelchair to sit alongside the driver or both front seats can swivel to aid transfer. This can be used both in Britain and continental Europe. Similar models are available for sale.

Pyehire
Ovangle Road, Morcambe LA3 3PF
- 01524 598641
- pye.hire@pye-motors.co.uk
- www.pyemotors.co.uk

Have a range of self-drive accessible vehicles that can carry between one and four passengers in wheelchairs and two to eight other people. These are available on daily or weekly hire.

Thorntrees Garage
Wigan Road, Leyland, Lancashire PR25 5SB
- 01772 622688
- julie@thorntreesgarage.co.uk
- www.thorntreesgarage.co.uk

Cars and vans that can carry passengers in wheelchairs are available for hire at daily, weekly and monthly rates. Thorntrees Garage is near the M6, M61 and M65 or customers can be picked up from Preston mainline rail station.

Wheelchair Travel Ltd
1 Johnston Green, Guildford GU2 9XS
- 01483 233640
- trevor@wheelchair-travel.co.uk
- www.wheelchairtravel.co.uk

A self-drive vehicle rental company with wheelchair accessible cars and minibuses available for any period of domestic and continental use by both UK and non-UK licence holders. Minibuses have lifts, wheelchair securing points and seatbelts. Fiat Doblo cars can carry one wheelchair only, driver and two passengers. Cars with hand controls also available. Vehicles can be delivered to home, hotel or airport. Also offered is a wheelchair taxi service, using luxury adapted minibuses.

Equipment

This section includes bodies that operate nationally or at least over a large part of the country. Some organisations that hire wheelchairs and other equipment to people living in or visiting their area are included in the regional sections of this guide. A full list can be obtained from:

British Healthcare Trades Association
Suite 4.06 New Loom House, 101 Back Church Lane, London E1 1LU
- 020 7702 2141
- bhta@bhta.com
- www.bhta.net

Regulating body with over 400 professional members who sell equipment such as scooters, wheelchairs, bath lifts and stair lifts. If a company is listed with them or on their website, it means they have passed a special code of practice and therefore met high quality standards.

ADVICE & GUIDANCE

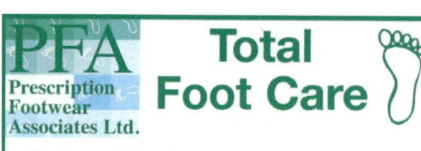

- **Footwear & Insoles**
  Comfort, Semi Bespoke, Made to Measure Shoes and Boots, Bespoke Insoles
- **Orthotics**
  Upper and Lower Limb Splints, Braces and Calipers, Spinal Braces and Corsets
- **Fracture and Soft Cast Bracing**
- **Podiatry/Chiropody**
  Complete Nail and Skin Care; Nail Surgery, Podiatric and Diabetic Assessments
- **Biomechanical Assessment**
  Plantar Pressure Mapping
- **Gait Assessment and Video Gait Analysis**
- **Medical Legal Orthotic Reports**
  Insurance and Rehabilitation Assessments
- **Multidisciplinary Team**

PRESCRIPTION FOOTWEAR ASSOCIATES
PFA House, Lake Lane, Barnham, Bognor Regis
PO22 0JB • Tel: 01243 554407
Email: info@prescriptionfootwear.co.uk
Website: www.prescriptionfootwear.co.uk

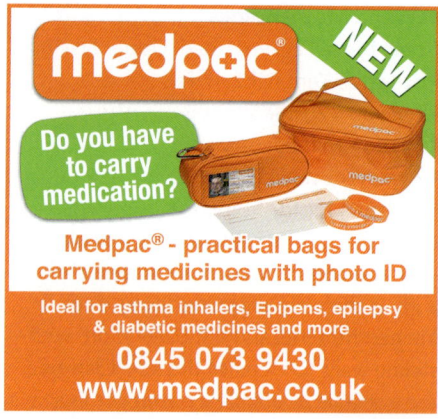

Medpac® - practical bags for carrying medicines with photo ID

Ideal for asthma inhalers, Epipens, epilepsy & diabetic medicines and more

0845 073 9430
www.medpac.co.uk

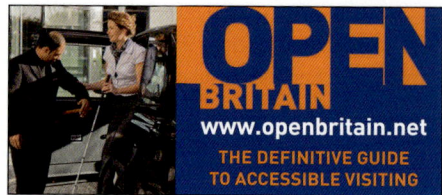

www.openbritain.net
THE DEFINITIVE GUIDE TO ACCESSIBLE VISITING

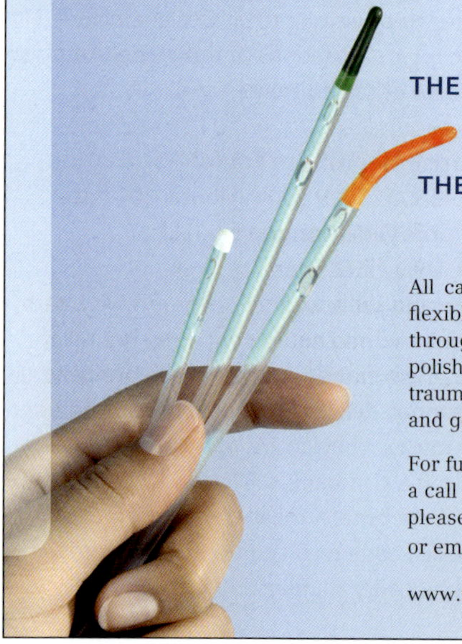

Intermittent catheters - with a very special Ergothan tip

LIQUICK® BASE-
THE READY TO USE HYDROPHYLIC CATHETER

LIQUICK PLUS-
THE READY TO USE HYDROPHILIC CATHETER WITH INTEGRAL COLLECTION BAG

All catheters benefit from the Ergothan® tip which is both flexible and strong, enabling it to glide smoothly and easily through the urethra and sphincter. The 'Soft Cat eyes' are polished inside and outside to effectively minimise any urethral trauma. The range offers uncoated, hydrophilic ready to use and gel based options. All are available on the Drug Tariff.

For further information or to arrange a call from a Territory Sales Manager, please call +44 1494 532761
or email info.uk@teleflex.com

www.teleflex.com

Teleflex

USEFUL RESOURCES

ABILITY AWARE LIMITED
We are a social enterprise company enabling independent living. We specialise in the everyday aids for daily living that help at home with leisure and with work.

As a social enterprise our twist is that any profits are reinvested to provide a social benefit. Our social benefit is to continually seek to improve the service we offer, and to provide excellent value and support to all our customers. We aim to be different to other retailers focusing on 'to serve' rather than 'to sell', this means that we listen and match products customers needs.

As part of our social commitment we:
- Are accredited Community Equipment Dispensers so are able to handle prescriptions from NHS and Local Authority prescribers.
- Provide our customers with a Made to Measure Service, which can be as simple as setting up a product to custom making our riser-recliner and fireside chairs to fit our customers specific measurements.
- Encourage customers to try before you buy. You can try our products in store or in your own home and bring it back if it does not fit. (Excludes continence, bathing and toileting products).
- Offer a range of bariatric, pediatric, visual and audio products.

For more information call our customer services team on 0845 3301144.

Ability2Travel
3 Mill Road, Kettering NN16 0RY
- T 01902 843 572
- E enquiry@ability2travel.co.uk
- W www.ability2travel.co.uk

Offer the services of travel companions/personal assistants to people with disabilities travelling in Britain or abroad. Assistance with making travel plans and arrangements can also be provided.

British Red Cross
44 Moorfields. London EC2Y 9AL
- T 0870 170 7000
- E information@redcross.org.uk
- W www.redcross.org.uk

Most branches can help people with disabilities in some or all of the following ways – referring people to other holiday facilities, providing voluntary assistance to disabled holiday-makers, and providing short-term loan of equipment such as wheelchairs. Enquiries should be made to the area office, addresses in local telephone directories or on their website above.

Direct Mobility Hire Ltd
Warren House, 201A Bury Street, Edmonton, London N9 9JE
- T 0800 092 9 322
- E info@directmobility.co.uk
- W www.directmobility.co.uk

Hire and sell a wide range of mobility, bath, toilet and bed equipment. Pressure relief and incontinence products also available. Next day delivery in area around London.

ADVICE & GUIDANCE

MEDPAC
Medpacs are practical bags specially designed for storing and carrying medicines safely and securely and come complete with a Photo ID Card for easy identification and a Treatment Card for all the essential information required to administer the medicine.

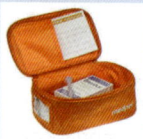
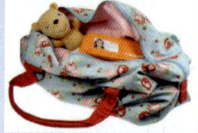

Medpacs come in two sizes and start at only £5.99, make these the essential addition to your holiday packing list!

www.medpac.co.uk

St John Ambulance
National Headquarters, 27 St Johns Lane, London EC1M 4BU
- 08700 10 49 50
- www.sja.org.uk

For road ambulance services, escorts, nursing and other care services in England, Wales and Northern Ireland apply to the County Headquarters listed in the telephone directory or on the website.

Theraposture Ltd
Kingdom Avenue, Northacre Industry Park, Westbury BA13 4WE
- 0800 834654
- info@theraposture.co.uk
- www.theraposture.co.uk

Offer a sale and rental scheme for adjustable beds for short-term use (two weeks minimum).

TELEFLEX
Teleflex is a global provider of medical devices used in hospital and home care. We serve healthcare providers in more than 130 countries with specialty devices for vascular access, general/regional anaesthesia, urology, respiratory, cardiac, surgery and the home care environment.

Continence care solutions
We are committed to making life easier and more manageable for people who use intermittent and Foley catheters for bladder control. We have developed a broad portfolio of urinary catheters and collection products to meet patient needs and offer clinical solutions. For information on intermittent catheters or to order free samples go to:
www.intermittent-catheters.co.uk

Homecare delivery solution
In addition to quality products, we offer a discreet, complimentary and confidential delivery service provided by an independent organisation with experience and expertise spanning many different clinical and product areas. They understand your needs which means they will provide you with an excellent home service. For more information go to the Home Delivery tab on our website www.intermittent-catheters.co.uk.

To contact Teleflex in relation to any of our products and services, call our friendly customer service team on 01494 532 761 or email info.uk@teleflex.com

www.teleflex.com

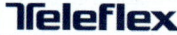

USEFUL RESOURCES

Walks With Wheelchairs
- www.walkswithwheelchairs.com

Online database of walks in the countryside of the UK that have been tried and tested by wheelchair users.

The Yellow Book
The National Gardens Scheme, Hatchlands Park, East Clandon, Surrey GU4 7RT
- 01483 211535
- webmaster@ngs.org.uk
- www.ngs.org.uk

The National Gardens Scheme's annual Guide to thousands of gardens, open for visiting by the public. Many are indicated in the Guide and on the website as being accessible to wheelchair users. Available from bookshops, by post or online from the addresses above. Price £9.99 (2013).

International holidays

This section includes details of companies and organisations that offer specialist holidays to destinations outside of the UK. Although this Guide is intended to cover the British Isles, the following details may be of use to you if you decide to travel further afield in the future.

Access Travel Ltd
6 The Hillock, Astley, Manchester M29 7GW
- 01942 888844
- office@access-travel.co.uk
- www.access-travel.co.uk

Offer a programme of holiday packages designed for disabled people in destinations around the Mediterranean, the Canaries and Florida. Holiday homes in France are also offered. A variety of self-catering and hotel accommodation options are available. ATOL protected.

Enable Holidays Ltd
39 Station Street, Walsall, West Midlands WS2 9JT
- 0871 222 4939
- info@enableholidays.com
- www.enableholidays.com

Offer overseas package holidays at selected resorts in the Mediterranean, Canaries and Florida at hotels chosen as being accessible. Powered wheelchairs and other equipment can be pre-booked, and adapted vehicles arranged for transfers and outings in many locations. All properties personally checked for accessibility.

Traveleyes
PO Box 511, Leeds LS5 3JT
- 08448 040 221
- www.traveleyes.co.uk

Travel company organising small group holidays for visually impaired and sighted people, with the latter acting as guides in exchange for a discounted price. Holidays have included walking trips in southern Spain and the Atlas mountains, visits to Tuscany, Sorrento, Greek Islands and Cuba with more destinations planned. Groups are kept to around 16 and the air holidays are ATOL protected.

Wings on Wheels
8 Cornfields, Church Lane, Tydd St Giles, Wisbech, Cambridgeshire PE13 5LX
- 01945 871111
- info@wingsonwheels.co.uk
- www.wingsonwheels.co.uk

Offer a programme of small escorted group holidays for disabled and non-disabled people throughout the year to overseas destinations and also tailored holidays for individuals and organisations in Britain, Europe and worldwide.

ENGLAND

> *The National Accessible Scheme is great – giving you the confidence to book somewhere which suits your specific needs.*

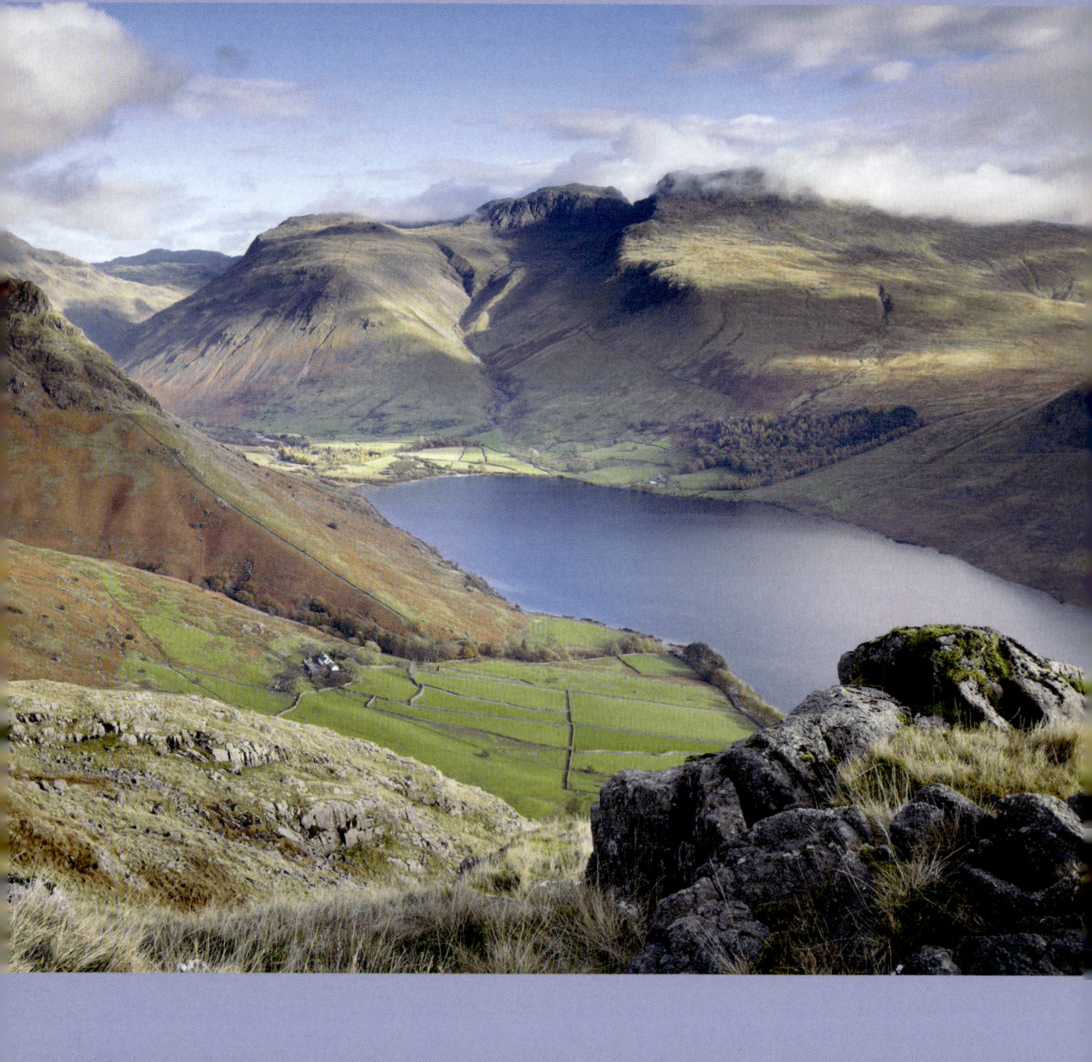

USEFUL RESOURCES

Publications & websites

Accessible Countryside for Everyone (ACE)
www.accessiblecountryside.org.uk
This site promotes accessibility to the countryside of England and Wales. Highlights walks suitable for wheelchair users of varying difficulties. The listed sites are selected for the physical access aspect however a number also have facilities for those with sight or hearing impairments. Site also lists accessible taxis, pubs and restaurants and links to specialist sites for accessible camping.

Access at Last
www.accessatlast.com
This website provides information on accessible holiday accommodation as well as suggestions for specialist equipment. The website is run by a disabled person and advertises only accommodation with at least one room with a level access shower. It includes detailed information and customer reviews.

Accessible Accommodation
www.accessibleaccommodation.com
This website helps you to find accessible accommodation in England, Ireland, Scotland, Wales and Northern Ireland. They aim to provide relevant information to those who need accessible accommodation when they travel, whether families with children, older people or those with reduced mobility and whether wheelchairs are required or not. Properties are not inspected and are classified by the property owner themselves. Requests for further information or to make a booking are made directly to the properties.

Caravanable
www.caravanable.co.uk
This website has been created by the mother of a wheelchair user. It lists caravan sites in the UK which have an adapted toilet, shower and basin with level or ramped access that are suitable for a disabled person.

Deaftravel
www.deaftravel.co.uk
This website has been launched for deaf people travelling independently abroad. As well as advice, information and local contacts, it includes travel stories both in written and signed video clip forms.

Direct Enquiries
www.directenquiries.com
This website holds the nationwide access register which gives information on the accessibility of a wide range of business premises around the country. It can be searched geographically, by type of business and by the nature of the access required. It also contains the list of toilets fitted with the National Key Scheme lock.

Disabled Holiday Directory
www.disabledholidaydirectory.co.uk
Online resource offering a large selection of holidays in the UK from country and coastal cottages to hotels, caravan sites and log cabins. Virtually all accommodation listed is wheelchair accessible with widened doorways. Some properties have equipment such as hoists and electric beds and facilities such as lowered kitchen and bathroom units and accessible wet rooms.

HOLIDAYS IN THE BRITISH ISLES

ADVICE & GUIDANCE

Disabled Holiday Information
PO. Box 186, Oswestry, Shropshire SY10 1AF
- info@disabledholidayinfo.org.uk
- www.disabledholidayinfo.org.uk

A website designed to give travellers with disabilities (whether they are wheelchair users or have other mobility issues) appropriate information on accessible holiday accommodation, attractions and activities in order to help them choose suitable accessible holidays. Properties bearing their logo on the site have been visited and assessed by their researchers for accessibility. Other properties are self-assessed.

Disability Now
- www.disabilitynow.org.uk

Online resource for disabled people. It includes regular features on holidays in Britain and abroad written by disabled people and holiday advertisements. The website also contains information on accessible holidays and accommodation rated by disabled people. A free e-newsletter is available.

Disability Rights UK
12 City Forum, 250 City Road, London EC1V 8AF
- 020 7250 3222
- enquiries@disabilityrightsuk.org
- www.disabilityrightsuk.org

Produce and stock a wide range of publications on matters affecting the lives of disabled people. Visit the website for a full list of all publications or to order online. The following may be particularly relevant to holiday-makers:
- *If Only I'd Known That A Year Ago* (2013)
- *National Key Scheme Guide* (2013)
- *Doing Transport Differently* (free to download, 2011)
- *Get Mobile: a guide to buying a scooter or powered wheelchair* (2012)
- *Get Motoring: a guide to buying a car* (2012)

DisabledGo
- www.disabledgo.info

The website gives access details on premises including shops, leisure facilities and catering establishments in an increasing number of towns and cities. The DisabledGo London App (available free from iTunes) provides information about access at venues and attractions across London with every venue assessed in person.

Disabled Holiday Directory
- www.disabledholidaydirectory.co.uk

Website giving detailed information on accessible holiday accommodation in the UK, Ireland and worldwide. The site also gives a useful list of questions that disabled people may wish to ask accommodation owners before making a booking.

English Heritage: Access Guide
- 0870 333 1181
  Textphone 0800 015 0516
- customers@english-heritage.org.uk
- www.english-heritage.org.uk/accessguide

An annual booklet giving information on accessibility and facilities for disabled people at around 100 historic buildings and sites owned by English Heritage. The booklet is available in alternative formats and can be picked up from any staffed property or from English Heritage

USEFUL RESOURCES

Customer Services Department, PO Box 569, Swindon SN2 2YP or downloaded for free from their website.

Farm Stay
National Agricultural Centre, Stoneleigh Park, Warwickshire CV8 2LG
- 024 7669 6909
- info@farmstayuk.co.uk
- www.farmstay.co.uk

The official guide listing holiday accommodation of all kinds on farms throughout the UK. Some information on accessibility is included. It can be obtained from Farm Stay (UK) Ltd.

Go Gluten-free, Wheat-free
- www.go-gluten-free-wheat-free.co.uk

An independent website giving information on accommodation and travel services in Britain and abroad suitable for coeliacs and others needing a gluten-free diet.

Good Beer Guide
230 Hatfield Road, St Albans AL1 4LW
- 01727 867201
- www.camra.org.uk/gbg

An annual publication with information on 4,500 pubs throughout the UK recommended by members of the Campaign for Real Ale (CAMRA). Those that are said to have easy access for wheelchair users to bars and toilets are indicated. Available, price £12.99 (2012), from bookshops or from CAMRA, a mobile phone based version of the guide is also now available for Smartphones.

The National Trust Access Guide
PO Box 39, Warrington WA5 7WD
- 0870 458 4000
  Textphone 0870 240 3207
- enquiries@nationaltrust.org.uk
- www.nationaltrust.org.uk

An annual book giving information on the accessibility and services for disabled visitors at National Trust properties throughout England, Wales and Northern Ireland. A free copy can be requested by post or email to the addresses above and is available in audio and Braille formats. The Access Guide is now available in smaller regional versions either by download from the website or in hard copy on request.

Rough Guide to Accessible Britain
- www.accessibleguide.co.uk

Produced in association with Motability, this book is packed with ideas for days out for disabled visitors. Includes details of things to do across Britain, from the arts to gondola trips on the Nevis Mountain range, with colour photos. All sites have been reviewed by writers with disabilities. The 2012 edition is available to download from the website.

Royal Society for the Protection of Birds
The Lodge, Potton Road, Sandy, Bedfordshire SG19 2DL
- 01767 680 551
- enquiries@rspb.org.uk
- www.rspb.org.uk

Welcomes disabled visitors to many of its nature reserves. Information on accessibility and facilities for disabled people is given on their website and in their monthly Bird Watching magazine.

HOLIDAYS IN THE BRITISH ISLES

ADVICE & GUIDANCE

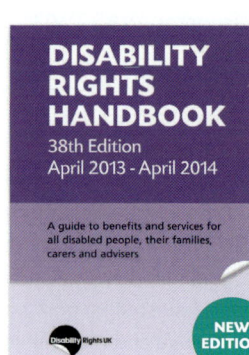

As comprehensive as ever
- How the benefit system works and how to make a claim
- Benefits for people with an illness, injury or disability
- Benefits for carers, young people and children and those looking for work, or in retirement
- Benefits for people injured at work or serving in the Armed Forces
- Challenging benefit decisions
- Getting and paying for care services

New in 2013
For people aged 16-64
- Personal Independence Payment: how to claim, what to do if you are turned down and what happens to people on Disability Living Allowance
- Extra information on Access to Work
- The new sanctions rules for Jobseeker's Allowance and Employment and Support Allowance
- The benefit cap: who will be affected and how it works

For families with disabled children
- Expanded guidance on Disability Living Allowance for children

For people 65 and over:
- Additional information on claiming Attendance Allowance

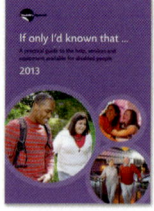

Personal Independence Payment is coming ...

From April 2013, Disability Living Allowance for people aged 16-64 will start to be replaced by a new benefit, the Personal Independence Payment. Over 2 million people will be affected.

The next two years will also see the biggest changes to the benefits system since the introduction of the welfare state. In this period of unprecedented change and benefits cuts, keeping up with the new rules is crucial.

Information and advice you can trust
The new edition of our Disability Rights Handbook, fully updated for 2013, provides in-depth information on the entire benefits system and comprehensive guidance on these critical changes.

The must-buy edition – out May 2013
Disability Rights Handbook 2013-2014 (38th Edition)
£29.99 inc P&P (£15.00 for people claiming benefits)
Order online at www.disabilityrightsuk.org

Stay informed – know your rights
This year's Handbook explains Personal Independence Payment and includes new additional guidance on Disability Living Allowance for children and Attendance Allowance (for people 65 and over) with tactics and tools to help make a successful claim.

It introduces Universal Credit which will replace several income-related benefits and tax credits and is planned to be phased in from April 2013.

All benefits explained in one book
Written in plain English by benefits specialists and legally referenced, it's the only user-friendly benefits guide designed specifically for both claimants and their advisers. It has the answers you need to help ensure the quality of your advice or to claim what you are entitled to.

Keep your Handbook up to date all year
Become a member of Disability Rights UK and we'll keep you up-to-date throughout the year with 'Disability and Welfare Rights Updates' our bi-monthly PDF magazine. 20+ pages of news and page-by-page Handbook updates. Download a free sample copy from our website.

If only I'd known that ...
Our companion guide, 'If only I'd known that a year ago' provides practical advice on accessing the help, services and equipment available for disabled people of all ages. See overleaf for more information.

Order your copy now at www.disabilityrightsuk.org

England

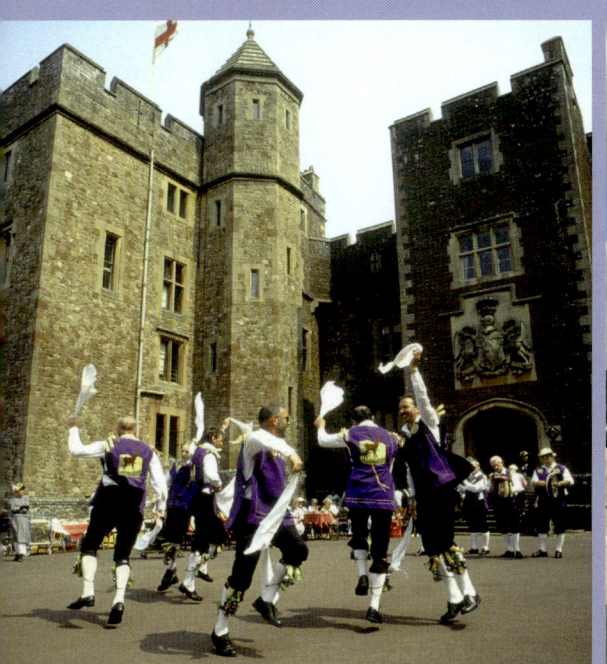

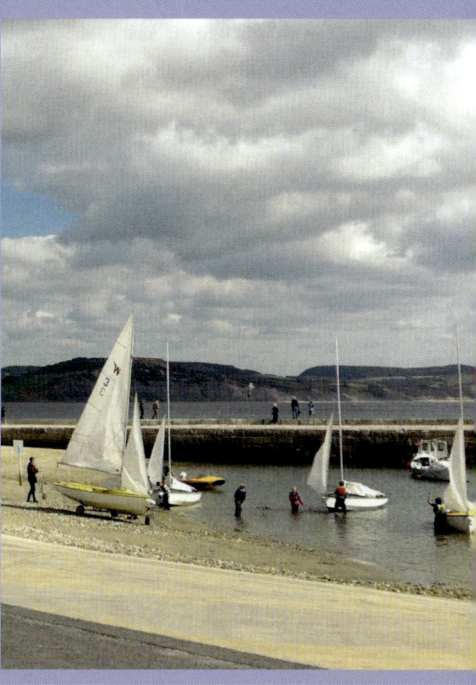

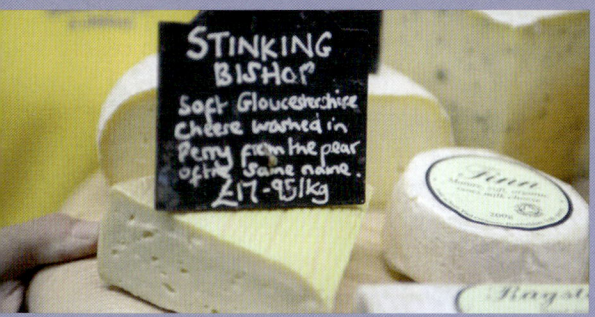

" *Exceptional accessible tourism venues are recognised and awarded through the VisitEngland Awards for Excellence.* "

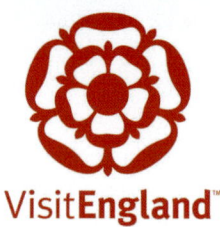

Visit England

England is a country of impressive diversity and variety. From the rolling hills of the Cotswolds and bustling city life of Manchester, to the charms of sleepy Cornish villages and the dramatic coastal splendour of the North East.

Importantly, England's tourism businesses are making it a top priority to ensure that their facilities and services are more accessible to their visitors. That means that holidays in England, with its plethora of exciting attractions and rich variety of accommodation, are becoming easier for everyone.

So whether The Great North Museum (Newcastle-upon-Tyne) takes your fancy, the National Theatre (London), Imperial War Museum North (Manchester), Windsor Castle (Berkshire) or the National Space Centre (Leicestershire), you are sure of a warm welcome.

Accessible England
VisitEngland runs a scheme to highlight those accommodation businesses which have improved their accessibility. The National Accessible Scheme (NAS) is great if you have a visual, hearing or mobility impairment giving you the confidence to book somewhere which suits your specific needs. A trained assessor has checked it out before you have checked in.

So remember – next time you book your accommodation in England – look out for the NAS logos. You can find information about NAS and the logos in the 'Advice and Guidance' part of this Guide.

Award-winning venues
Exceptional accessible tourism venues are recognised and awarded through the VisitEngland Awards for Excellence. The awards are the highest accolade in English tourism. The 'Access for All Award' is given to those who show a strong commitment to access resulting in excellent facilities.

The Great North Museum in Newcastle (2012 Gold Winner) houses premier collections of archaeology, natural history, geology and world cultures. With excellent accessibility for visitors with a range of access needs you can rest assured that your visit to the planetarium or life-sized T-Rex dinosaur skeleton will be a comfortable one.

At The Curve Theatre in Leicester (2012 Gold Winner) you can enjoy not only complete physical access but a range of assisted performances, including BSL, audio description and screen captioning. The Beacon museum in Whitehaven (Highly Commended 2012) equally excels in offering a warm welcome with the needs of disabled visitors a top priority.

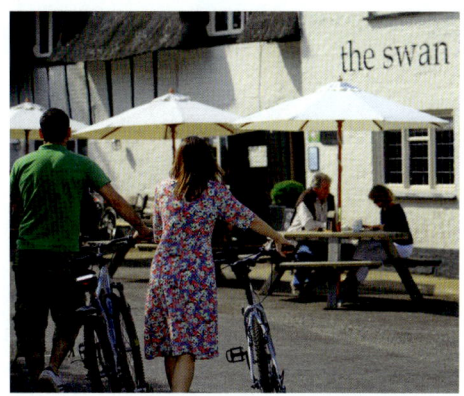

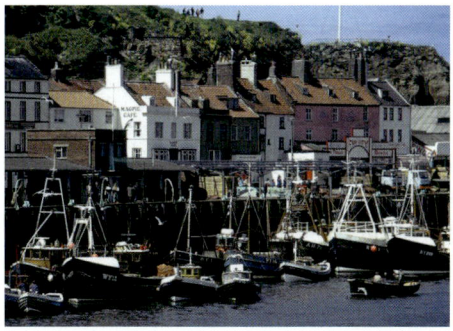

Information is key

All VisitEngland star rated accommodation and quality assured attractions are now required to provide information on their facilities and services to help you 'know before you go'. This information is presented as an Access Statement, which is simply a document that tells you lots of useful details about the premises and its surroundings.

Typical information may include, for example, the frequency of buses, useful telephone numbers, the number of steps to the front door and the availability of subtitles on televisions.

So, when you are next researching which accommodation to stay at and attractions to visit, ask to see their Access Statements. Help to raise awareness of this important document amongst England's tourism businesses.

The national tourist board website has a dedicated information section for people with physical or sensory needs. To make your travels around England easier and more enjoyable for you, we've put together some practical information and links to other useful websites, which we hope you'll find useful.

Find out more at
www.visitengland.com/accessforall

ENGLAND

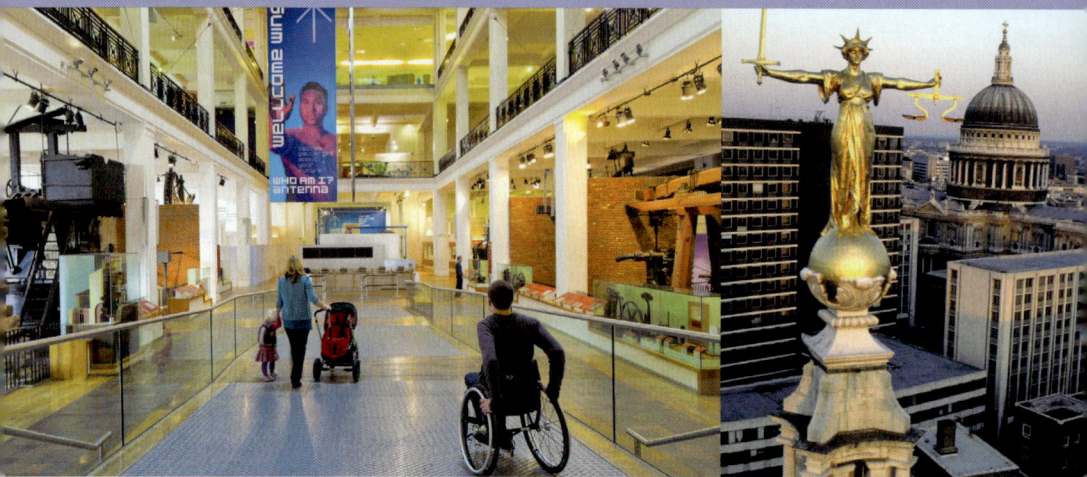

About London

London is one of the world's most important tourist destinations as well as hosting more British visitors than any other city or area. Whether your trip is for pleasure or business, for a particular event or general sightseeing, London will have something for you.

Many of London's major sights are well known – Buckingham Palace, Trafalgar Square, Marble Arch, Piccadilly Circus, Westminster Abbey, St Paul's Cathedral, Tower Bridge and the Tower of London. The Olympic Stadium and other aspects of the Olympic Park in Stratford will doubtless be added to the list of London's iconic sites.

London is the home of many internationally important museums and art collections including the British Museum, the National Gallery and the National Portrait Gallery both off Trafalgar Square. The national British Art collection is in Tate Britain near Westminster. The Victoria and Albert, the Natural History and the Science Museums are clustered in South Kensington. Other accessible attractions include the London Transport Museum in Covent Garden, the Imperial War Museum in Kennington and Somerset House between the river and the Strand.

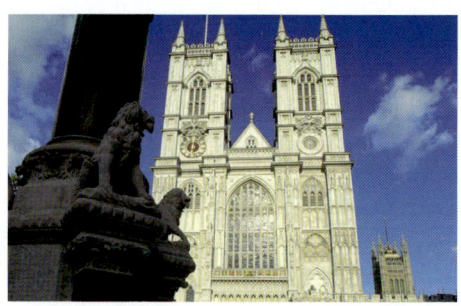

HOLIDAYS IN THE BRITISH ISLES

A string of attractions exist along the riverfront. The most dramatic are the London Eye opposite Westminster and the Tate Modern at Bankside with its international collection of 20th Century art. Nearby Southwark Cathedral has a recently opened visitor centre as does The Globe, a reconstructed Elizabethan theatre. Families may enjoy a visit to the London Aquarium in the old County Hall while adults can explore the history and taste of wine at Vinopolis near London Bridge.

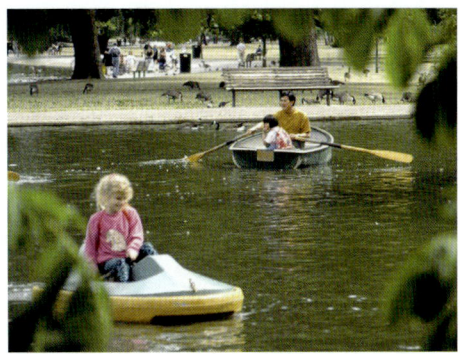

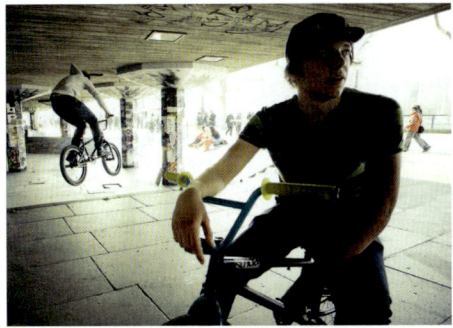

Central London has more open spaces, large and small, than many comparable cities and these are home to attractions such as the Serpentine Gallery in Hyde Park and London Zoo in Regents Park. In the outer areas there are large open areas at Hampstead Heath to the north, Epping Forest in the east and Richmond Park in West London. Also to the west, the London Wetlands Centre is at Barnes across the river from Hammersmith and Kew Gardens is a designated World Heritage Site.

There is much to see outside London too. The accessible Docklands Light Railway serves the centre of Greenwich with its many historic buildings. An access leaflet covering the National Maritime Museum, the Queen's House and the Royal Observatory is available. Newly restored, the Cutty Sark and its visitor centre are fully wheelchair accessible.

English Heritage premises include the home of Charles Darwin at Down House in the extreme south east of Greater London and Eltham Palace with its restored 1930's interior.

Shopping opportunities include famous retail streets, stores and markets in both central London and major suburban centres. For live entertainment, London offers an enormous variety of theatre and concerts, many in venues with recently improved access. Visitors to London may well encounter an event, be it pageantry like the Changing of the Guard or a State Visit, celebrations such as the Lord Mayor's Show or the Chinese New Year, a colourful demonstration or a major exhibition or sports fixture.

Hitchin
Buntingford
Halstead
Bishop's Stortford
Great Dunmow
Braintree
Luton
Stevenage
Buzzard
Dunstable
Luton Airport
Stansted Airport
Hertford
Witham
Hemel Hempstead
St Albans
Harlow
Maldon
Chelmsford
Princes Risborough
Hatfield
Potters Bar
Epping
Chipping Ongar
High Wycombe
Amersham
Barnet
Brentwood
Billericay
Watford
Harrow
Finchley
Rayleigh
Ilford
Beaconsfield
Maidenhead
LONDON
Dagenham
Basildon
Slough
Canvey Island
Grays
Thames
Tilbury
Grain
Heathrow
Dartford
Richmond
Rochester
Bracknell
Gravesend
Staines
Orpington
Chatham
Sutton
Esher
Croydon
Woking
Leatherhead
Maidstone
Farnborough
Sevenoaks
Dorking
Redhill
Yalding
Guildford
Reigate
Charing
Godalming
Surrey Hills
Tonbridge
Gatwick
Royal Tunbridge Wells
Bordon
Crawley
East Grinstead
Tenterden
Haslemere
Hawkhurst
High Weald
Horsham
Crowborough
Southwater
Haywards Heath
Billingshurst
Uckfield
Northiam
Heathfield
Rye
Burgess Hill
Pulborough
SOUTH DOWNS
Ashington
Battle
Storrington
Steyning
Lewes
Hailsham
Hastings
Worthing
Arundel
Bexhill
Brighton
Littlehampton
Newhaven
Eastbourne
Bognor Regis
Beachy Head
Selsey Bill
0
10
20 Km
0
10
Miles

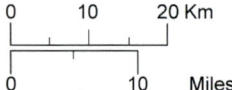

Resources
Tourism

Visit London
London and Partners, 2 More London Riverside, London SE1 2RR
- 020 7234 5800
- partnersales@londonandpartners.com
- www.visitlondon.com

Organisation representing the tourist industry in London. Some information for disabled people is included on their website.

Artsline
C/O 21 Pine Court, Wood Lodge Gardens, Bromley BR1 2WA
- ceo@artsline.org.uk
- www.artsline.org.uk

Free online-based advice service for disabled people on arts and entertainment venues in London. Full details are provided on access and provision for disabled people at London theatres, cinemas and other venues. Access guides are available in print, on tape and on the website.

Transport

Transport for London
TfL Customer Services, 4th Floor, 14 Pier Walk, London SE10 0ES
- Customer Services 0843 222 1234
  Travel Information 020 7918 3015
- www.tfl.gov.uk

Historically the public transport networks in London were not designed for wheelchair users or people with mobility problems. Although considerable barriers still exist, a range of developments have made it easier for disabled people to use at least parts of London's public transport system.

London Buses
All bus routes regulated by Transport for London use buses that have low-level floors with improved circulation, space for a wheelchair user and entrance ramps. Along some routes work has been carried out to adjust the kerbs at bus stops. However, accessibility to wheelchair users may be limited due to the bus being unable to draw up close to the pavement at bus stops.

THINGS TO SEE OR DO

Tate Britain
Home to the national collection of British art from the 16th century. Wheelchair access is available throughout, and touch tours are organised for visually impaired visitors. Large print and Braille floor plans and large print captions in exhibitions are also available. The gallery also offers a range of free talks and workshops for visitors with learning disabilities.
- www.tate.org.uk/visit/tate-britain

London Underground
All stations on the Jubilee Line Extension from Westminster to Stratford have lifts between street and platform levels with only a small gap between platform and train. There are a number of other stations with step-free access to platforms either at the outer parts of the network or where there has been substantial work carried out. Transport for London has a long-term programme to create a network of 100 accessible Underground stations and carry out other improvements. A map showing which stations are accessible for wheelchair users is available from the TFL website.

ENGLAND

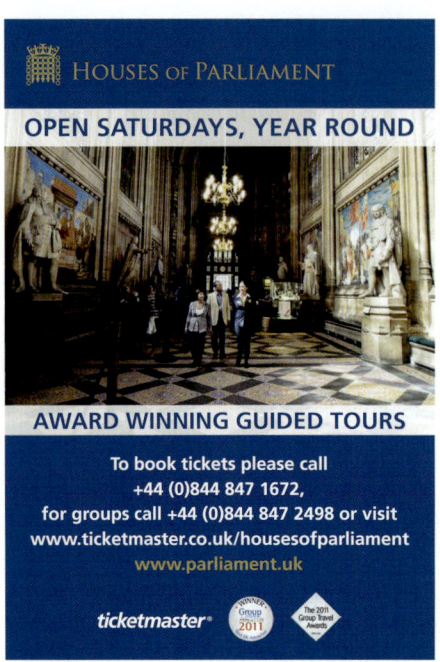

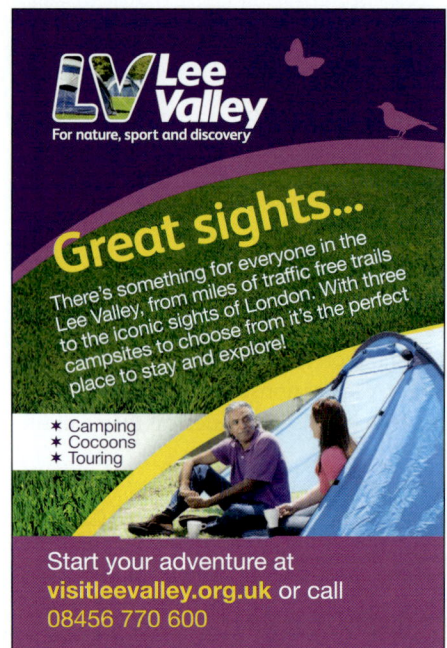

MIC hotel & conference centre

An award-winning central London social enterprise venue, MIC is the first UK accredited ethical hotel with the Social Enterprise Mark providing affordable quality hotel rooms, hospitality and meeting facilities all year round.

MIC Hotel and Conference Centre
81-103 Euston Street London NW1 2EZ
www.micentre.com
tel +44 (0)207 380 0001 | fax +44 (0)207 387 5300

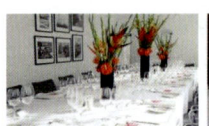
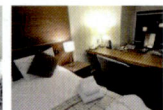
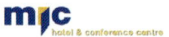

Riverside chalets

Situated in the heart of Lee Valley Park at Broxbourne, on a back-water of the River Lee, this 6 berth chalet is suitable for disabled people.

Including a double bed with bunk beds in separate rooms and a double sofa bed in the living area. A large bathroom with battery-operated seat over bath or shower and handrails. The kitchen is equipped with a 4-burner hob, microwave oven and fridge. There is a table and chairs along with a TV and electric heaters to keep you warm in the colder months.

Tel: 01992 462085
www.leevalleyboats.co.uk

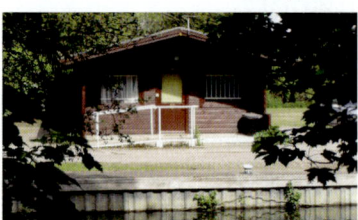

LONDON

Docklands Light Railway
Customer Services, Serco Docklands, Castor Lane, London E14 0DS
- 020 7363 9700
  Textphone 020 7093 0999
- cservice@dlr.co.uk
- www.tfl.gov.uk

Runs from Tower Hill and Bank to Stratford, Beckton, the Isle of Dogs, Greenwich, Lewisham, Woolwich Arsenal and London City Airport. There are wheelchair accessible lifts or ramps to all station platforms and level access onto the trains.

The Congestion Charge
Discount Registration, Congestion Charging, PO Box 4780, Worthing BN11 9PQ
- www.tfl.gov.uk/roadusers/congestioncharging

Blue Badge holders are eligible to register for a 100 per cent discount, even if they do not own a vehicle or drive. Two vehicles can be registered that would normally be used to travel within the charging zone. This could be an owned vehicle, or the one travelled in. Therefore for disabled visitors to London it would be worth registering for the discount if they are going to be using a car in central London for more than 2 weekdays. The Registration Pack can be obtained by calling 0845 900 1234, textphone 020 7649 9123. Vehicles exempt from Vehicle Excise Duty are automatically exempt from the charge.

Journey Planner
- journeyplanner.tfl.gov.uk

Transport for London's internet travel planner. It can be searched for routes using accessible vehicles and step-free stations and interchanges.

Taxis
All licensed public hire taxis (London Black Cabs) in London have space for a passenger in a manual wheelchair and carry or are equipped with a ramp.

Tramlink
- Customer Services 084 3222 1234
  Travel Information 020 7918 3015

A network running through Croydon to Beckenham and Wimbledon in South London. Designed to be accessible for disabled passengers.

THINGS TO SEE OR DO

The Original Bus Tour
A trip in an open top bus to tour London's most famous landmarks with the city's largest bus tour provider. Recorded and live commentaries available in English and many other languages and the ability to get on and off at places of interest. 85 per cent of the company's vehicles are wheelchair accessible – and they invite passengers to email or call to ensure a suitable bus and support if you need it is available when you want to travel.
- 020 8877 2120
- info@theoriginaltour.com

ENGLAND

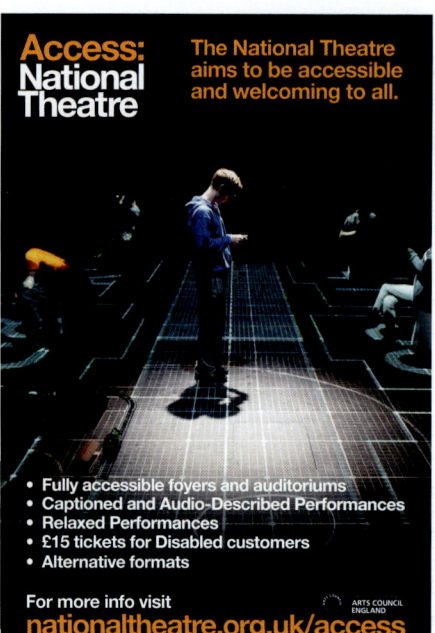

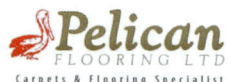

Pelican Flooring
178 Stoke Newington Road
London, N16 7UY

Tel/Fax: (020) 7254 7955
Email: pelicanflooringltd@xln.co.uk
www.pelicanflooring.co.uk

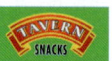

Quality packaged snacks, catering products and bar sundries supplied to the licensed trade. Regular, reliable van-sales service via a fleet of 14 trucks to London and South East England.

Unit 2 Anchorage Point, 90 Anchor & Hope Lane, London SE7 7SQ. Tel: 020 8858 4339
Email: info@tavernsnacks.com
www.tavernsnacks.com

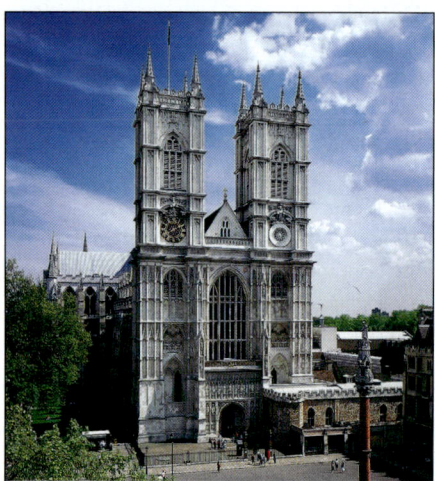

WESTMINSTER ABBEY
Open for visiting throughout the year.
For details visit **www.westminster-abbey.org**

Westminster Abbey is pleased to support the work of Disability Rights UK and wish them every success with this publication.

For information about Public Conveniences in the Royal Borough of Kensington and Chelsea, please telephone Streetline on **020 7361 3001** or visit our website at **www.rbkc.gov.uk**

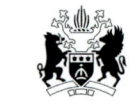

THE ROYAL BOROUGH OF
KENSINGTON AND CHELSEA

LONDON

Information & advice

DIAL

DIAL offers free, impartial and confidential information and advice by telephone to disabled people, their relatives and professionals. Local branches of DIAL are constantly changing but at the time of writing, the following groups were members of DIAL UK and may be able to help visitors in their areas. Please call before travelling to check whether the service and organisation is still available.

DIAL Barking and Dagenham
Boundary Road, Barking, Essex IG11 7JR
☎ 020 8594 4119

Disability Advice Service Lambeth
336 Brixton Road, Lambeth, London SW9 7AA
☎ 020 7738 5656

Disability and Social Care Advice Service (Wandsworth)
64 Altenburg Gardens, Battersea, London SW11 1JL
☎ 020 7978 7306

Disability Coalition Tower Hamlets
Disability Resource Centre, 40 - 50 Southern Grove, Tower Hamlets E3 4PX
☎ 020 8980 2200

Disability Network Hounslow
63-65 Bell Road, Hounslow, TW3 3NX
☎ 020 8577 0956

Equalities National Council
123 Star Lane, Newham, London E16 4PZ
☎ 020 7474 9812

Greenwich Association of Disabled People
Trafalgar Road, Greenwich SE10 9EQ
☎ 020 8305 2221

Hammersmith and Fulham Action on Disability
Greswell Street, London SW6 6PX
☎ 020 7471 8510

Havering Association For People With Disabilities
1a Woodhall Crescent, Hornchurch, Essex RM11 3NN
☎ 01708 476 554

Inspire Community Trust
20 Whitehall Lane, Slade Green, Bexley, Kent DA8 2DH
☎ 020 3045 5100

Lewisham Disability Coalition
2 Catford Broadway, Catford, London SE6 4SP
☎ 020 8314 1414

POhWER (London and The South Coast)
Loman Street, Southwark SE1 0EH
☎ 0300 456 2370

Richmond Advice and Information on Disability
4 Waldegrave Road, Teddington, Richmond-upon-Thames, Kingston upon Thames TW11 8HT
☎ 020 8831 6070

Westminster Action Network on Disability
96 Bourne Terrace, Westminster, London W2 5TH
☎ 0845 604 6442

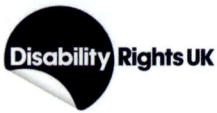

Visit our online shop
For products and books that open doors to independent living.

www.disabilityrightsuk.org

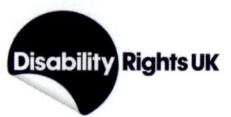

Become a member
Help us realise our vision and make your voice count.

www.disabilityrightsuk.org

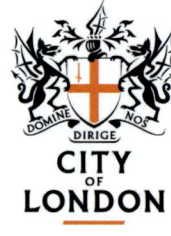

CITY OF LONDON

Working to achieve an Accessible and Inclusive Environment in the City of London

LEIGH ADAMS LLP

CHARTERED ACCOUNTANTS
& LICENSED INSOLVENCY
PRACTITIONERS

Brentmead House
Britannia Road
London N12 9RU

Telephone: 020 8446 6767
Facsimile: 020 8446 6864
Email: mail@leighadams.co.uk

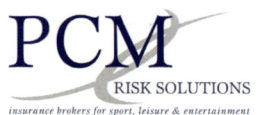

Disability sports clubs our speciality
Contact us today on
Tel: 020 8288 3501
Fax: 020 8288 3507
www.pcmrisksolutions.com

Ticino Bakery Ltd

Is pleased to support
Disability Rights UK

LONDON

Equipment hire

SHOPMOBILITY
The National Federation of Shopmobility UK (NFSUK), PO Box 6641, Christchurch BH23 9DQ
- 0844 4141 850
- info@shopmobilityuk.org
- www.shopmobilityuk.org

Scheme which lends manual wheelchairs, powered wheelchairs and powered scooters to members of the public with limited mobility to shop and to visit leisure and commercial facilities within the town, city or shopping centre. You can find the nearest Shopmobility scheme to you through their on-line directory. Contact specific Shopmobility Schemes to make equipment bookings or find out more information.

City Mobility
16 Enterprise House, Warrington WA2 0SQ
- www.citymobility.co.uk

Manual and electric wheelchairs and scooters are available to rent on daily, weekly or monthly rates.

Direct Mobility Hire
Warren House, 201a Bury Street, Edmonton London N9 9JE
- 0800 092 93 22
- info@directmobility.co.uk
- www.directmobility.co.uk

Hire and sell a wide range of mobility, bath, toilet and bed equipment. Pressure relief and incontinence products also available. Next day delivery in London and surrounding areas.

Keep Able
615-619 Watford Way, Apex Corner, Mill Hill, London NW7 3JN
- 020 8201 0810
- apex@hearingandmobility.co.uk

Wheelchairs may be hired through the above store where a wide range of equipment is also available.

Opt4Mobility
9/11 The Causeway, Teddington, Middlesex TW11 0HA
- 0800 1955 803
- info@opt4mobility.com
- www.opt4mobility.com

As well as selling a wide range of mobility and daily living equipment, offer a hire service for transit and manual wheelchairs.

THINGS TO SEE OR DO

Cutty Sark
Moored at Greenwich, this newly restored sailing ship and visitor centre situated underneath its bow are fully wheelchair accessible. A lift takes wheelchair users to the deck of the clipper, where most areas are suitable for wheelchair users.
- www.rmg.co.uk/cuttysark

HOLIDAYS IN THE BRITISH ISLES

ENGLAND

Publications

Access to London
Access Project, 39 Bradley Gardens, West Ealing, London W13 8HE
- accessinlondon@gmail.com
- www.accessinlondon.org

Gives information on getting around the London area, accommodation, attractions, entertainment, sports venues, shopping, places to eat and pubs. Copies of any of the PHSP (Pauline Hephaistos Survey Projects) guides can be ordered by sending your address via email or post to the above address. The guides are distributed without charge but a donation of £10 to £15 is asked to help fund the cost of research, printing and postage.

Access London Theatre
- 020 7557 6700
- enquiries@solttma.co.uk

The *Access London Theatre Guide*, published three times a year, gives details on audio-described, sign-interpreted, captioned and signed performance listings, access and facilities at more than 70 London theatres. The guide is available in print, audio tape, CD, Braille or large print. To order a free issue contact Access London Theatre on the details above. To order or download the Guide together with listings of assisted performances, visit:
- www.officiallondontheatre.co.uk/access

Access for Disabled People in the City of London
- 020 7332 1995
  Textphone 18001 020 7332 1995
- access@cityoflondon.gov.uk
- www.cityoflondon.gov.uk

Regularly revised booklet listing parking bays for Blue Badge holders, public accessible toilets and places of interest in The City and information on Congestion Charging. Also available in alternative formats, it can be obtained from the Access Team, Department of the Built Environment, City of London, PO Box 270, Guildhall, London EC2P 2EJ or downloaded from their website.

Accommodation

NAS ASSESSED ACCOMMODATON

BROMLEY

Best Western Bromley Court Hotel
Hotel
- 020 8461 8600
- patrickwall@bromleycourthotel.co.uk
- www.bw-bromleycourthotel.co.uk

HOLBORN

SACO London – Holborn
Four star serviced apartments
- 0845 1220 405
- janejones@sacoapartments.co.uk
- www.sacoapartments.co.uk

DOCKLANDS

Radisson Blu Edwardian Providence Wharf
Four star hotel
- 0208 7577 900
- vanderwm@radisson.com

LONDON

ROTHERHITHE
YHA London Thameside
Two star hostel
- 0162 9592 686
- margaretgibson@yha.org.uk
- www.yha.org.uk

KENSINGTON
Meininger Hotel London Hyde Park
Four star hotel
- 020 7590 6907
- ine.scharse@meininger-hotel.com
- www.meininger-hotels.com

TOWER HILL
Mint Hotel Tower Of London
Hotel
- 0845 601 3009
- toweroflondon.reservations@minthotel.com
- www.minthotel.com

WESTMINSTER
Tune Hotel – Westminster
Accredited budget hotel
- 0207 244 4100
- enquiry@tunehotels.com
- www.tunehotels.com

YHA London Central
Four star hostel
- 0162 9592 686
- margaretgibson@yha.org.uk
- www.yha.org.uk

OTHER ACCOMMODATION

KENSINGTON
Copthorne Tara Hotel
Scarsdale Place, London W8 5SR
- 020 7937 7211
- reservations.tara@millenniumhotels.co.uk
- www.millenniumhotels.co.uk

Hotel off Kensington High Street in West London.

ENGLAND

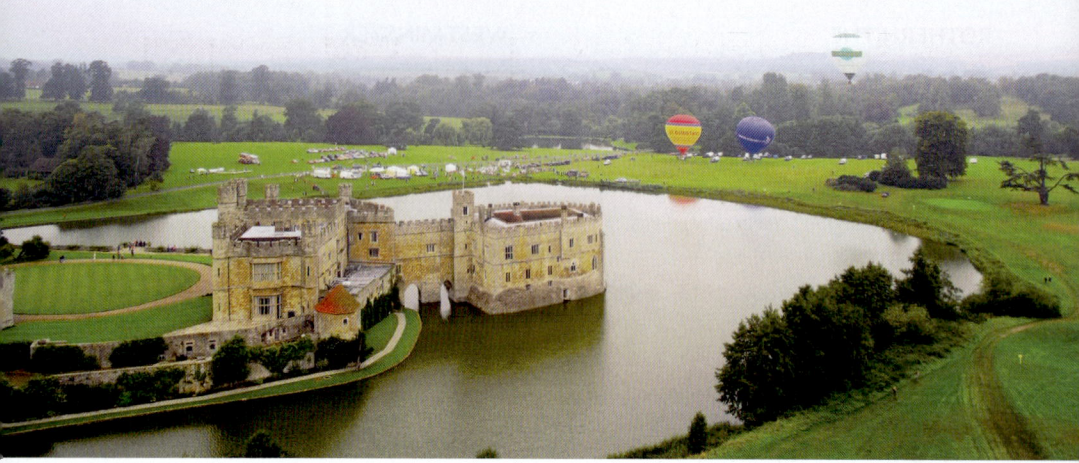

About South East England

Although sometimes over-shadowed by London, the counties of Kent, Surrey and East and West Sussex have their own special features and many attractions for holiday makers and day visitors.

Resorts large and small are found around the coast. Brighton with its distinctive Royal Pavilion and a thriving arts and entertainment scene can claim to be Britain's first seaside resort. Eastbourne has a long level seafront but is close to the South Downs, England's newest National Park, and the cliffs of Beachy Head. Other resorts include Hastings, Worthing, Littlehampton, Bognor Regis and Margate, home to the new Turner Contemporary Gallery.

Historically, the area has always been important. The Romans landed here and among the many reminders of their civilisation is Fishbourne Palace near Chichester. At the site of the Battle of Hastings, at Battle north of Hastings, English Heritage have opened a new visitor centre, although access difficulties remain for the battlefield itself.

Since 1066, the military emphasis on the area has been to repel invasions.

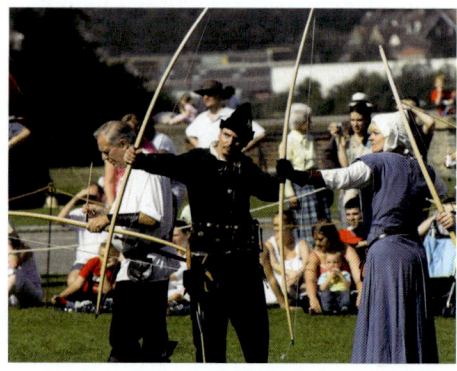

SOUTH EAST ENGLAND

Evidence of this includes Dover Castle, the Military Aviation Museum at the Battle of Britain airfield at Tangmere in West Sussex and a cluster of attractions in north Kent including the Chatham Historic Dockyard. Also at Chatham, Dickens World is a family attraction bringing to life the work of the region's leading literary figure.

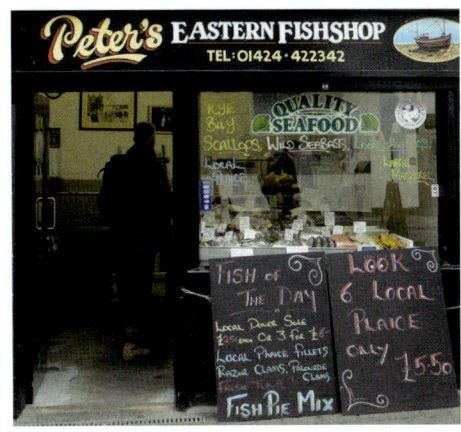

At Canterbury, disabled people can access most parts of the great Cathedral. There are also historic Cathedrals in Chichester and Rochester and a more modern one at Guildford. Historic secular buildings include the beautiful Leeds Castle near Maidstone, the imposing 17th century Petworth House in West Sussex owned by the National Trust and the modernist De La Ware Pavilion at Bexhill.

Before the Industrial Revolution the forested Weald was a major centre for iron manufacture. A variety of old industrial and transport buildings are on display at the Amberley Museum north of Arundel. The several heritage railways in the area include the Bluebell Railway, which has a coach for wheelchair users. More modern industries are represented at Mercedes-Benz World and the Brooklands Museum of motor racing and aviation at Weybridge and at The Body Shop Tour in Littlehampton.

Animal attractions in the area include the WWT Wetlands Centre at Arundel, Wildwood north of Canterbury, Birdworld near Farnham and the South of England Rare Breeds Centre near Ashford, which is run by people with learning disabilities. Noted gardens include Painshill Landscape Garden near Cobham. Other outdoor attractions include the award-wining Seven Sisters Country Park in East Sussex and Capstone Farm Country Park near Gillingham. Thorpe Park in north west Surrey is a destination for family outings. There is also the possibility of a shopping trip to Bluewater near Dartford or a day trip to France by ferry from Dover or through the Channel Tunnel.

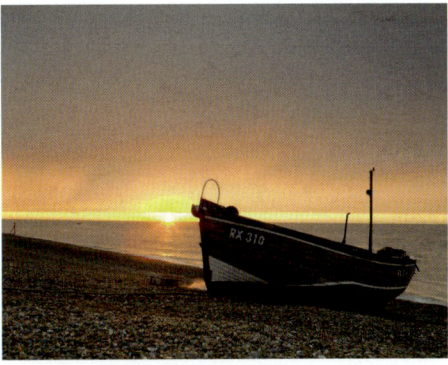

HOLIDAYS IN THE BRITISH ISLES

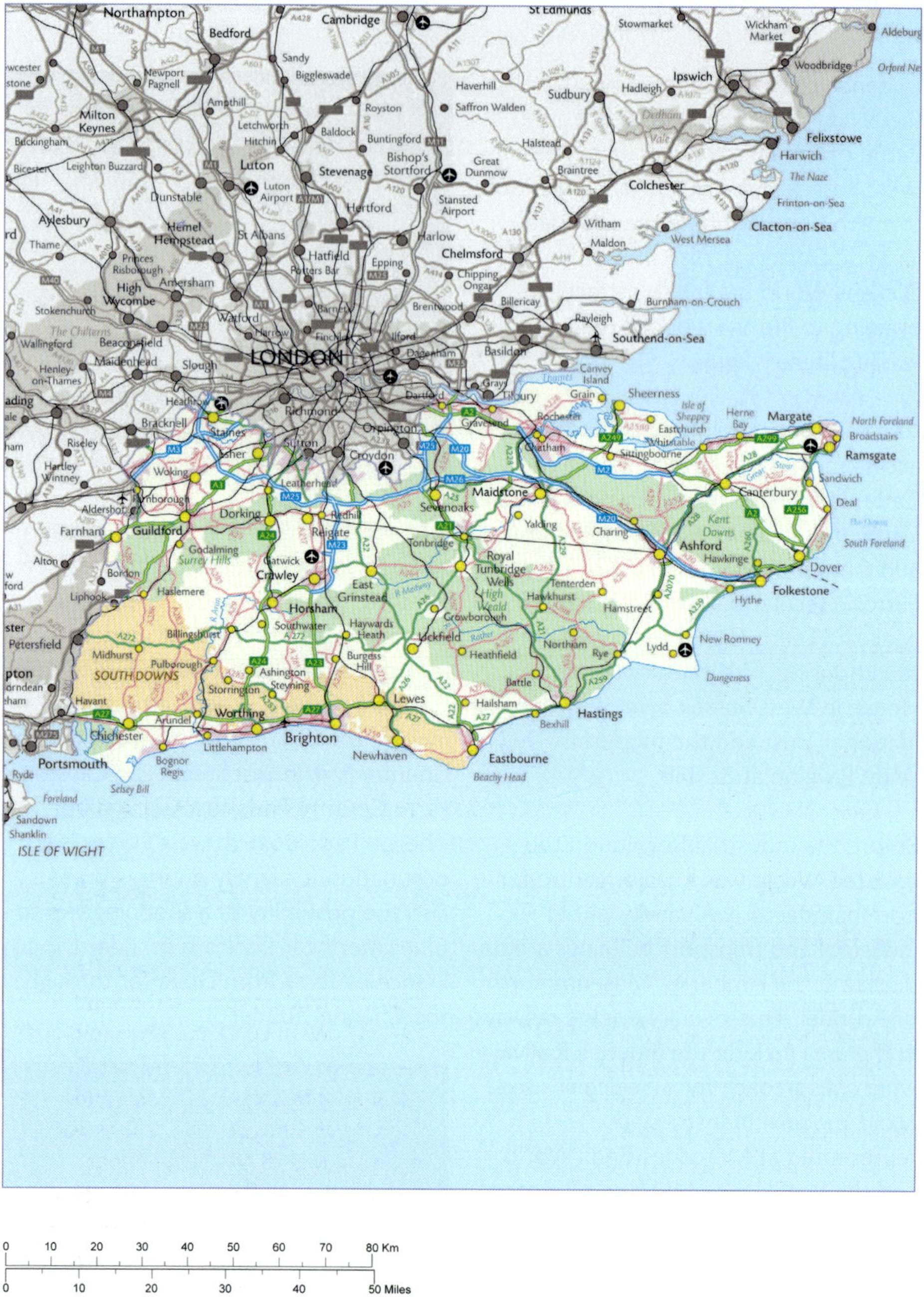

ENGLAND

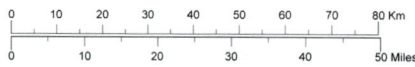

HOLIDAYS IN THE BRITISH ISLES

SOUTH EAST ENGLAND

Resources
Tourism

Tourism South East
40 Chamberlayne Road, Eastleigh
Hampshire SO50 5JH
- ☎ 023 8062 5400
- ✉ enquiries@tourismse.com
- 🌐 www.visitsoutheastengland.com

Issue a number of publications on accommodation and attractions in the region.

Information & advice

East Sussex Disability Association
1 Faraday Close, Eastbourne BN22 9BH
- ☎ 01323 514500
- ✉ info@esda.org.uk
- 🌐 www.esda.org.uk

Provide a wide variety of services including advice on equipment, welfare rights and an information service.

Kent Association for Disabled People
The Chequers Centre Management Suite, Pads Hill, Maidstone ME15 6AT
- ☎ 01622 756444
- 🌐 www.kadp.org.uk

Organise three one-week holidays for disabled people at hotels on the south coast. Voluntary helpers provide some care but no medical or night care is available.

Voluntary Association for Surrey Disabled
10 Havenbury Estate, Station Road, Dorking RH4 1ES
- ☎ 01372 841148
- ✉ info@vasd.org.uk
- 🌐 www.vasd.org.uk

Two adapted vehicles and manual wheelchairs can be hired by individuals and organisations in Surrey. Self catering properties are available in Bognor Regis and Bracklesham Bay.

DIAL
DIAL offer free, impartial and confidential information and advice by telephone to disabled people, their relatives and professionals. Local branches of DIAL are constantly changing but at the time of writing, the following groups were members of DIAL UK and may be able to help visitors in their areas. Please call before travelling to check whether the service and organisation is still available:

Brighton & Hove DAC
Montague Place, Brighton BN2 1JE
- ☎ 01273 203016 (also textphone)

DIAL North West Kent
7 The Hive, Northfleet, Kent DA11 9DE
- ☎ 01474 356962

> **THINGS TO SEE OR DO**
>
> **Turner Contemporary**
> This new art gallery in Margate is the largest exhibition space in the South East outside of London, with sensational views over the North Kent Coast. The gallery is fully accessible, with a ramp to the main entrance and café, as well as an internal lift to all upper floor galleries. Seven disabled parking spaces are available on the piazza at the front of the gallery. Wheelchairs are available to hire.
> - ☎ 01843 233000.
> - 🌐 www.turnercontemporary.org

ENGLAND

THE GENERAL ESTATES CO LTD

Holiday caravans for sale and rent in East Sussex

Seaviews at
Sunnyside Caravan Park
Marine Parade, Seaford

Country location at
Orchard View Park
Victoria Road, Herstmonceux
Nr Hailsham

Call Mary
01323 892825

Holiday Homes for sale
Hayling Island

Call Chris
02380 843011

www.general-estates.co.uk
managers@sunnyside-caravan-park.co.uk

For more information on public facilities, why not telephone for more details before you travel?

Please telephone for all enquiries: 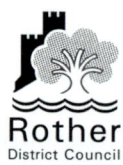 Rother District Council

01424 787 000

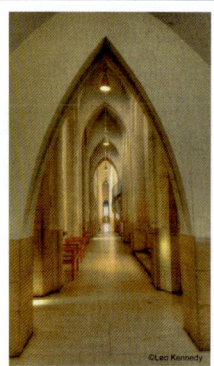
©Leo Kennedy

Experience the modern beauty of Guildford Cathedral

Open daily
Admission free

Guided Tours (pre-booked)

Daily services, including choral evensong

Restaurant and gift shop

Wide-ranging programme of concerts, events and art exhibitions

Full facilities for disabled visitors

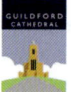

For more details call
01483 547860 or visit
www.guildford-cathedral.org

Guildford Cathedral, Stag Hill, Guildford, Surrey GU2

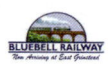

SUSSEX BY STEAM!

STEAM HAULED TRAIN SERVICES EVERY DAY APRIL-OCTOBER AND EVERY WEEKEND THROUGHOUT THE YEAR

DISABLED FACILITIES AT SHEFFIELD PARK AND KINGSCOTE STATIONS, LEVEL ACCESS ONTO PLATFORM AND WHEELCHAIR ACCESSIBLE CARRIAGE AVAILABLE ON SOME SERVICES

FOR MORE INFORMATION PLEASE CONTACT

CUSTOMER SERVICES

BLUEBELL RAILWAY

SHEFFIELD PARK STATION

EAST SUSSEX TN22 3QL

01825 720800 *www.bluebell-railway.com*

Voice for Disability

7 St Johns Parade, Alinora Crescent,
Goring-by-Sea, West Sussex BN12 4HJ
☎ 01903 219482

Equipment hire

SHOPMOBILITY

The National Federation of Shopmobility
UK (NFSUK), PO Box 6641, Christchurch
BH23 9DQ
☎ 0844 41 41 850
✉ info@shopmobilityuk.org
🌐 www.shopmobilityuk.org
Scheme which lends manual wheelchairs, powered wheelchairs and powered scooters to members of the public with limited mobility to shop and to visit leisure and commercial facilities within the town, city or shopping centre. You can find the nearest Shopmobility scheme to you through their on-line directory. Contact specific Shopmobility Schemes to make equipment bookings or find out more information.

Southern Mobility Centres

Mobility House, 2A Cavendish Avenue,
Eastbourne BN22 8EN
☎ 01323 645067
✉ sales@southernmobility.com
🌐 www.southernmobility.com
Manual wheelchairs and of hoists are available to hire at weekly and monthly rates.

Weald Mobility Care Centre

330 Seasied, Eastbourne, East Sussex BN22 7RH
☎ 01323 431455
🌐 www.wealdmobility.co.uk

Scooters and manual wheelchairs are available for hire for two days and over. Free local delivery and collection.

Publications

Access to places in and around Eastbourne

☎ 0871 663 0031
🌐 www.visiteastbourne.com
Published annually, this booklet provides information on accessible places in and around Eastbourne and includes a wheelchair route map. The wheelchair route map can also be downloaded from their website. The booklet is available free of charge from Eastbourne Tourist Information Centre, Cornfield Road, Eastbourne, East Sussex BN21 4QA.

Accessible Worthing – An Access Guide

☎ 01903 221066
🌐 www.visitworthing.co.uk
Available from Worthing Tourist Information Centre, Chapel Road, Worthing, West Sussex BN11 1HL.

THINGS TO SEE OR DO
Beachy Head With a height of 152 metres (530ft) above sea level, it is the highest chalk sea cliff in Britain, with panoramic views from the cliff top. The Peace Path is a circular 'easy access' route starting opposite the main Beachy Head car park and leading to a viewpoint on the Head. Suitable for people with impaired mobility, wheelchair users and those with mobility scooters and push chairs. 🌐 www.nationalparks.gov.uk

ENGLAND

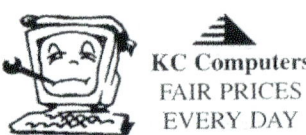

KC Computers
FAIR PRICES EVERY DAY

*Please find us at: Edgewood Electrical
261 London Road, St Leonards-on-Sea*

Does your computer need a boost?

For the best value computers & components on the South Coast

We also stock CD media and Original HP, Epsom & Lexmark Inks

www.kccomputers.co.uk
Tel: 01424 714713

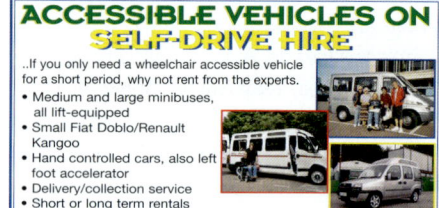

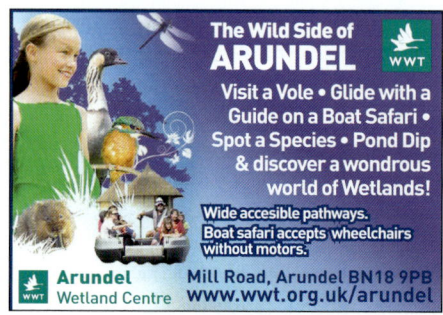

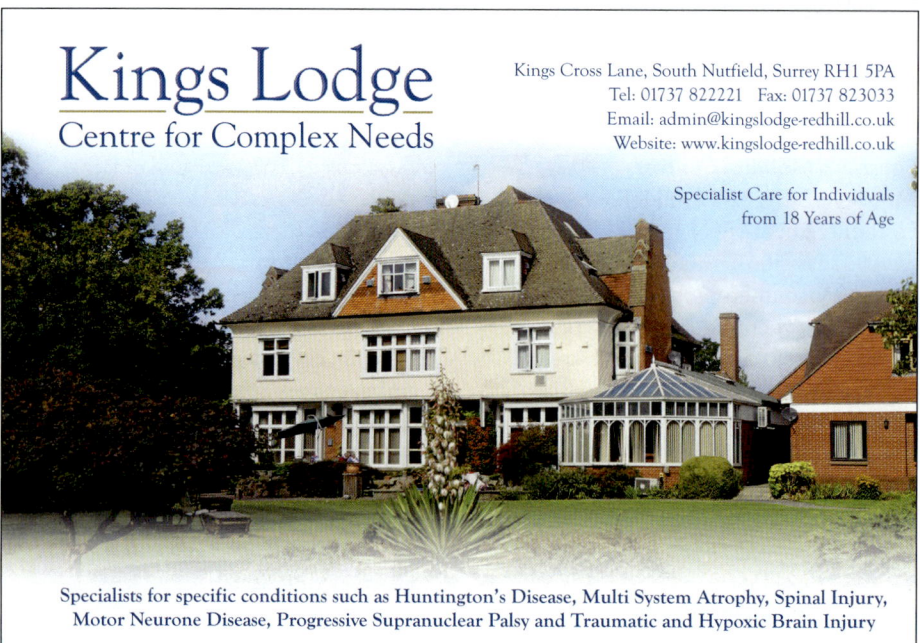

Kings Lodge
Centre for Complex Needs

Kings Cross Lane, South Nutfield, Surrey RH1 5PA
Tel: 01737 822221   Fax: 01737 823033
Email: admin@kingslodge-redhill.co.uk
Website: www.kingslodge-redhill.co.uk

Specialist Care for Individuals
from 18 Years of Age

Specialists for specific conditions such as Huntington's Disease, Multi System Atrophy, Spinal Injury, Motor Neurone Disease, Progressive Supranuclear Palsy and Traumatic and Hypoxic Brain Injury

SOUTH EAST ENGLAND

Walks for All in Kent & Medway
- ☎ 08458 247 247
- 🌐 www.kent.gov.uk/explorekent

Gives detailed information for disabled people on 16 country routes in the area. Free to download from their website.

Maidstone: a Disabled Person's Guide to the Town Centre
- ☎ 01622 602169
- ✉ tourism@maidstone.gov.uk

A map showing the location of dropped kerbs, reserved parking bays and toilets for disabled people. Available from Maidstone Visitor Information Centre, Maidstone Museum & Bentlif Art Gallery, St Faith's Street, Maidstone, Kent ME14 1LH.

Accommodation

NAS ASSESSED ACCOMMODATON

BRIGHTON, Sussex
Myhotel Brighton
Four star metro hotel
- ☎ 01273 900 365
- ✉ benferrer@myhotels.com
- 🌐 www.myhotels.com

Jurys Inn Brighton Hotel
Accredited hotel
- ☎ 0127 3862 121
- ✉ suzanne_cannon@jurysinns.com
- 🌐 http://brightonhotels.jurysinns.com/

CANTERBURY, Kent
Iffin Farmhouse
Four star self-catering
- ☎ 01227 462776
- ✉ info@iffin.co.uk
- 🌐 www.iffin.co.uk

CHICHESTER, Sussex
Bishop Otter Campus – University Of Chichester
Two and Three star campus accommodation
- ☎ 01243 812120
- ✉ conference@chi.ac.uk
- 🌐 www.chi.ac.uk/conference

Chichester Park Hotel
Three star hotel
- ☎ 01243 817 400
- ✉ dean@chichesterparkhotel.com
- 🌐 www.chichesterparkhotel.com

Eastmere House
Four star bed & breakfast
- ☎ 01243 544204
- ✉ bernardlane@hotmail.com
- 🌐 www.eastmere.com

George Bell House
Five star guesthouse
- ☎ 01243 813 581
- ✉ gmenterprises@hichestercathedral.org.uk
- 🌐 www.chichestercathedral.org.uk

THINGS TO SEE OR DO

The Bluebell Railway
Historic steam trains departing from Sheffield Park Station in Sussex. Most trains carry at least a couple of wheelchairs, with some trains featuring an extensively modified 'open saloon' carriage to allow for wheelchair access and to accommodate larger parties with flexible seating and a panoramic view from the windows.
- ☎ 01825 720800
- 🌐 www.bluebell-railway.com

HOLIDAYS IN THE BRITISH ISLES

ENGLAND

Knight James Commercial

Is pleased to support Disability Rights UK

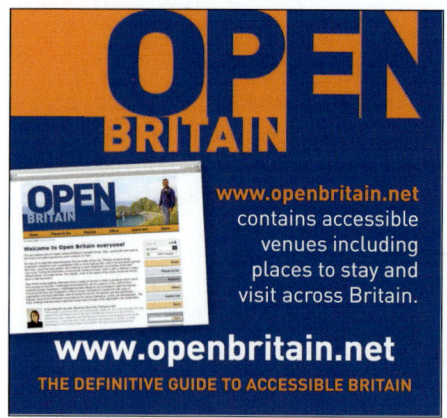

www.openbritain.net contains accessible venues including places to stay and visit across Britain.

www.openbritain.net

THE DEFINITIVE GUIDE TO ACCESSIBLE BRITAIN

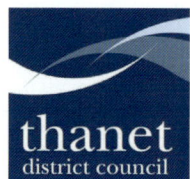

Is pleased to support Disability Rights UK

Pekes
Manor House and cottages
Golden Cross, near Hailsham, Sussex

Set in the peaceful and secluded grounds of our Tudor manor house, Mounts View is a stunning eco friendly cottage with 5 bedrooms, 3 bathroooms (one with wet room), private sauna, good kitchen and an exceptional sitting room with dining alcove and brilliant views.

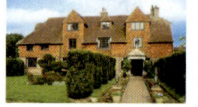

Contact: Eva Morris
Tel: 020 7352 8088
Sat-Mon: 01825 872 229
e.mail: pekes.afa@virgin.net
www.pekesmanor.com

Distinctly different, unique self catering holidays

Taken in support of Disability Rights UK

S.E.T.S. *Electrical Wholesaler*

Unit 1, Manor Industrial Estate, Newton Road,
Hove, East Sussex BN3 7BA

Telephone: (01273) 724288 Fax: (01273) 321416

SOUTH EAST ENGLAND

CHIDDINGSTONE, Kent
Hay Barn & Straw Barn
Four star self-catering
- T: 0189 2510 117
- E: admin@gardenofenglandcottages.co.uk
- W: gardenofenglandcottages.co.uk

EASTBOURNE, Sussex
Best Western York House Hotel
Three star hotel
- T: 0170 3255 301
- E: info@yorkhousehotel.co.uk
- W: www.yorkhousehotel.co.uk

Hydro Hotel
Three star hotel
- T: 01323 720643
- E: martin.hollands@hydrohotel.com
- W: www.hydrohotel.com

EASTRY, Kent
The Old Dairy
Four star self-catering
- T: 01843 841656
- E: info@montgomery-cottages.co.uk
- W: www.montgomery-cottages.co.uk

FARNHAM, Surrey
High Wray
Two star self-catering
- T: 01252 715589
- E: alexine@highwray73.co.uk
- W: www.highwray73.co.uk

FOLKESTONE, Kent
Shuttlesfield Barn
Four star self-catering
- T: 0130 3862 729
- E: geoffs.hirst@btinternet.com
- W: www.shuttlesfieldbarn.co.uk

HASTINGS, Sussex
Seaspray
Four star guest accommodation
- T: 01424 436583
- E: jo@seaspraybb.co.uk
- W: www.seaspraybb.co.uk

MAIDSTONE, Kent
Coldblow Farm
Three and Four star camping and holiday park
- T: 01622 730439
- E: dora@coldblowfarm.co.uk
- W: www.kentdownsecolodge.co.uk

Village Maidstone
Accredited hotel
- T: 01925 578310
- E: kim.brining@village-hotels.com
- W: www.village-hotels.com

MARDEN, Sussex
Pitlands Barns
Five star self-catering
- T: 0239 2631 263
- E: info@pitlandsbarns.co.uk
- W: www.pitlandsbarns.co.uk

West Marden Farm
Four and Five star self-catering
- T: 0239 2631 382
- E: carole@westmardenfarm.com
- W: www.barleycottage.co.uk

PEACEHAVEN, Sussex
Little Haven
Four star self-catering
- T: 0127 3587 365
- E: juliette.payne@yahoo.co.uk

ENGLAND

PLUMPTON GREEN, Sussex
Heath Farm
Four star self-catering
- 01273 890712
- hanbury@heath-farm.com
- www.heath-farm.com

ROBERTSBRIDGE, Sussex
Poppinghole Farm Cottages
Four star holiday cottages
- 0158 0830 622
- cottages@poppingholefarm.co.uk
- www.poppingholefarm.co.uk/cottages

ROYAL TUNBRIDGE WELLS, Kent
Alconbury Guest House
Five star bed & breakfast
- 0189 2511 279
- camilla.robinson@live.co.uk
- www.alconburyguesthouse.com

STANWELL, Surrey
The Stanwell
Three star hotel
- 0178 4262 389
- grn@thestanwell.com
- www.thestanwell.com

TENTERDEN, Kent
Little Silver Country Hotel
Three star hotel
- 01233 850321
- enquiries@little-silver.co.uk
- www.little-silver.co.uk

TUNBRIDGE WELLS, Kent
Smart and Simple Hotel
Two star hotel
- 0189 2552 700
- reception@sshtw.co.uk
- www.smartandsimple.co.uk

WADHURST, Sussex
Bardown Farm
Five star self-catering
- 0129 7324 63
- jenny.trice@premiercottages.co.uk
- www.bardownfarm.co.uk

OTHER ACCOMMODATION

BOGNOR REGIS, West Sussex
Invicta Warren
Elmer Sands, Middleton, Near Bognor Regis, West Sussex
- 01306 741500
- www.vasd.org.uk
Self-catering bungalow designed for wheelchair users run by the Voluntary Association for Surrey Disabled.

Farrell House
27 Nelson Road, Bognor Regis, West Sussex PO21 2RY
- 08456 584478
- info@livability.org.uk
- www.livability.org.uk
Self-catering chalet-bungalow adapted and equipped for disabled people.

Russell Hotel
King's Parade, Bognor Regis PO21 2QP
- 01243 871300
- russell.hotel@actionforblindpeople.org.uk
Hotel near the seafront and park designed for blind and partially sighted people and their companions.

SOUTH EAST ENGLAND

BRACKLESHAM BAY, West Sussex
Tamarisk
Farm Road, Bracklesham Bay, West Sussex
- ☎ 020 7452 2087
- ✉ info@livability.org.uk
- 🌐 www.livability.org.uk

Self-catering bungalow near the beach adapted and equipped for disabled people. Contact Livability (see voluntary organisations in Useful resources).

Voluntary Association for Surrey Disabled Holiday Chalet
Sussex Beach Holiday Village, Earnley, Bracklesham Bay, West Sussex
- ☎ 01306 741500
- ✉ info@vasd.org.uk
- 🌐 www.vasd.org.uk

Chalet designed for wheelchair users on a holiday park by the beach is Sussex, run by the Voluntary Association for Surrey Disabled.

EAST PRESTON, West Sussex
Bradbury Hotel
Station Road, East Preston BN16 3AL
- ☎ 01903 770339
- 🌐 www.royalblindsociety.org.uk

Small hotel for visually impaired people and their companions near the West Sussex coast.

FARNHAM, Surrey
High Wray
73 Lodge Hill Road, Farnham GU10 3RB
Contact: Mrs Alexine Crawford
- ☎ 01252 715589
- ✉ crawford@highwray73.co.uk
- 🌐 www.highwray73.co.uk

'Rose' is a purpose-built, self-catering flat for disabled people a mile from town.

FELPHAM, West Sussex
Beach Lodge
Strand Way, Felpham, Near Bognor Regis PO22 7LH
- ☎ 020 7452 2087
- ✉ info@livability.org.uk
- 🌐 www.livability.org.uk

Detached house facing the sea – east of Bognor. Contact Livability (see voluntary organisations in Useful resources).

HERNE BAY, Kent
Strode Park Foundation
Strode Park House, Herne CT6 7NE
- ☎ 01227 373292
- ✉ info@strodepark.org.uk
- 🌐 www.strodepark.org.uk

Two self-catering holiday bungalows designed for disabled people and their companions.

HORLEY, Surrey
Brambles MS Respite Care Centre
Suffolk Close, Massetts Road, Horley RH6 7DU
- ☎ 01293 771644
- 🌐 www.brambles.org.uk

Purpose-built centre for respite care for people with multiple sclerosis.

SOUTH NUTFIELD, Surrey
Kings Lodge Centre For Complex Needs
Kings Cross Lane, South Nutfield, Surrey RH1 5PA
- ☎ 01737 822221
- ✉ admin@kingslodge-redhill.co.uk
- 🌐 www.kingslodge-redhill.co.uk

Provides long or short-term care, respite and day care as well as palliative care for people aged 18 and over, who have a physical or cognitive disability resulting from neurological condition.

ENGLAND

About the South of England

This is a large and varied region stretching from Buckinghamshire and Oxfordshire, through Berkshire and Hampshire to eastern Dorset and the Isle of Wight. It includes much of the Chiltern and Cotswold hills and the Thames Valley as well as the New Forest and stretches of attractive coastline.

There are many opportunities for seaside holidays in the south. The largest resort is Bournemouth where there are entertainments and attractions for young and old. Other resorts include Poole and Southsea and Ryde, Sandown and Shanklin on the Isle of Wight.

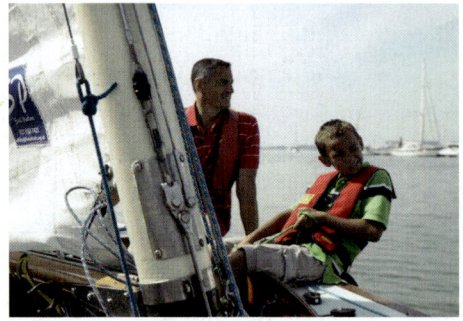

At Portsmouth, many attractions in the Historic Dockyard depict the military and naval heritage of the city including the Royal Naval Museum, the Mary Rose display and the HMS Victory. An access trail has been laid out around the site and a panoramic view can be obtained from the Spinnaker Tower. The D-Day Museum and Overlord Embroidery are elsewhere in the city. There are other military museums in the region in Aldershot and Winchester.

There is also a full range of urban amenities in Reading and Southampton where part of the harbour has been redeveloped as Ocean City with waterfront restaurants, bars and shops. In Oxford, guided walks are open to disabled people around the historic university buildings, while the world's first university museum, the Ashmolean, is fully accesible. Other historic towns in the region include the cathedral city of Winchester, the Royal Borough of Windsor dominated by the castle, the old port of Poole and market towns such as Banbury and Aylesbury. Riverside towns along the Thames include Marlow,

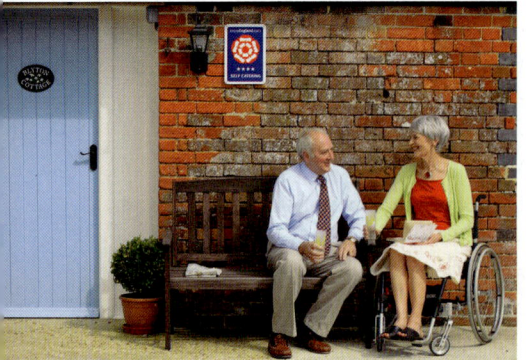

SOUTHERN ENGLAND

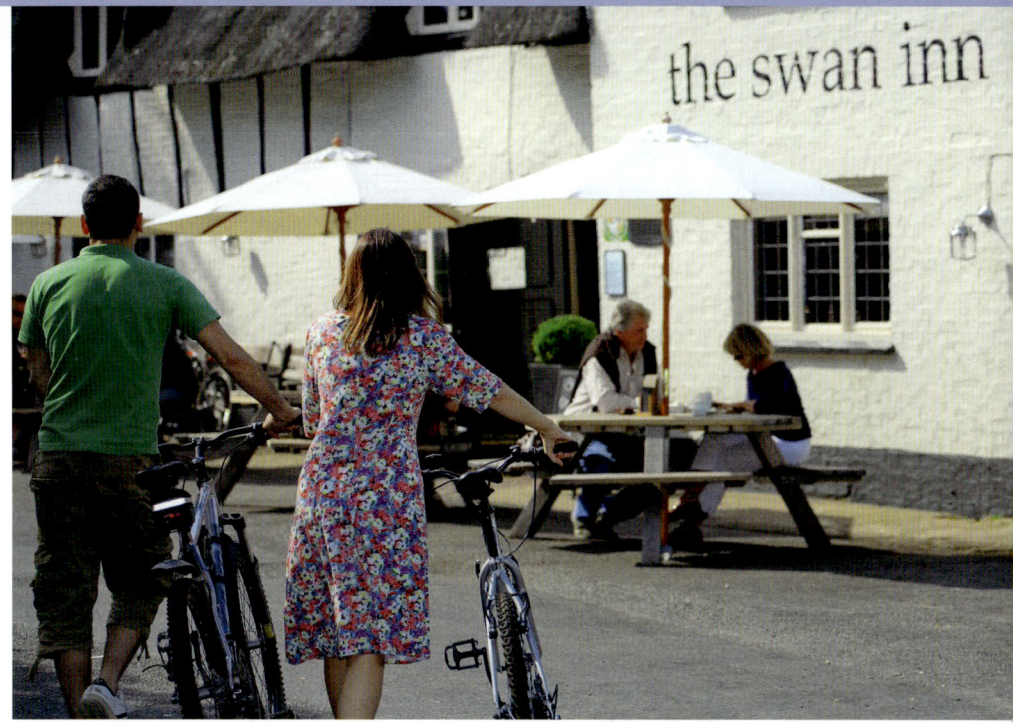

Maidenhead and Henley, home of the River & Rowing Museum.

Two areas have their own specific characteristics – the New Forest National Park, and the Isle of Wight. A good starting point to learn more about the natural and human history of the former is the New Forest Museum and Visitor Centre at Lyndhurst. The Isle of Wight has been a tourist destination since the middle of the 19th century when Queen Victoria made her home at Osborne House near Cowes. This is now run by English Heritage and offers a two mile walk around the grounds that is suitable for wheelchair users. The many other attractions on the Island include the Isle of Wight Steam Railway, Needles Park overlooking Alum Bay and simply watching the boats in the Solent.

Historic houses that can be visited elsewhere in the region include the National Trust's Basildon Park near Reading and Blenheim Palace at Woodstock in Oxfordshire. Beaulieu Abbey in the New Forest houses a large collection of veteran and classic cars. Outdoor attractions include the restored Greenham Common near Newbury, Marwell Zoo and Old Winchester Hill National Nature Reserve both in Hampshire and the Cotswold Wild Life Park at Burford. Most children, and many adults, will enjoy Legoland outside Windsor.

HOLIDAYS IN THE BRITISH ISLES

ENGLAND

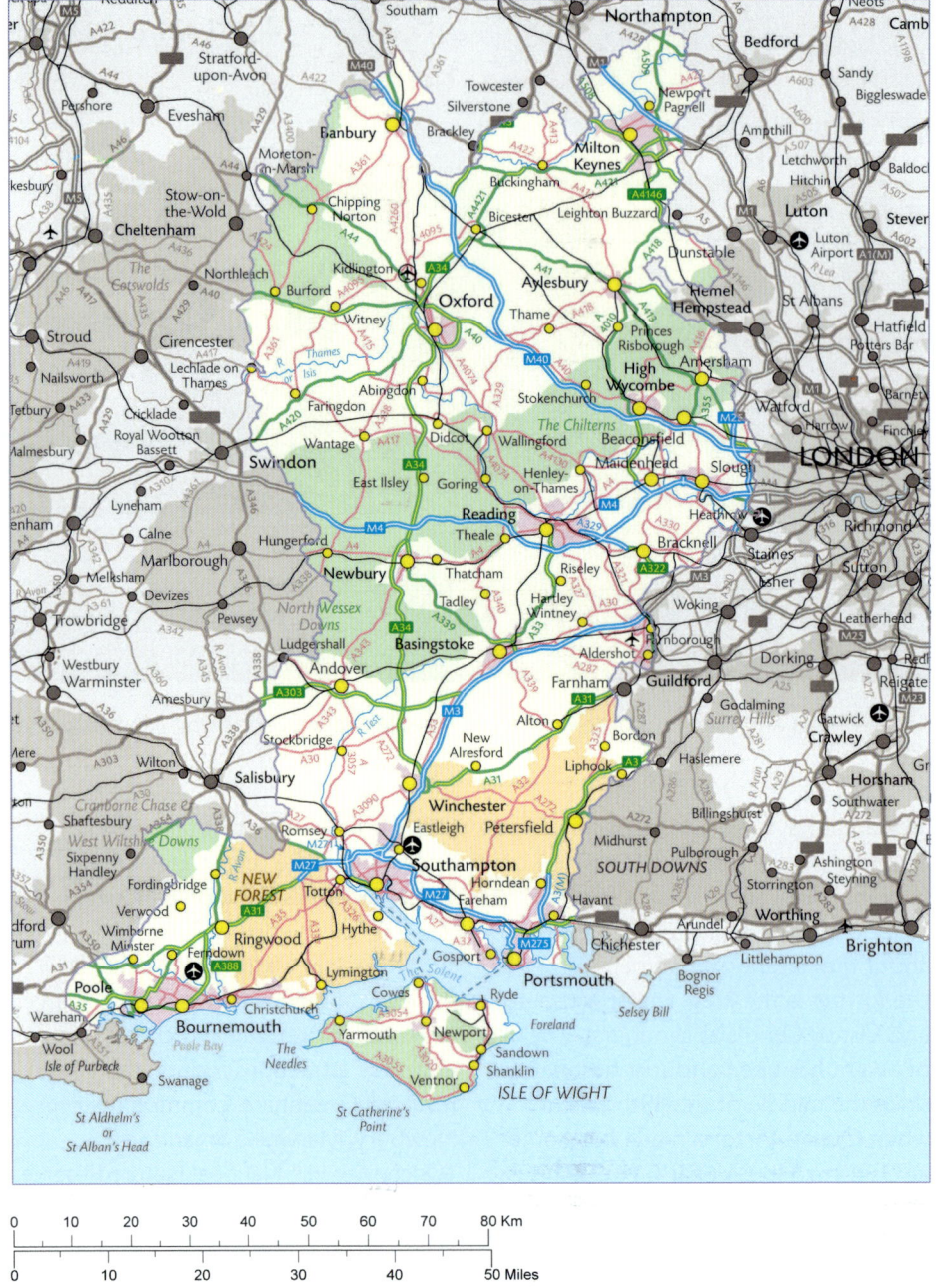

Resources

Tourism

Tourism South East
40 Chamberlayne Road, Eastleigh
Hampshire SO50 5JH
- 023 8062 5400
- enquiries@tourismse.com
- www.visitsoutheastengland.com

Issue a number of publications and online information on accommodation and attractions in the region.

Transport

Hovertravel Ltd
Quay Road, Ryde, Isle of Wight PO33 2HB
- 08434 87 88 87
- www.hovertravel.co.uk

Operate a fast crossing for foot passengers by hovercraft between Portsmouth and Ryde on the Isle of Wight. A lift and space for a wheelchair are available on all crossings. Visit:
- www.hovertravel.co.uk/accessibility-information.php

Red Funnel Ferries
12 Bugle Street, Southampton SO14 2JY
- 0844 844 2699
- post@redfunnel.co.uk
- www.redfunnel.co.uk

Operate car ferries and high speed passenger services between Southampton and Cowes on the Isle of Wight. Ferries have lifts and there are toilets for disabled passengers on board and at terminals.

Wightlink Isle of Wight Ferries
PO Box 59, Portsmouth PO1 2XB
- 0871 376 1000
- www.wightlink.co.uk

Operate car ferries between Portsmouth and the Isle of Wight and fast catamaran services for foot passengers only between Portsmouth and Ryde. The vessels on the Portsmouth-Fishbourne service are equipped with lifts and toilets for disabled passengers. Wheelchairs are available at all terminals. A Wightlink Disabled Persons Card is available giving discounted fares. For assistance call:
- 023 9281 2011

Ferry travel concessions
Several schemes may reduce the cost of ferry travel for patients and their carers attending hospital appointments on the mainland. For more information:
- www.redfunnel.co.uk/ferry-travel/healthcare-travel-scheme/
- www.iwight.com

THINGS TO SEE OR DO

Ashmolean Museum
The world's first university museum situated in the centre of Oxford, containing antique coins, books, engravings, geological and zoological specimens and a large collection of ancient egyptian mummies. The museum is fully accessible including various interactive exhibits.
- 01865 278000
- www.asmol.ox.ac.uk

ENGLAND

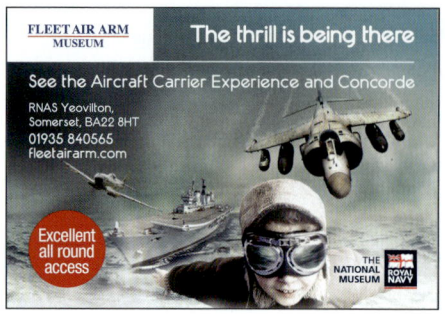

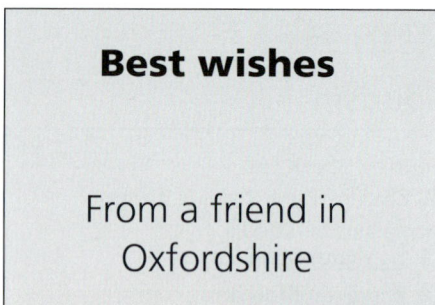

Best wishes

From a friend in Oxfordshire

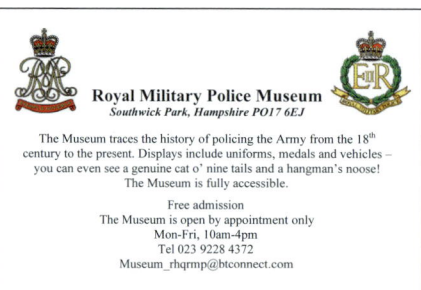

Royal Military Police Museum
Southwick Park, Hampshire PO17 6EJ

The Museum traces the history of policing the Army from the 18th century to the present. Displays include uniforms, medals and vehicles – you can even see a genuine cat o' nine tails and a hangman's noose! The Museum is fully accessible.

Free admission
The Museum is open by appointment only
Mon-Fri, 10am-4pm
Tel 023 9228 4372
Museum_rhqrmp@btconnect.com

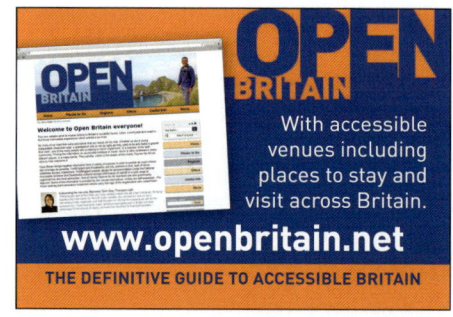

With accessible venues including places to stay and visit across Britain.

www.openbritain.net

THE DEFINITIVE GUIDE TO ACCESSIBLE BRITAIN

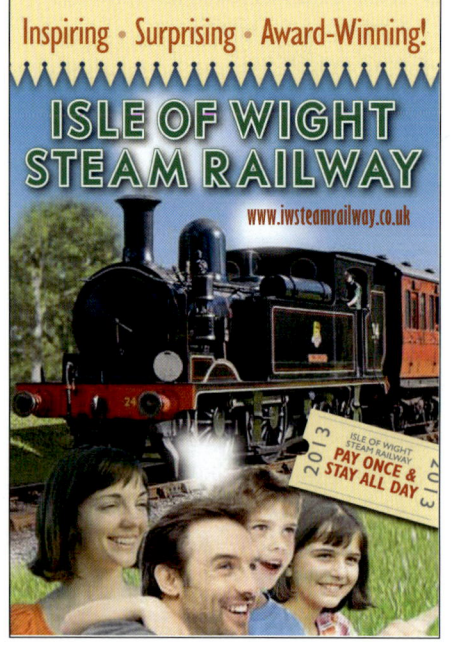

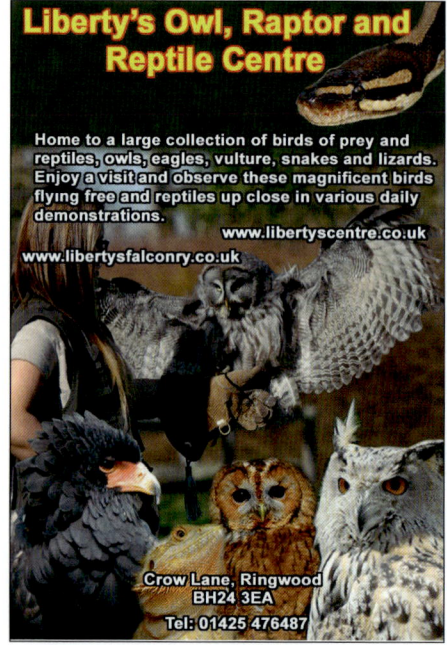

Information & advice

The Ark and Dis:Course
The Ark Studio, Nine Mile Ride, Ravenswood Village, Crowthorne, Berkshire RG45 6BQ
- 01344 755 528
- nigel@theark.org.uk
- www.theark.org.uk

A charity that enhances the lives of people with disabilities through access to the arts and new media. It also houses Dis:Course, which provides information, advice and support for people with disabilities.

British Red Cross Berkshire Branch
John Nike House, 90 Eastern Avenue, Reading RG1 5SF
- 08444 122 750
- www.redcross.org.uk

Provide some information on holidays for disabled and elderly people and may be able to provide transport for groups and individuals.

Disability Wessex, Bournemouth
- 01202 589999

Has a small team of experienced advisers, with extensive knowledge, relevant training and qualifications and the majority have personal experience of living with a health condition or impairment. Aim to provide advice and assistance, to enable disabled people and families to understand and secure their rights and entitlements.

Green Island Holiday Trust
- 01202 842880
- organiser@greenislandholidaytrust.com
- www.greenislandholidaytrust.com

Organise holidays for disabled people with volunteer helpers at Holton Lee on the shore of Poole Harbour. Activities include birdwatching, painting, boat trips and barbecues. Priority will be given to people living in Dorset and Hampshire.

DIAL
Offer free, impartial and confidential information and advice by telephone to disabled people, their relatives and professionals. Local branches of DIAL are constantly changing but at the time of writing, the following groups were members of DIAL UK and may be able to help visitors in their areas. Please call before travelling to check whether the service and organisation is still available:

DIAL Isle of Wight
- 01983 522 823

Milton Keynes CIL
- 01908 231 344

Portsmouth Disability Forum
- 02392 824 853

THINGS TO SEE OR DO

Osborne House
The Ring Walk in the Isle of Wight is a two-mile circular walk suitable for wheelchair users around the grounds of Osborne House, Queen Victoria's summer residence. The palace itself has wheelchair access to the ground floor with a lift to the first floor.
- www.walkswithwheelchairs.com
- 01983 200 022

ENGLAND

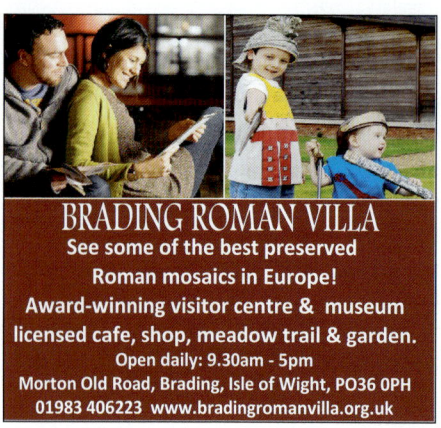

K&B Marketing Ltd

Is pleased to support Disability Rights UK

Majestic Transformer Co.

Best Wishes From Everyone At

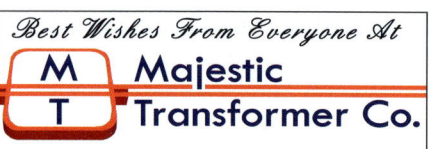

TRANSFORMERS & CHOKES
- Custom made to 125kVA
- Manufactured in 7/10 Days
- Established over 70 years
- Enquiries Invited

245, Rossmore Road, Poole,
Dorset BH12 2HQ
Email: info@transformers.uk.com
Web Site: www.transformers.uk.com

P.A. MEECHAM

Craft member British Horological Institute

Antique Clocks repaired and restored
Established 35 years

Longcase and Bracket Clocks, Wall Clocks,
French Clocks and Carriage Clocks

Malthouse Cottage, Shipton Road,
Milton-under-Wychwood,
West Oxfordshire. OX7 6JT

Telephone: 01993830215
Email: peter.meecham@zen.co.uk

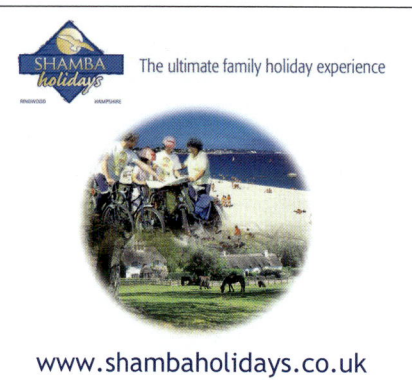

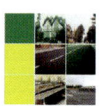

Wilson & Scott

One of the UK's leading independent road marking, antiskid and coloured surfacing contractors.

www.wilsonandscott.co.uk

HOLIDAYS IN THE BRITISH ISLES

Equipment hire

SHOPMOBILITY
The National Federation of Shopmobility UK (NFSUK), PO Box 6641, Christchurch BH23 9DQ
- ☎ 0844 41 41 850
- ✉ info@shopmobilityuk.org
- 🌐 www.shopmobilityuk.org

Scheme which lends manual wheelchairs, powered wheelchairs and powered scooters to members of the public with limited mobility to shop and to visit leisure and commercial facilities within the town, city or shopping centre. You can find the nearest Shopmobility scheme to you through their on-line directory. Contact specific Shopmobility Schemes to make equipment bookings or find out more information.

British Red Cross, Isle of Wight Branch
Red Cross House, Winnall Close, Winchester, Hampshire SO23 0LB
- ☎ 0845 0547 222

Can lend wheelchairs, walking and bathing equipment for holidaymakers. Advance booking required.

Dunbar Dean Electric Transport Ltd
31 St Catherine's Road, Southbourne, Bournemouth BH6 4AE
- ☎ 01202 426135

Electric and manual wheelchairs and scooters are available for hire. Delivery can be arranged.

Island Mobility
32 Dodnor Lane, Newport, Isle of Wight PO30 5XA
- ☎ 01983 530000
- ✉ info@islandmobility.co.uk
- 🌐 www.islandmobility.co.uk

Manual wheelchairs, walkers and mobile hoists for hire on daily or weekly terms. Powered scooters available for experienced users on a weekly basis. A range of other equipment is stocked. Collection and delivery service offered throughout the Isle of Wight.

Publications

Bournemouth: Accessibility Guide
- ☎ 0845 051 1700
- ✉ accessibility@bournemouth.gov.uk
- 🌐 www.bournemouth.co.uk

Regularly updated guide giving information on accommodation, attractions, places to eat & drink and entertainment. Available free of charge from Bournemouth Tourism, Westover Road, Bournemouth BH1 2BU.

Accessible Portsmouth – A Guide for Visitors with Disabilities
- ☎ 023 9282 6722
- ✉ vis@portsmouthcc.gov.uk
- 🌐 www.visitportsmouth.co.uk

Access guide produced by the City Council working with disabled people. The guide is available in print, audio, Braille and large print formats from ECCS, Portsmouth City Council, Civic Offices, Guildhall Square, Portsmouth PO1 2AD.

ENGLAND

Winchester: Visitor Trail by Wheelchair
- 01962 840500
- tourism@winchester.gov.uk
- www.visitwinchester.co.uk

A leaflet for visitors to the city prepared by Winchester Shopmobility and Winchester City Council. Available from the Tourist Information Centre, Guildhall, High Street, Winchester SO23 9GH.

Online resources

www.visitthames.co.uk
This website, managed by the Environment Agency, gives information on activities, attractions and places to stay along the Thames from its source in the Cotswolds to Teddington.

THINGS TO SEE OR DO

Thames Path Walks for All
Organisation who offer walks in the Thames Valley, with the Chiltern Hills on one side and the Berkshire Downs on the other, starting in Goring-on-Thames, Oxfordshire. Walks are likely to be suitable for people with impaired mobility and users of wheelchairs, mobility scooters and pushchairs. Facilities include NKS toilets, refreshments and picnic tables.
- www.chilternsaonb.org

Accommodation

NAS ASSESSED ACCOMMODATION

ABINGDON, Oxfordshire
Abbey Guest House
Four star house
- 01235 537020
- info@abbeyguest.com
- www.abbeyguest.com

BORTHWOOD, Isle of Wight
Borthwood Cottages
Four star self-catering
- 01983 403967
- anne@borthwoodcottages.co.uk
- www.borthwoodcottages.co.uk

BRACKNELL, Berkshire
SACO Bracknell
Four star serviced apartments
- 0845 1220 405
- janejones@sacoapartments.co.uk
- www.sacoapartments.com

BRIGHSTONE, Isle of Wight
Yafford Mill Barn
Five star self-catering cottages
- 0192 9481 555
- honor.vass@islandcottageholidays.com
- www.islandcottageholidays.com

COGGES, Oxfordshire
Swallows Nest
Four star self-catering
- 01993 704919
- jan@strainge.fsnet.co.uk

SOUTHERN ENGLAND

EAST BOLDRE, Hampshire
Ivy Roost Cottage
Five star cottage
- 0208 7474899
- karen.rogers1@btopenworld.com
- www.ivyretreats.com

HAMPSTEAD NORREYS, Berkshire
Manor Farm Courtyard Cottages
Four star cottages
- 01635 201276
- stayatmanorfarm@gmail.com

LECKHAMPSTEAD, Buckinghamshire
Weatherhead Farm
Four star farmhouse
- 01280 860502
- weatherheadfarm@aol.com
- www.weatherheadfarm.co.uk

LISS, Hampshire
The Jolly Drover
Four star inn
- 01730 893237
- thejollydrover@googlemail.com
- www.thejollydrover.co.uk

MAIDENHEAD, Berkshire
Holiday Inn Maidenhead
Hotel
- 08719 429053
- jackie.duncan@ihg.com
- www.holidayinn.co.uk

MARLOW, Buckinghamshire
Granny Anne's
Four star bed & breakfast
- 01628 473086
- roger@grannyannes.co.uk
- www.marlowbedbreakfast.co.uk

MILTON KEYNES, Buckinghamshire
South Lodge
Five star bed & breakfast
- 01908 582946
- info@culturevultures.co.uk
- www.culturevultures.co.uk

NEWCHURCH, NEAR SANDOWN, Isle of Wight
Mulberry Rest
Five star self-catering
- 0198 3400 096
- donnadempsey@me.com

OXFORD, Oxfordshire
YHA Oxford
Four star hostel
- 0162 9592 686
- margaretgibson@yha.org.uk
- www.yha.org.uk

SANDOWN BAY, Isle of Wight
Sandown Bay Holiday Park, No 6 & No 113
Three star self-catering
- 01825 723998
- afton@phonecoop.coop
- www.visitsoutheastengland.com/accommodation/chalet-6-and-113 sandown-bay-holiday-park-p732501

Fort Holiday Park
Three star holiday park
- 01983 402858
- bookings@fortholidaypark.co.uk
- www.fortholidaypark.co.uk

ENGLAND

SHANKLIN, Isle of Wight
Sunny Bay Apartments
Four star apartments
- 01983 861 555
- rda7376401@aol.com
- www.sunnybayaprtments.com

The Marine Villa
Five star self-catering
- 0168 9606 060
- mowe@totalise.co.uk
- www.greentiles.co.uk

STOKE MANDEVILLE, Buckinghamshire
Olympic Lodge
Three star guest accommodation
- 0129 6484 848
- stoke.mandeville@harpersfitness.co.uk
- www.olympic-lodge.co.uk

Accommodation in Stoke Mandeville Stadium complex owned by British Wheelchair Sports Foundation on the outskirts of Aylesbury.

OTHER ACCOMMODATION

ABINGDON, Oxfordshire
Kingfisher Barn
Rye Farm, Abingdon, Oxfordshire OX14 3NN
- 01235 537538
- info@kingfisherbarn.com
- www.kingfisherbarn.com

Bed & breakfast in barn conversion close to town centre.

FRESHWATER, Isle of Wight
Brambles Chine Bungalow
194 Brambles Chine, Monks Lane, Freshwater, Isle of Wight PO40 9SQ
Contact: Mrs S. C. Griffiths, Chalet Secretary, 3 Western Road, Shanklin, Isle of Wight
- 01983 863658
- www.iwasbah.co.uk

Chalet on holiday park at the west of Island.

LYMINGTON, Hampshire
Garden Bench, Bench Cottage & Little Bench
Pennington, Near Lymington SO41 8HH
- 01590 673141
- enquiries@ourbench.co.uk
- www.ourbench.co.uk

Cottages designed for wheelchair users in grounds of owners' home near New Forest. Contact: Mrs Mary Lewis, Our Bench, Lodge Road, Pennington, Lymington SO41 8HH.

NEW MILTON, Hampshire
Holiday Homes Trust Caravan
New Milton, Hampshire
- 020 8433 7290
- scout.holiday.homes@scouts.org.uk
- www.holidayhomestrust.org

Adapted units in New Milton, south west Hampshire.

Smugglers View Chalets
New Milton, Hampshire
Chalets adapted for wheelchair users.
Contact: Livability
- 020 7452 2067
- info@livability.org.uk
- www.livability.org.uk

SOUTHAMPTON, Hampshire
Vitalise Netley Waterside House
Abbey Hill, Netley Abbey, Southampton
SO31 5FA
- 0303 303 0145
- bookings@vitalise.org.uk
- www.vitalise.org.uk

Centre by Southampton Water purpose-built for breaks for people with disabilities.

ENGLAND

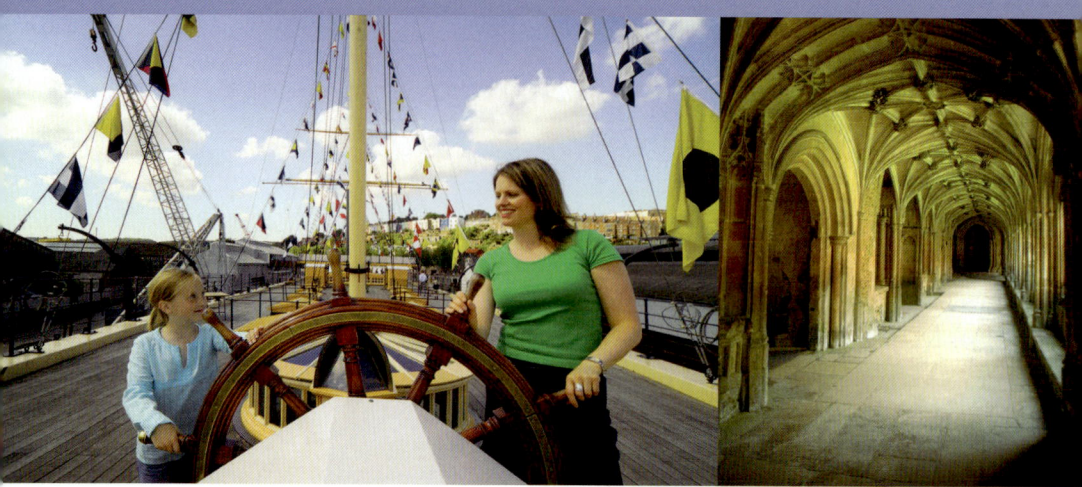

About the West Country

This region comprises Somerset, Wiltshire, Gloucestershire, much of Dorset and the area around Bristol. It includes the rolling chalk uplands of the Salisbury Plain in the east, part of the Exmoor National Park in the west, the Mendip Hills, the Forest of Dean, much of the Cotswolds, the Somerset Levels and two distinctive coastlines.

Many of the most important signs of prehistoric Britain can be found in the area. Stonehenge in Wiltshire is world famous. Perhaps of equal significance are the stone rings of Avebury and there are several examples of ancient figures cut into chalk hillsides, such as the Cerne Abbas Giant in Dorset. Much of the Dorset and East Devon 'Jurassic coast' has been declared a World Heritage Site because the many fossils found in the area were vital in the development of knowledge of early life on Earth.

The region's leading city is Bristol. As well as a history that equals any other major town, there are a range of modern museums, theatrical and music performances, shops and a thriving nightlife. The docks in the heart of the city now contain many attractions including the SS Great Britain, the M Shed displaying the history of the city and its people and At-Bristol with its interactive displays of science and wildlife.

The city of Bath has attracted visitors since the Romans bathed in its thermal springs, a practice that today's visitors can replicate. Its status as a World Heritage Site comes from the later tourist development at the end of the 18th Century when it was the smartest resort in the country. The hilly nature of the town means that there are restrictions for some disabled people, but a number of attractions are accessible, including the Assembly Rooms and medieval Abbey, and the massed Georgian architecture which can all be appreciated by disabled visitors.

Other towns to visit include Salisbury with its famed Cathedral and Close. Wells boasts a magnificent Cathedral and the oldest continuously populated street in Europe. Gloucester Cathedral, made famous in the Harry Potter films and the city's docks that now house a waterways museum are also worth a visit. Also in Gloucestershire, Cheltenham has developed as a Georgian spa town. Dorchester, the historic county town of Dorset, was Thomas Hardy's Casterbridge. In part of the old railway works at Swindon is Steam, a museum that depicts the history of the Great Western Railway and its workers.

On the Bristol Channel coast the largest resort is Weston-Super-Mare with a long, level seafront and a wide range of entertainment. Other resorts on this coast include Minehead on the edge of Exmoor and Burnham-on-Sea. The Dorset coast includes Weymouth on a sheltered bay behind Portland Bill and picturesque Lyme Regis.

Other attractions in the area with facilities for disabled visitors include the Tank Museum at Bovington in Dorset and Longleat House and Safari Park in Wiltshire. The West Somerset Railway has coaches adapted to carry wheelchair users between Minehead and the outskirts of Taunton.

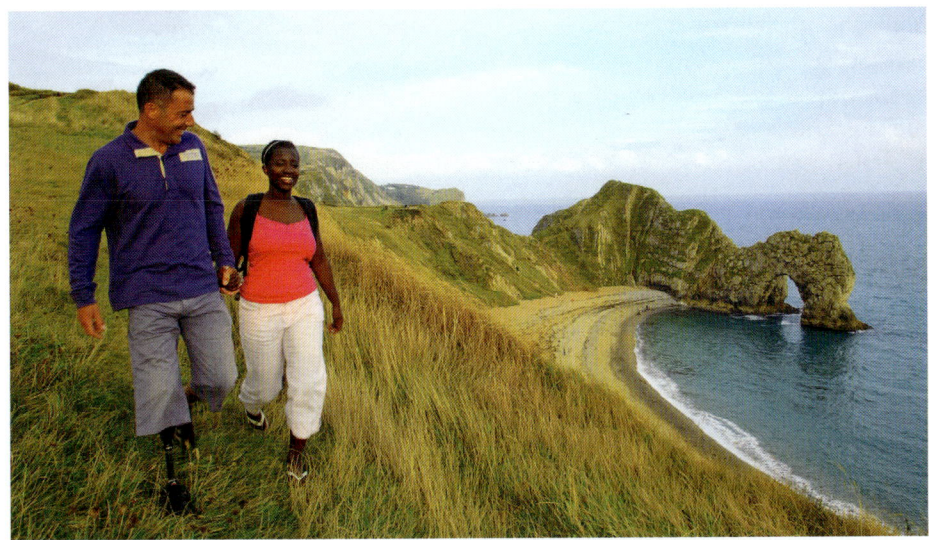

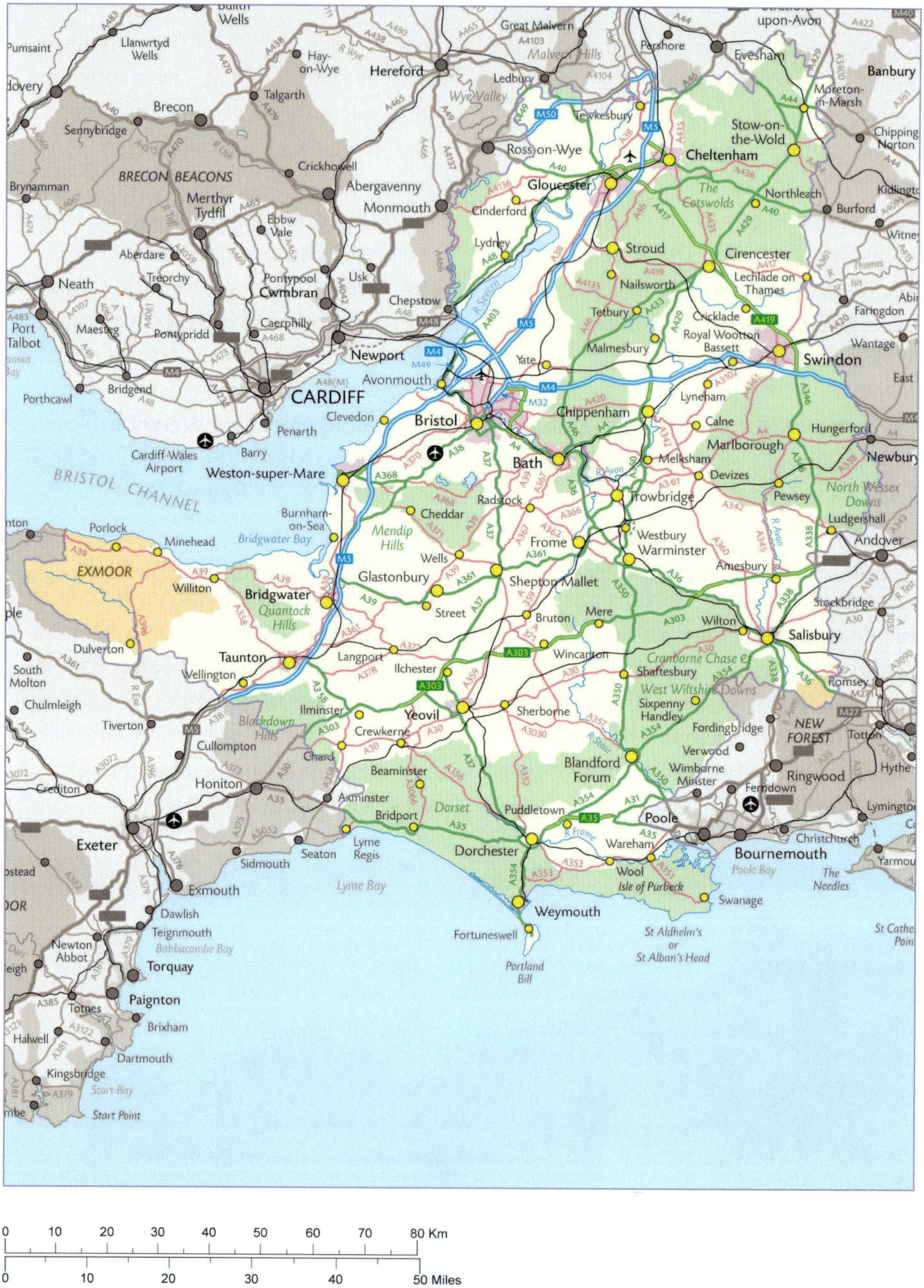

ENGLAND

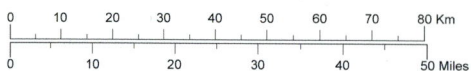

HOLIDAYS IN THE BRITISH ISLES

Resources
Tourism

South West Tourism
Woodwater Park, Exeter EX2 5WT
- T 0870 442 0880
- E post@swtourism.co.uk
- W www.visitsouthwest.co.uk

General tourist information is given on their website. Specific information for disabled people is provided at:
- W www.accessiblesouthwest.co.uk

Information & advice

Dorset Association for the Disabled
Unit 18a, Enterprise Park, Piddlehinton, Dorchester DT2 7UA
- T 01305 849122
- E dad.hq@tesco.net

Provide holidays for Association members and can respond to enquiries.

Disability Wessex, Bournemouth
- T 01202 589999

Has a small team of experienced advisers, with extensive knowledge, relevant training and qualifications and the majority have personal experience of living with a health condition or impairment. Aim to provide advice and assistance, to enable disabled people and families to understand and secure their rights and entitlements.

Independent Living Centre Semington
- T 01380 871007

Offer wheelchair hire and equipment advice and assessments. Also provides information regarding accessible holidays.

Nailsea Disability Initiative
- T 01275 812183
- E team@nailseadisability.org
- W http://nailseadisability.wordpress.com

Run a drop in centre for members of the public which is open between 10.00 a.m. and 3.00 p.m. Monday to Thursday.

DIAL
Offer free, impartial and confidential information and advice by telephone to disabled people, their relatives and professionals. Local branches of DIAL are constantly changing but at the time of writing, the following groups were members of DIAL UK and may be able to help visitors in their areas. Please call before travelling to check whether the service and organisation is still available:

DIAS Bristol
- T 0117 983 2828 (also Textphone)

NORDIS Gillingham
- T 01747 821010

THINGS TO SEE OR DO

Cotswold Water Park
Britain's largest water park with 132 lakes, covering over 30 square miles. The park offers free accessible parking, accessible toilets and a designated accessible picnic site and viewpoint. There are also angling terraces and accessible lakeside paths. A disabled sailing club is located at Whitefriars and a riding club catering for disabled riders is based at South Cerney.
- T 01793 752413
- W www.waterpark.org

ENGLAND

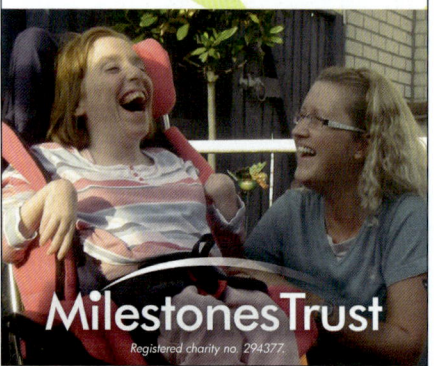

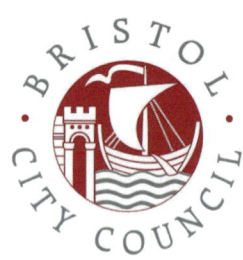

Bristol City Council
fully supports
Disability Rights UK

0117 922 2100
www.bristol.gov.uk

Double-Gate Farm
Near Wells, Somerset

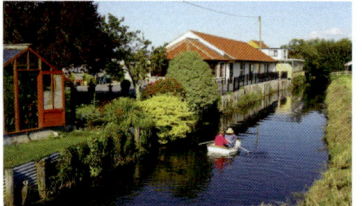

Listed Georgian Farmhouse and Riverside Suites
nestling in a pleasant position
on the Somerset Levels.
Central location ideal for exploring Somerset.

Choice of B&B and Self-Catering.
Multiple night discounts available.

Ground floor area and Games Room
all wheelchair accessible.

Double-Gate Farm, Godney,
Near Wells, Somerset, BA5 1RZ
Phone: 01458 832217
Fax: 01458 835612
E-mail: doublegatefarm@aol.com
www.doublegatefarm.co.uk

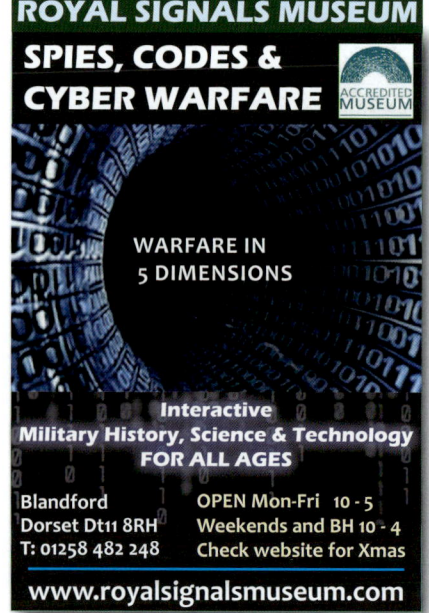

HOLIDAYS IN THE BRITISH ISLES

WEST COUNTRY

Weston and North Somerset DIAL
- 01934 419426
- www.westondial.co.uk

Gives detailed advice and information on subjects such as welfare rights, access and holidays. Open Tuesdays between 11.00a.m and 1.30 p.m. and Thursdays between 11.00 a.m. and 3.00 p.m.

Equipment hire

SHOPMOBILITY
The National Federation of Shopmobility UK (NFSUK), PO Box 6641, Christchurch BH23 9DQ
- 0844 41 41 850
- info@shopmobilityuk.org
- www.shopmobilityuk.org

Scheme which lends manual wheelchairs, powered wheelchairs and powered scooters to members of the public with limited mobility to shop and to visit leisure and commercial facilities within the town, city or shopping centre. You can find the nearest Shopmobility scheme to you through their on-line directory. Contact specific Shopmobility Schemes to make equipment bookings or find out more information.

Purbeck Mobility Limited
Mobility Centre, St Johns Hill, Wareham, Dorset BH20 4NB
- 01929 552623
- enquiries@purbeckmobility.com
- http://purbeckmobility.com

Provide wheelchairs and scooters to visitors to the Purbeck area on daily and weekly rates.

Weston Mobility Centre
215 Milton Road, Weston-super-Mare BS22 8EG
- 01934 642071
- miltonmobility@gmail.com
- www.westonmobilitycentre.co.uk

In addition to hiring wheelchairs, they supply a wide range of other disability equipment, including spare parts.

Publications

South Somerset: a Guide for People with Disabilities
- 01935 462462
- tourism@southsomerset.gov.uk

Published by the South Somerset District Council. A booklet giving information for disabled people on attractions, accommodation, car parking, public toilets and organisations. Available from information centres in the area or from Tourism Unit, South Somerset District Council, Brympton Way, Yeovil BA20 2HT.

THINGS TO SEE OR DO

Stonehenge
Just outside Amesbury in Wiltshire stands one of the most famous prehistoric sites in the world. At the centre of the most dense complex of Neolithic and Bronze Age monuments in England, including several hundred burial mounds. Wheelchair loan, accessible toilets and disabled parking are available. Tactile models and exhibitions of the standing stones are available for visually impaired visitors.
- www.english-heritage.org.uk/daysout/properties/stonehenge
- 0870 333 1181

ENGLAND

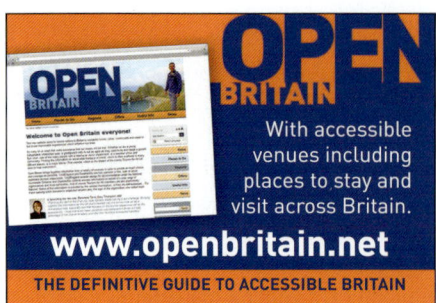

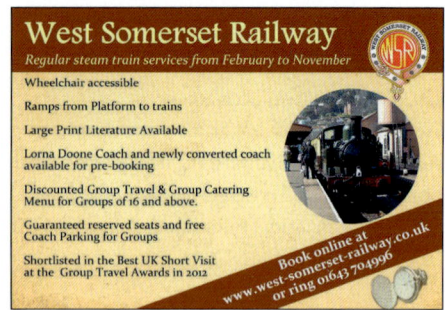

COTSWOLD CHARM—CHIPPING CAMPDEN

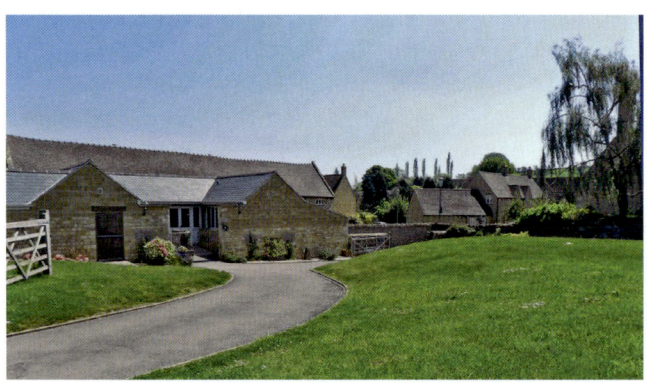

3 Four Star Cottages with level access
Ewe Pen sleeps M3i - en suite wetroom, sleeps 5
Lower Chapter— sleeps 2
George Barn—en suite wetroom, sleep 4, available April '13

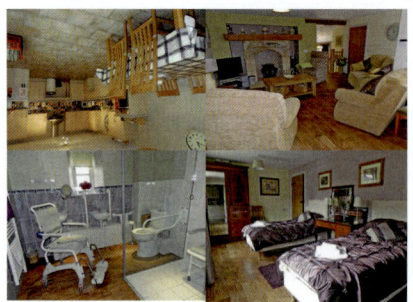
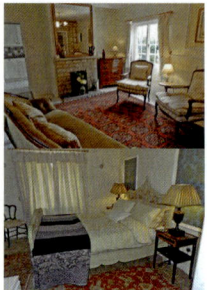

T: (01386) 840164 Mob/Text: 0788 964 9812
E: info@cotswoldcharm.com   www.cotswoldcharm.com
Contact: Michael Haines

WEST COUNTRY

West Dorset for Visitors with Special Needs
- tourism@westdorset-dc.gov.uk
- www.westdorset.com

A free booklet published by West Dorset District Council. It gives information on visiting the towns of Dorchester, Bridport, Sherborne, Beaminster and Lyme Regis. Available from Tourist Information Centres in the area or from West Dorset District Council, Community Enabling Division, Stratton House, High West Street, Dorchester DT1 1UZ.

Online resources

www.accessiblesouthwest.co.uk
A website giving information on accessible accommodation and attractions in the region. Includes sections on equipment hire, services and accessible public toilets.

www.visitforestofdean.co.uk
Contains 'Facilities and Information for those with disabilities visiting the Forest of Dean', with information regularly updated by Forest of Dean Council.

www.visitsomerset.co.uk
- 01934 750833
- somersetvisitorcentre@somerset.gov.uk

The website of Somerset Tourism includes information for disabled visitors to the county including accommodation that has been inspected for accessibility and attractions that are said to have facilities for disabled visitors, a county wide list of unisex public toilets and organisations that can provide further information. General advice on the area is also available from the Somerset Visitor Centre.

Accommodation

NAS ASSESSED ACCOMMODATION

AWRE NEAR NEWNHAM ON SEVERN, Gloucestershire
Priory Cottages
Four star self-catering
- 0174 7828 170
- enq@hideaways.co.uk
- www.hideaways.co.uk

BATH, Somerset
SACO Bath
Four star serviced apartments
- 0845 1220 405
- janejones@sacoapartments.co.uk
- www.sacoapartments.co.uk

THINGS TO SEE OR DO

Montacute House
Montacute, Somerset TA15 6XP
Mansion built in the late 16th century. The formal gardens include a collection of roses, mixed borders and 'wobbly hedges'. Ground floor (including great hall, lower Maybank corridor, parlour and drawing room), cafe and gardens are fully accessible to wheelchair users and wheelchairs are available to hire. Accessible toilets are located by the ticket entrance and designated accessible parking is available 40 yards from the entrance.
- 01935 823289
- www.nationaltrust.org.uk/montacute-house

HOLIDAYS IN THE BRITISH ISLES

ENGLAND

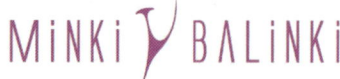
Visionary creative hub

www.minkibalinki.com

The Old Stables
3 self-catering units in Britford, Salisbury

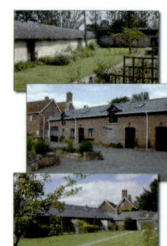

The ground floor has excellent facilities for elderly or disabled people.

For more information:
The Old Stables
Lower Road,
Britford, Salisbury,
Wiltshire SP5 4DY
T: +44 (0)1722 349002
E: mail@old-stables.co.uk
www.old-stables.co.uk

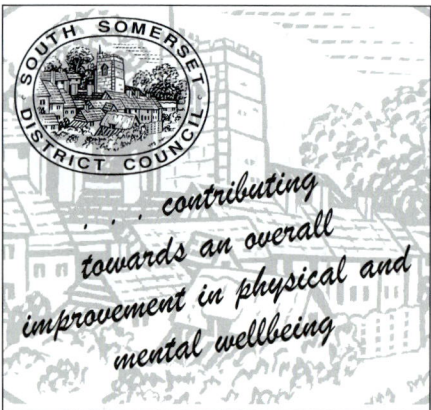
...contributing towards an overall improvement in physical and mental wellbeing

The Coppleridge Inn
A traditional family run country inn

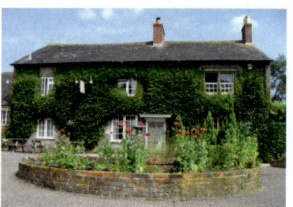

10 luxurious ground floor rooms
Set in 15 peaceful acres of Dorset
www.coppleridge.com

Luxurious wood cabin as featured on ITV's 'Great little escapes'

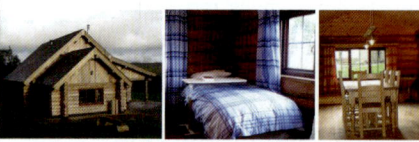

Tamarack Lodge . Fyfett Farm . Otterford
Near Chard . Somerset TA20 3QP UK
Telephone 01823 601 270

www.tamaracklodge.co.uk

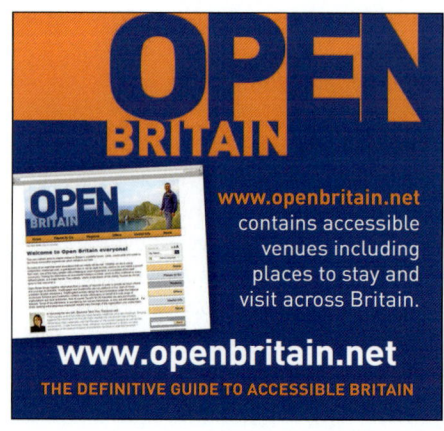

HOLIDAYS IN THE BRITISH ISLES

WEST COUNTRY

University of Bath
Three and Four star campus accommodation
- T: 0122 5384 869
- E: K.F.McCormick@bath.ac.uk
- W: www.bath.ac.uk/salesandevents

Carfax Hotel
Two star townhouse
- T: 0122 546 2089
- E: sylvia.back@carfaxhotel.co.uk
- W: www.carfaxhotel.co.uk

BEAMINSTER, Dorset
Stable Cottage
Four star self-catering
- T: 01308 862305
- E: meerhay@aol.com
- W: www.meerhay.co.uk

BOOKHAM, ALTON PANCRAS, Dorset
Bookham Court
Four and Five star self-catering
- T: 01300 345511
- E: andy.foot1@btinternet.com
- W: www.bookhamcourt.co.uk

BOURNEMOUTH, Dorset
BOD
Four star self-catering
- T: 01202 423046
- E: admin@afash.co.uk
- W: www.afash.co.uk

BROAD QUAY, Bristol
SACO Bristol – Broad Quay
Four star serviced apartments
- T: 0845 1220 405
- E: janejones@sacoapartments.co.uk
- W: www.sacoapartments.co.uk

BURTON BRADSTOCK, Dorset
Norburton Hall
Four and Five star self-catering
- T: 0130 8897 007
- E: info@norburtonhall.com
- W: www.norburtonhall.com

CHEDDAR, Somerset
YHA Cheddar
Three star hostel
- T: 0162 9592 686
- E: margaretgibson@yha.org.uk
- W: www.yha.org.uk

CHEW MAGNA, Somerset
Woodbarn Farm Cottages
Three and Four star cottages
- T: 01275 332599
- E: woodbarnfarm@hotmail.com
- W: www.woodbarnfarmcottages.co.uk

CHICKERELL, Dorset
Tidmoor Self Catering Cottages
Four star self-catering
- T: 0130 578 7867
- E: sarah@tidmoorstables.co.uk
- W: www.tidmoorstables.co.uk

The Lugger Inn
Three star inn
- T: 0130 5766 611
- E: ralph@theluggerinn.co.uk
- W: www.theluggerinn.co.uk

CORFE CASTLE, Dorset
Mortons House Hotel
Three star hotel
- T: 01929 480988
- E: bev@mortonshouse.co.uk
- W: www.mortonshouse.co.uk

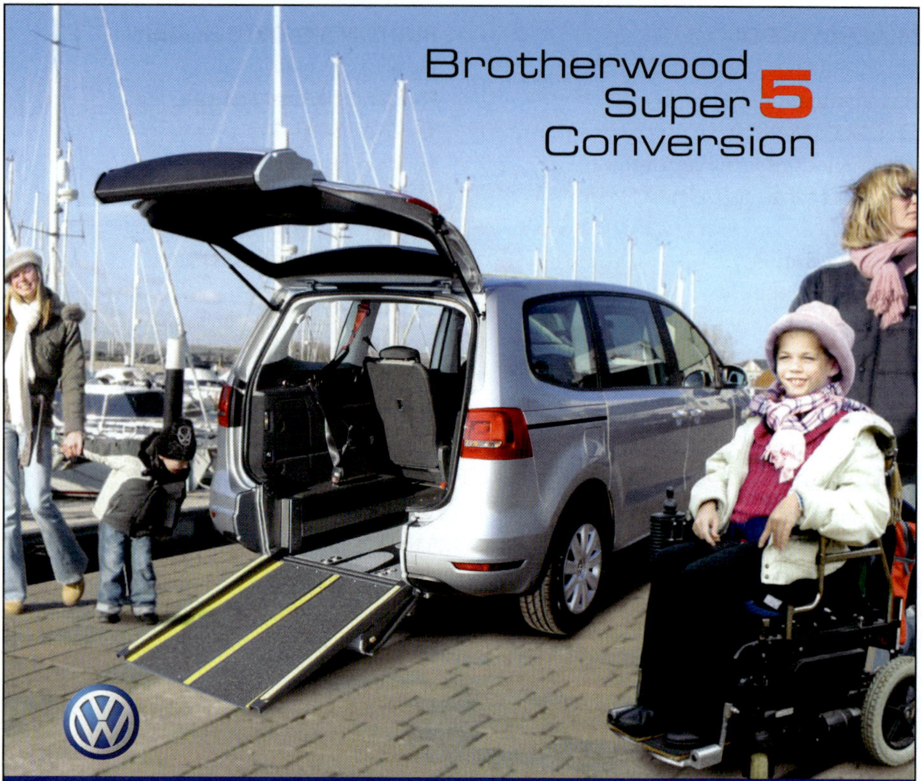

ENGLAND

Brotherwood Super 5 Conversion

At the heart of a Brotherwood conversion is seating for all the family

The Brotherwood converted Sharan offers compact transport for five adults, including the driver and one wheelchair passenger.

The optional centre Quick Fold Seat can be simply tilted to transform the car in seconds without any lifting or storing, hence the title - SUPER FIVE.

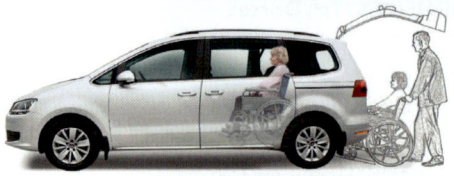

BROTHERWOOD
Automobility Limited
BEER HACKETT, SHERBORNE, DORSET DT9 6QP

phone: 01935 872603   or visit
www.brotherwood.com

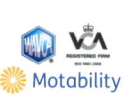
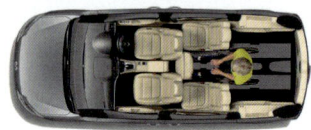

For comprehensive details of new and previously owned conversions, long or short term hire and Motability options

WEST COUNTRY

DORCHESTER, Dorset
Aquila Heights
Four star guest accommodation
- 01305 267145
- enquiries@aquilaheights.co.uk
- www.aquilaheights.co.uk

EXFORD, Somerset
Westermill Farm
Three star self-catering
- 01643 831238
- holidays@westermill-exmoor.co.uk
- www.westermill.com

FERNDOWN, Dorset
Birchcroft
Four star self-catering
- 07889 090773
- holidayinndorset@btinternet.com
- www.holidayindorset.org

GLOUCESTER, Gloucestershire
Deerhurst Cottages
Four star self-catering
- 01684 275845
- enquiries@deerhurstcottages.co.uk
- www.deerhustcottages.co.uk

GODNEY, Somerset
Double-Gate Farm
Four star farmhouse
- 01458 832217
- doublegatefarm@aol.com
- www.doublegatefarm.com

GORWELL, Dorset
Gorwell Farm Cottages
Four star self-catering
- 01305 871401
- mary@gorwellfarm.co.uk
- www.gorwellfarm.co.uk

HIGH LITTLETON, Somerset
Greyfield Farm Cottages
Four and Five star self-catering
- 0176 1471 132
- june@greyfieldfarm.com
- www.greyfieldfarm.com

HORSINGTON, Somerset
Half Moon Inn
Three star inn
- 01963 370140
- halfmoon@horsington.co.uk
- www.horsington.co.uk

HUNTWORTH, Somerset
Lakeview Holiday Cottages
Four star self-catering
- 0127 866 1584
- jayne@snotaroholdings.co.uk
- www.lakeviewholidaycottages.co.uk

LANGTON HERRING / RODDEN, Dorset
Character Farm Cottages
Four star self-catering
- 01305 871347
- ann@characterfarmcottages.co.uk
- www.characterfarmcottages.co.uk

LITTLEDEAN, Gloucestershire
Orchard Barn & Meadow Byre
Four and Five star self-catering
- 01594 827311
- geoff@searanckes.com
- www.forestbarnholidays.co.uk

LONG BREDY, Dorset
Stables Cottage
Four star self-catering
- 0130 5789 000
- shane@dream-cottages.co.uk
- www.dream-cottages.co.uk

ENGLAND

LYDNEY, Gloucestershire
2 Danby Cottages
Four star self-catering
- 0117 9422301
- glawes@talktalk.net
- www.danbycottages.co.uk

The Lodge
Four star self-catering
- 01594 843745
- allaston-lodge@hotmail.co.uk

LYTCHETT MINSTER, Dorset
South Lytchett Manor Caravan & Camping Park
Five star holiday, touring and camping park
- 01202 622 577
- info@southlytchettmanor.co.uk
- www.southlytchettmanor.co.uk

MALMESBURY, Wiltshire
Best Western Mayfield House Hotel
Three star hotel
- 0166 657 409
- reception@mayfieldhousehotel.co.uk
- www.mayfieldhousehotel.co.uk

MINEHEAD, Somerset
Woodcombe Lodges
Four star self-catering
- 01643 702789
- nicola@woodcombelodge.co.uk
- www.woodcombelodge.co.uk

NEWENT, Gloucestershire
Leadon View Barn
Four star self-catering
- 0153 1821868
- ianbrownnewent@tiscali.co.uk
- www.leadonviewbarn.com

The Moorhens
Four and Five star holiday cottages
- 0159 4827 311
- lynda@forestbarnholidays.co.uk
- www.forestbarnholidays.co.uk

POOLE, Dorset
The New Beehive Hotel
Three star small hotel
- 0120 270 1531
- info@thenewbeehive.co.uk
- www.thenewbeehive.co.uk

RADSTOCK, Somerset
The Garden House
Five star self-catering
- 0176 124 1080
- jclayton@janeclayton.co.uk
- www.lilycombe.co.uk

SOUTH BARROW, Somerset
The Stables
Four star self-catering
- 0196 3440 421
- a-nixon@btconnect.com

SALISBURY, Wiltshire
Old Stables
Four star self-catering
- 07794 403111
- mail@old-stables.co.uk
- www.old-stables.co.uk

STOKE ABBOTT, Dorset
Lewesdon Farm Holidays
Four star cottages
- 01308 868270
- lewesdonfarmcottages@tiscali.co.uk
- www.lewesdonfarmholidays.co.uk

WEST COUNTRY

TAUNTON, Somerset
Holly Farm Cottages
Four star self-catering
- 0182 349 0828
- robhembrow@btinternet.com
- www.holly-farm.com

TINCLETON, Dorset
Tincleton Lodge and Rose Cottage
Five star self-catering
- 01305 848391
- enquiries@dorsetholidaycottages.net
- www.dorsetholidaycottages.net

TYTHERINGTON, Somerset
The Lighthouse
Four star guest accommodation
- 01373 453585
- reception@lighthouse-uk.com
- www.lighthouse-uk.com

UPWEY, Dorset
Millspring
Four star self-catering
- 0130 5789 000
- shane@dream-cottages.co.uk
- www.dream-cottages.co.uk

WEST MILTON, Dorset
Lancombes House
Four star self-catering
- 01308 485375
- info@lancombes-house.co.uk
- www.lancombes-house.co.uk

WESTON-SUPER-MARE, Somerset
The Royal Hotel
Three star bed & breakfast
- 0193 4423 100
- jonathan@royalhotelweston.com
- www.royalhotelweston.com

Spreyton Guest House
Four star guest accommodation
- 0193 4416 887
- info@spreytonguesthouse.com
- www.spreytonguesthouse.com

WEYMOUTH, Dorset
Jubilee View Apartment
Three star self-catering
- 0238 0770 301
- info@jubileeview.com
- www.jubileeview.webeden.co.uk

WINFORD, Somerset
Winford Manor Hotel
Three star hotel
- 0127 5472 292
- traceybeck@winfordmanor.co.uk
- www.winfordmanor.co.uk

WINSLEY, Wiltshire
Church Farm Country Cottages
Four star self-catering
- 01225 722246
- stay@churchfarmcottages.com
- www.churchfarmcottages.com

WOOLLAND, Dorset
Ellwood Cottages
Four star self-catering
- 01258 818 196
- admin@ellwoodcottages.co.uk
- www.ellwoodcottages.co.uk

HOLIDAYS IN THE BRITISH ISLES

OTHER ACCOMMODATION

BLANDFORD FORUM, Dorset
The Ellwood Centre
Wooland, Blandford Forum DT11 0ES
- 01258 818196
- admin@ellwoodcottages.co.uk
- www.ellwoodcottages.co.uk

Single storey self-catering cottages designed for disabled people.

BURNHAM-ON-SEA, Somerset
BPF Bungalow
Contact: British Polio Fellowship, Eagle Office Centre, The Runway, Ruislip HA4 6SE
- 0800 018 0586
  01903 529057
- holidays@britishpolio.org.uk
- www.britishpolio.org.uk

Purpose-built bungalow on the seafront in Burnham-on-Sea.

Holiday Homes Trust Caravan
Burnham-on-Sea Holiday Village, Burnham-on-Sea TA8 1LA
- 020 8433 7290
- scout.holiday.homes@scouts.org.uk
- www.holidayhomestrust.org

Adapted units on holiday park near the town centre.

CHRISTCHURCH, Dorset
Number 31
c/o 40 Walcott Avenue, Christchurch, Dorset BH23 2NG
- 01202 481597
- info@31aha.co.uk
- www.31aha.co.uk

Self-catering bungalow originally adapted for wheelchair using owner, a mile from centre of coastal town.
Contact: Liz Cox

MINEHEAD, Somerset
Promenade Hotel
The Esplanade, Minehead TA24 5QS
- 01643 702572
- promenadehotel@livability.org.uk
- www.livability.org.uk

Hotel owned by Livability specially adapted for disabled guests.

POOLE, Dorset
Holton Lee
East Holton, Poole BH16 6JN
- 01202 625632
- admin@holtonlee.co.uk
- www.holtonlee.co.uk

Purpose-built centre for disabled people and carers in countryside overlooking Poole Harbour.

Orton Rigg Hotel
53 Cliff Drive, Canford Cliffs, Poole BH13 7JF
- www.ortonrigghotel.co.uk

Hotel adapted for disabled guests in secluded setting.

Holiday Homes Trust Caravan
Rockley Park, Hamworthy, Poole BH15 4LZ
- 020 8433 7290
- scout.holiday.homes@scouts.org.uk
- www.holidayhomestrust.org

Adapted unit on holiday park overlooking Poole Harbour.

WEST COUNTRY

SALISBURY, Wiltshire

Websters
11 Hartington Road, Salisbury SP2 7LG
- 01722 339779
- enquiries@websters-bed-breakfast.com
- www.websters-bed-breakfast.com

Bed & breakfast house in the city of Salisbury.

WESTON-SUPER-MARE, Somerset

The Lauriston Hotel
6-12 Knightsbridge Road, Weston-super-Mare BS23 2AN
- 01934 620758
- lauriston@visionhotels.co.uk

Hotel in grounds near the seafront for blind and partially sighted people and their companions.

WEYMOUTH, Dorset

Anchor House
3 Holland Road, Weymouth, Dorset DT4 0AL
- 08456 584478
- info@livability.org.uk
- www.livability.org.uk

Victorian house owned by Livability, adapted for wheelchair users.

Wimborne & Ferndown Lions Club Caravans
Littlesea Holiday Park, Near Weymouth. Contact: Frank Fortey, 23 Egdon Drive, Wimborne BH21 1TY
- 01202 886022
- www.lions.org.uk/wimborne-ferndown

Caravan designed for disabled people. Sited on Haven holiday park by Chesil Beach.

THE ROYAL SIGNALS MUSEUM

Dorset's Hidden Gem!

From semaphore to high tech cyber space, and electronic warfare: discover the rapidly evolving story of the British Army's dynamic cutting edge ... The Royal Signals.

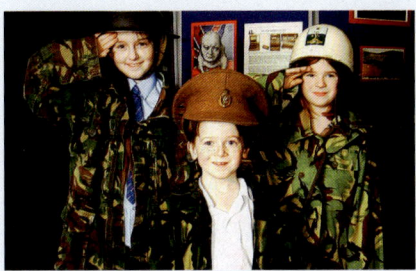

The modern museum is nestled in the beautiful countryside of North Dorset, in the attractive Edwardian town of Blandford Forum.

It traces the history of the British Army's battlefield communications experts from the introduction of the telegraph in the Crimea to the secretive story of cryptography and cyber warfare via espionage and satellites!

A voyage of discovery through hands-on, family-friendly interactive displays: guide a laser beam, "direction find" the enemy, set up satellite networks, break codes, practice Morse more!

Adults must bring photo ID.

www.royalsignalsmuseum.co.uk

HOLIDAYS IN THE BRITISH ISLES

ENGLAND

About Devon & Cornwall

The two counties of England's south west peninsula have long been a major holiday destination and offer a wide range of attractions for visitors.

You are never far from the sea in this region and there is a series of resorts around the coast. The towns of Torquay and Paignton are known as the English Riviera because of their mild climate and high-class entertainment. Parts of the coast are hilly, although east Devon resorts such as Exmouth and Sidmouth are fairly level as is Penzance in the far west. At other resorts such as Ilfracombe, St Ives, Newquay or Falmouth a car may be needed away from the seafront itself.

Much of the coastal scenery is dramatic. Among the places where this can be experienced are at the cliff-top National

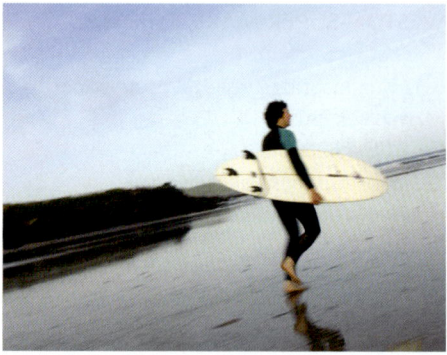

Trust car park at Wheel Coates near St Agnes, with its view over the North Cornwall cliffs and old tin mines, and Lands End. Marine life can be experienced at the National Seal Sanctuary near Helston and the National Marine Aquarium at Plymouth.

Inland, the countryside can also be wild, particularly in the National Parks of Dartmoor and Exmoor and areas such as Bodmin Moor in Cornwall. However, there are plenty of opportunities to experience the countryside and its activities at attractions such as Mount Edgcumbe Country Park overlooking Plymouth Sound, or the Crealy Farm Adventure Park in east Devon. At the Eden Project, outside St Austell, a dramatic global garden has been

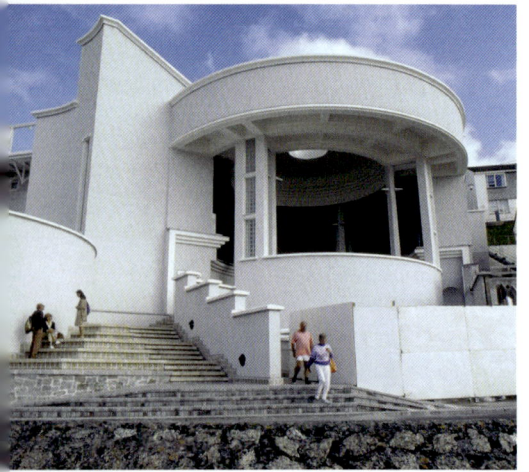

DEVON & CORNWALL

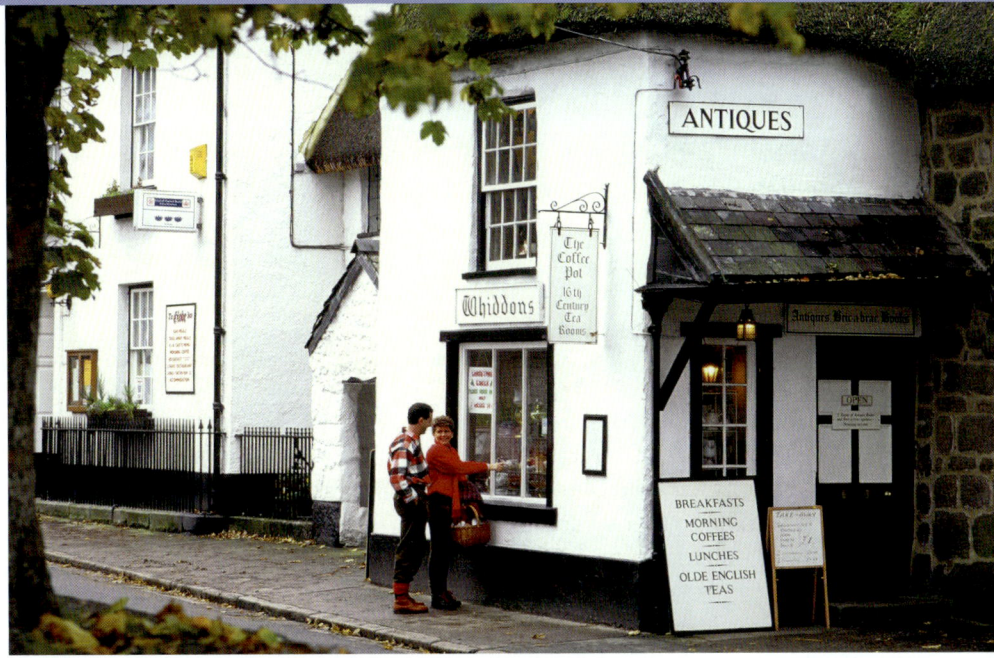

developed in a disused china clay pit. Longer established planting can be enjoyed at the Royal Horticultural Society's Rosemoor Garden at Torrington.

Historic buildings in the area include Okehampton Castle in Devon owned by English Heritage, Buckfast Abbey and a number of National Trust properties such as Saltram House and Killerton House and Garden both near Exeter.

In Plymouth, the region's largest city, the National Marine Aquarium is a major attraction and the Plymouth Dome, on the Hoe, uses multi-media displays to show the civic and maritime history of the area. Exeter, county town of Devon, still has many old buildings especially in the area around the Cathedral. Truro is the location of the Royal Cornwall Museum. Other attractive towns include Barnstaple and Bideford in north Devon.

For family outings there is Flambards Theme Park near Helston or a trip on the Seaton Tramway in East Devon, both having facilities for disabled visitors. Finally, this is a region with distinctive food to be sampled, be it genuine Cornish Pasties, fresh caught fish or the widely available cream teas.

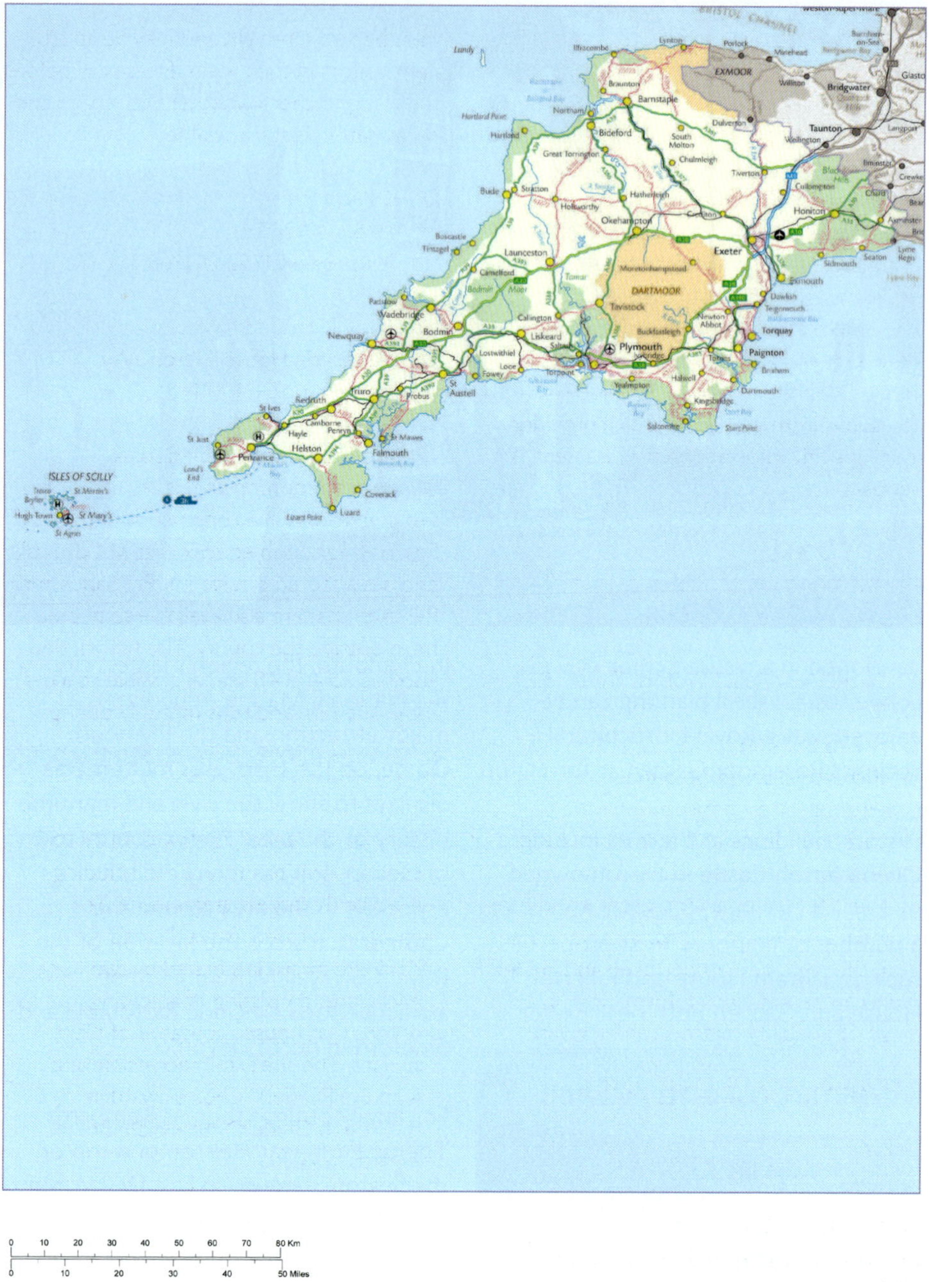

ENGLAND

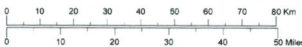

HOLIDAYS IN THE BRITISH ISLES

Resources

Tourism

Visit South West
Woodwater Park, Exeter EX2 5WT
- 013 9222 9168
- info@swtourismalliance.org.uk
- www.visitsouthwest.co.uk

The official tourist board for the South West. General tourist information is provided on their website. See also www.accessiblesouthwest.co.uk which provides more specific information for disabled people.

Transport

Richard Willson Accessible Transport Services
49 Carne View Road, Probus, Truro TR2 4HZ
- 01726 883460
- Richard.willson@btconnect.com

A well-established transport provider offering ambulance and accessible minibus services for wheelchair users, with or without their companions. Escorts and care attendants can be supplied. Journeys to and from the region are undertaken and guided tours can be arranged. Information on a range of disability matters can be given.

Information and Advice

DIAL
Offer free, impartial and confidential information and advice by telephone to disabled people, their relatives and professionals. Local branches of DIAL are constantly changing but at the time of writing, the following groups were members of DIAL UK and may be able to help visitors in their areas. Please call before travelling to check whether the service and organisation is still available.

DIAC Plymouth
- 01752 201065
  Textphone 01752 201766

Cornwall Disabled Association
1a, 1 Riverside House, Heron Way, Newham, Truro TR1 2XN
- 01872 273518
- info@cornwalldisabled.co.uk
- www.freedomonwheels.org.uk

Provide holidays, in conjunction with Social Services, for disabled residents of Cornwall and has adapted caravans at Par Sands and Rejerrah that are also available to people from outside the county. The Association also has 20 and 48 seat accessible coaches for group hire and runs monthly outings.

THINGS TO SEE OR DO

The Eden Project
Bodelva, St Austell, Cornwall, PL24 2SG
Ecological visitor attraction, including the world's largest greenhouse. The complex, located in a reclaimed Kaolinite pit, is dominated by two huge enclosures consisting of adjoining domes that house thousands of plant species. The site is fully accessible and won the Readers' Choice award at the Rough Guide to Accessible Britain Awards in 2010.
- 01726 811911
- www.edenproject.com

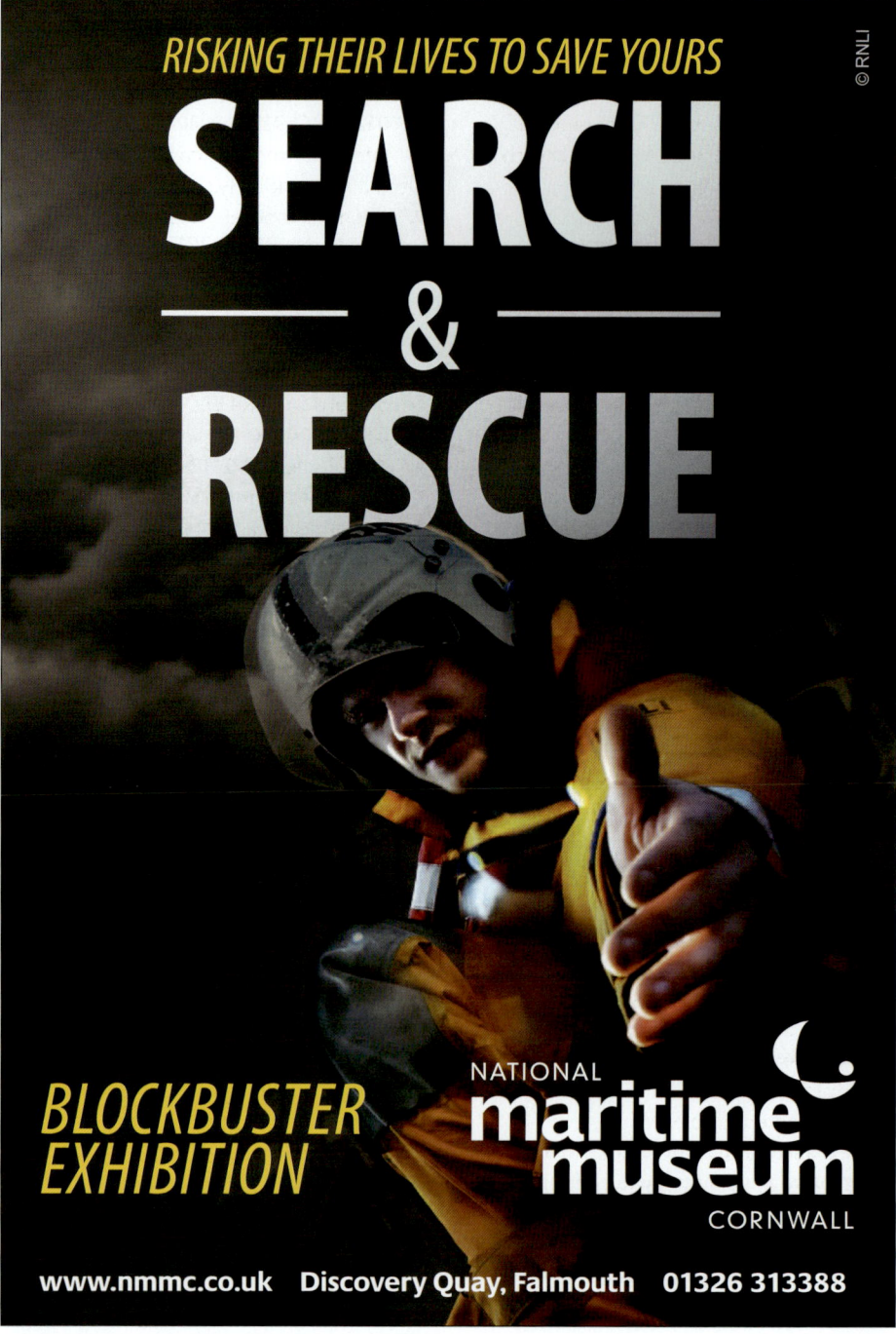

DEVON & CORNWALL

Equipment hire

SHOPMOBILITY
The National Federation of Shopmobility UK (NFSUK), PO Box 6641, Christchurch BH23 9DQ
- ☎ 0844 41 41 850
- ✉ info@shopmobilityuk.org
- 🌐 www.shopmobilityuk.org

Scheme which lends manual wheelchairs, powered wheelchairs and powered scooters to members of the public with limited mobility to shop and to visit leisure and commercial facilities within the town, city or shopping centre. You can find the nearest Shopmobility scheme to you through their on-line directory. Contact specific Shopmobility Schemes to make equipment bookings or find out more information.

Braunton Mobility Centre
3 Cross Tree Centre, Braunton, Devon EX33 1AA
- ☎ 01271 814577
- 🌐 www.mobilityinbraunton.co.uk

Manual wheelchairs and scooters are available for hire as well as a wide range of equipment for sale.

Exeter Community Transport Association
8-10 Paris Street, Exeter EX1 1GA
- ☎ 01392 494001
- ✉ info@exetercta.co.uk
- 🌐 www.exetercta.co.uk

In association with Exeter Shopmobility there is a long term loan service for both residents and visitors for use anywhere. They have manual wheelchairs at £2.50 a day and two portable scooters at £5 per day.

HSC Mobility
Unit 16, Mobility House, Marsh Lane Industrial Park, Hayle, Cornwall TR27 5JR
- ☎ 01736 755927
- ✉ info@hsc-mobility.co.uk
- 🌐 www.hsc-mobility.co.uk

Wheelchairs, scooters, hoists, adjustable beds and other equipment are available for hire.

Tremorvah Industries
Unit 8, Threemilestone Industrial Estate, Truro, Cornwall TR4 9LD
- ☎ 01872 324340
  Textphone 01872 324364
- ✉ enquiries.tremorvah@cornwall.gov.uk
- 🌐 www.tremorvah.co.uk

Hire and sell manual and powered wheelchairs, scooters, commodes, hoists and a range of other equipment. Deliveries can be made throughout Cornwall.

> ### THINGS TO SEE OR DO
>
> #### Geevor Tin Mine Museum
> Pendeen, Penzance, Cornwall TR19 7EW
>
> One of the largest preserved mine sites in the country. There is wheelchair access to the museum, a number of the mine buildings, and many surface areas. Specialist guided tours around the site and underground are provided for visually impaired visitors and guide dogs are permitted everywhere on site, including underground.
> - ☎ 01736 788662
> - 🌐 www.geevor.com

HOLIDAYS IN THE BRITISH ISLES

ENGLAND

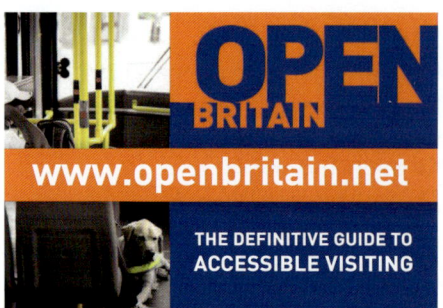

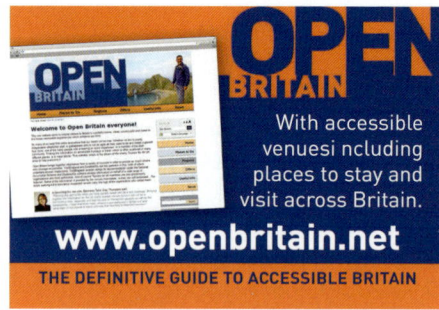

Trenona Farm, Truro, Cornwall.
- quality holiday cottages with great access for wheelchair users
- located on a peaceful working farm near Truro and St Mawes
- sleep 4-6 people
- parking
- wifi
- children and pets welcome

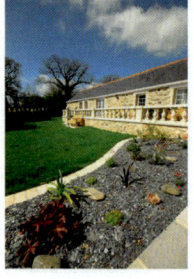

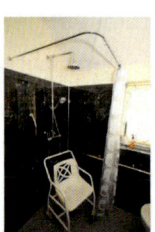

- spacious open plan kitchen/diner/lounge
- en suite bedrooms with wet floor showers/baths
- enclosed garden with patio and barbecue

Contact:
Mrs Pamela Carbis
01872 501339

www.trenonafarmholidays.co.uk

Brookfields Bed & Breakfast

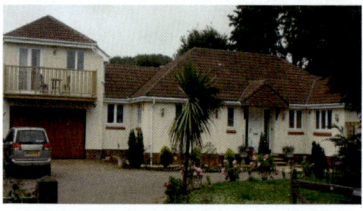

- Brookfields B&B is at ground level with wide doors, suited to the young, elderly & disabled. Ramps available. Nothing is too much trouble.
- Choice of Double or Twin rooms, all with en-suite bathrooms.
- Use of lounge, landscaped gardens, patio & BBQ, children's play area.
- Close to Bus, Pub & Restaurants plus 3 miles from beach.
- Affordable luxury personalised service, free Wi-Fi. Experienced with disabilities.
- Cost from £65 a night per room including breakfast

Contact David & Rosemary on:
Telephone: 01395 567430 or 07802 755411
Email: d.zirker@btinternet.com
Website: www.brookfieldsbandb.co.uk

Brookfields, Venn Ottery Road, Newton Poppleford,
Sidmouth EX10 0BU

BEST WISHES TO DISABILITY RIGHTS UK FROM

FIC (UK) LTD

TEL: 01736 366 962 FAX: 01736 351198

Publications

Easy-Going Dartmoor
- 01822 890414
- www.dartmoor-npa.gov.uk

A guide giving information on walks, driving routes, viewpoints and access information to Dartmoor towns and villages suitable for disabled people. Produced by Dartmoor National Park Authority, The High Moorland Visitor Centre, Old Duchy Hotel, Princetown, Yelverton PL20 6QF. Also available to download from the website.

The English Riviera: Access for All
Regularly updated leaflet for Torquay, Paignton and Brixham. Available free at Tourist Information Centres in each town or from English Riviera Tourist Board, The Tourist Centre, Vaughan Parade, Torquay TQ2 5JG.
- 01803 211211 or 084 4474 2233
- holiday@englishriviera.co.uk
- www.englishriviera.co.uk

Online resources

www.accessiblesouthwest.co.uk
A website providing information on accessible accommodation, attractions, places of interest, places to eat, public toilets, and beaches in the region. There is also information on disability groups and organisations that can assist the disabled traveller whilst staying away from home, as well as local suppliers of accessibility equipment to hire.

www.dartmoor.co.uk
Dartmoor's official tourism website contains information about places to stay, things to do and routes to further information. Information about accommodation grading can be found at:
- www.dartmoor.co.uk/where-to-stay/grading

THINGS TO SEE OR DO

Accessible beaches
Marazion beach near Penzance, Hayle Bay near Polzeath and Preston beach near Paignton all offer at least partial access for wheelchair users. Saunton Sands, near Braunton, North Devon, is currently the only beach in the region to offer an all-terrain wheelchair for hire. It is able to traverse all areas of the beach and can even be used in the shallows of the sea. It is available for hire on a half day, daily or weekly basis. Advance booking is recommended during the summer period and school holidays, contact Saunton beach shop:
- 01271 890771
- info@sauntonbeach.info

Dartmoor iPhone app
Updated regularly, the app provides a comprehensive and interactive guide to Dartmoor National Park and surrounding towns. Information on where to stay, what to do, eating out and what's on. Maps show you where you are in relation to nearby hotels, activities, attractions, shops and events. Search and refine results for prices, opening times, directions and descriptions. The app can be downloaded at:
- www.dartmoor.co.uk/plan-your-visit/dartmoor-iphone-app

ENGLAND

Bocaddon Holiday Cottages

Three cottages, specially designed to accommodate the needs of disabled people.

Accessible throughout, fitted with large bathrooms with level flooring, roll-in shower seats and plenty of hand rails.

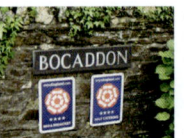

Contact: Mrs Alison Maiklem
Bocaddon Farm,
Lanreath,
Looe,
Cornwall PL13 2PG.

www.bocaddon.com

Telephone: 01503 220192   Email: holidays@bocaddon.com

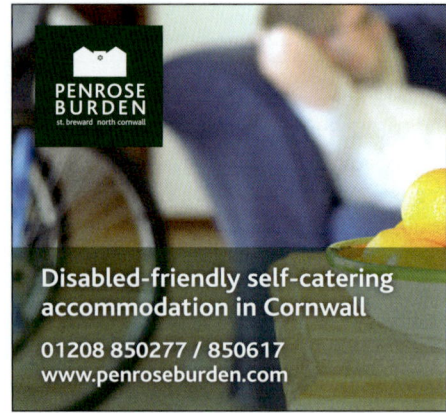

Wooda Farm five star Holiday Park
In the countryside – beside the sea

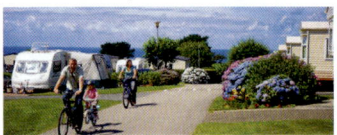

Wooda Farm Holiday Park
Poughill, Bude, Cornwall EX23 9HJ
Tel: 01288 352069   Fax: 01288 355258
Email:enquiries@wooda.co.uk
www.wooda.co.uk

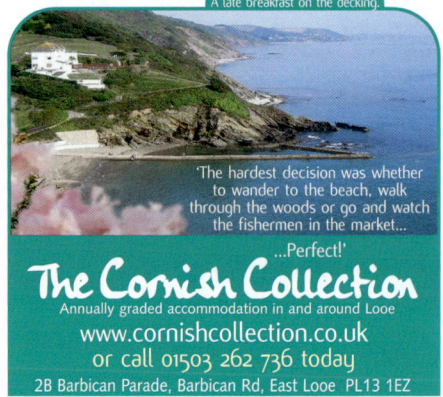

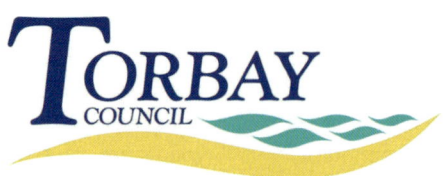

is committed to being accessible to all
www.torbay.gov.uk/disability

Accommodation

NAS ASSESSED ACCOMMODATION

AXMINSTER, Devon
Goodlands
Five star self-catering
- 0129 7320 36
- info@hedgehogcorner.co.uk
- www.hedgehogcornerholidaylets.co.uk

BARNSTAPLE, Devon
Calvert Trust Exmoor
Five star activity centre
- 01598 763221
- marketingexmoor@calvert-trust.org.uk
- www.calvert-trust.org.uk/exmoor

BODMIN, Cornwall
Lanhydrock Hotel and Golf Club
Three star hotel
- 01208 262570
- clare@lanhydrockhotel.com
- www.lanhydrockhotel.com

BOSCASTLE, Cornwall
The Old Coach House
Four star guest accommodation
- 0184 025 0398
- info@old-coach.co.uk
- www.old-coach.co.uk

Reddivallen Farmhouse
Five star guest accommodation
- 01840 250854
- liz@redboscastle.com
- www.redboscastle.com

BRAUNTON, Devon
Phoenix Retreat
Four star self-catering
- 0127 1816 577
- carol@phoenixcareathome.co.uk
- www.phoenixholidayretreat.co.uk

BUCKLAND BREWER, Devon
West Hele
Three and Four star self-catering
- 01237 451044
- lorna@westhele.co.uk
- www.westhele.co.uk/

BUDLEIGH SALTERTON, Devon
Badgers Den
Four star self-catering
- 0139 544 3282
- mandydickinson3@btinternet.com
- www.holidaycottagedevon.com

CHAPEL AMBLE, Cornwall
The Olde House
Three and Four star self-catering
- 01208 813 219
- info@theoldehouse.co.uk
- www.theoldehouse.co.uk

CREDITON, Devon
Creedy Manor
Four star self-catering
- 01363 772684
- sandra@creedymanor.com
- www.creedymanor.com

ENGLAND

CROWS-AN-WRAY, Cornwall
Tredinney Farm Holiday Cottage
Four star self-catering
- 01736 810352
- rosemary.warren@btopenworld.com

DAVIDSTOW, Cornwall
Pendragon Country House
Five star guest accommodation
- 01840 261131
- enquiries@pendragoncountryhouse.com
- www.pendragoncountryhouse.com

EXETER, Devon
Hue's Piece
Four star self-catering
- 01392 466720
- annahamlyn@paynes-farm.co.uk
- www.visitwestcountry.com/huespiece

GOLANT, Cornwall
South Torfrey Farm
Four and Five star self-catering
- 01726 833126
- debbieandrews@southtorfreyfarm.com
- www.southtorfreyfarm.com

Penquite Farm
Five star self-catering
- 0172 6833 319
- ruth@penquitefarm.co.uk
- www.penquitefarm.co.uk

GOLBERDON, NEAR CALLINGTON, Cornwall
Berrio Mill
Four star self-catering
- 01579 363252
- enquiries@berriomill.co.uk
- www.berriomill.co.uk

GUNNISLAKE, Cornwall
Todsworthy Farm Holidays
Four star self-catering
- 01822 834744
- jon@todsworthyfarmholidays.co.uk
- www.todsworthyfarmholidays.co.uk

HARLYN BAY, Cornwall
Yellow Sands Cottages
Three and Four star self-catering
- 01637 881548
- yellowsands@btinternet.com
- www.yellowsands.co.uk

HAYLE, Cornwall
Rowan Barn
Four star farmhouse
- 0173 685 1223
- info@rowanbarn.co.uk
- www.rowanbarn.co.uk

HOLCOMBE ROGUS, Devon
Whipcott Water Cottages
Four star self-catering
- 01823 672339
- bookings@oldlimekiln.freeserve.co.uk

HONITON, Devon
Stonehayes Farm Cottages
Four and Five star cottages
- 0129 7443 550
- lymebaycottages@btconnect.com
- www.stonehayesfarm.co.uk

ILFRACOMBE, Devon
Mullacott Farm
Four star guest accommodation
- 0127 1866 877
- relax@mullacottfarm.co.uk
- www.mullacottfarm.co.uk

DEVON & CORNWALL

Wildercombe House
Five star bed & breakfast
- 01271 865765
- askus@wildercombehouse.com
- www.wildercombehouse.com

KILKHAMPTON, Cornwall
Forda Lodges & Cottages
Four and Five star self-catering
- 0128 832 1413
- info@forda.co.uk
- www.forda.co.uk

LANREATH, LOOE, Cornwall
Bocaddon Holiday Cottages
Four star self-catering
- 0150 3220 192
- holidays@bocaddon.com
- www.bocaddon.com

LIZARD, Cornwall
YHA Lizard Point
Four star hostel
- 0162 9592 686
- margaretgibson@yha.org.uk
- www.yha.org.uk

LOOE, Cornwall
Lesquite
Bed & breakfast and self-catering apartments
- 01503 220315
- stay@lesquite.co.uk
- www.lesquite.co.uk

MORETONHAMPSTEAD, Devon
Budleigh Farm
Three star self-catering
- 01647 440235
- judith@budleighfarm.co.uk
- www.budleighfarm.co.uk

MORVAL, Cornwall
Tudor Lodges
Four star self-catering
- 01503 241290
- mollytudor@aol.com

MOUNT HAWKE, Cornwall
Ropers Walk Barns
Four star self-catering
- 01209 891632
- peterandliz@roperswalkbarns.co.uk
- www.roperswalkbarns.co.uk

MYLOR, Cornwall
Mylor Yacht Harbour – Admiralty Apartments
Four star self-catering
- 0132 637 2121
- culum@mylor.com
- www.mylorharbourside.com

NEWQUAY, Cornwall
The Park
Four and Five star self-catering
- 0163 7860 322
- info@mawganporth.co.uk
- www.mawganporth.co.uk

NORTHLEIGH, Devon
Smallicombe Farm
Four star guest accommodation and self-catering
- 01404 831310
- maggie_todd@yahoo.com
- www.smallicombe.com

OKEHAMPTON, Devon
Beer Farm
Four star self-catering
- 01837 840265
- info@beerfarm.co.uk
- www.beerfarmcottages.com

HOLIDAYS IN THE BRITISH ISLES

ENGLAND

PENZANCE, Cornwall
Hotel Penzance
Four star townhouse
- 01736 363117
- enquiries@hotelpenzance.com
- www.hotelpenzance.com

PILLATON, Cornwall
Kernock Cottages
Five star self-catering
- 0129 7324 63
- jenny.trice@premiercottages.co.uk
- www.kernockcottages.com

POLZEATH, Cornwall
Manna Place
Four star self-catering
- 01208 863258
- anniepolzeath@hotmail.com
- www.mannaplace.co.uk

PORTHTOWAN, Cornwall
Rose Hill Lodges
Five star self-catering
- 0129 7324 63
- jenny.trice@premiercottages.co.uk
- www.rosehilllodges.com

PORTREATH, Cornwall
Gwel an Mor Lodges
Self-catering holiday lodges
- 02380 251992
- sandy@landish.co.uk
- www.gwelanmor.com

PORTSCATHO, Cornwall
Pollaughan Cottages
Four and Five star self-catering
- 0129 7324 63
- jenny.trice@premiercottages.co.uk
- www.pollaughan.co.uk

REDMOOR, Cornwall
Chark Country Holidays
Four star self-catering
- 01208 871118
- charkholidays@tiscali.co.uk
- www.charkcountryholidays.co.uk

RUAN HIGH LANES, Cornwall
Trenona Farm Holidays
Four star self-catering
- 0187 250 1339
- pam@trenonafarmholidays.co.uk
- www.trenonafarmholidays.co.uk

SANDFORD, Devon
Ashridge Farm
Four star bed & breakfast
- 01363 774292
- jill@ashridgefarm.co.uk
- www.ashridgefarm.co.uk

SIDMOUTH, Devon
Boswell Farm Cottages
Four star cottages
- 0139 5514 162
- dillon@boswell-farm.co.uk
- www.boswell-farm.co.uk

ST CLETHER, Cornwall
Ta Mill
Three and Four star self-catering
- 01840 261797
- helen@tamill.co.uk
- www.tamill.co.uk

ST ENDELLION, Cornwall
Tolraggott Farm Cottages
Four star self-catering
- 01208 880927
- enquiries@tolraggottfarm.co.uk
- www.rock-wadebridge.co.uk

DEVON & CORNWALL

ST MARTINS, Cornwall
Bucklawren Farm
Four and Five star self-catering
- 01503 240738
- bucklawren@btopenworld.com
- www.bucklawren.com

ST MARY'S, Isles of Scilly
Isles of Scilly Country Guest House
Three star guest house
- 01720 422 440
- scillyguesthouse@hotmail.co.uk
- www.scillyguesthouse.co.uk

The Atlantic
Three star hotel
- 0845 2411 133
- neil.roberts@staustellbrewery.co.uk
- atlantichotelscilly.co.uk

ST VEEP, Cornwall
A Little Bit Of Heaven
Four star self-catering
- 01208 873295
- daphne@alittlebitofheaven.co.uk
- www.alittlebitofheaven.co.uk

STRATTON, BUDE, Cornwall
Oak Lodge Bed and Breakfast
Four star bed & breakfast
- 0128 8354 144
- julie@oaklodgebude.com
- www.oaklodgebude.com

TORQUAY, Devon
Atlantis Holiday Apartments
Four star self-catering
- 01803 607929
- enquiry@atlantistorquay.co.uk
- www.atlantistorquay.co.uk

Crown Lodge
Four star guest accommodation
- 01803 298772
- stay@crownlodgehotel.co.uk
- www.crownlodgehotel.co.uk

WHITNAGE, Devon
West Pitt Farm
Three, Four and Five star self-catering
- 01884 820296
- susannewestgate@yahoo.com
- www.westpittfarm.co.uk

WIDECOMBE-IN-THE-MOOR, Devon
Wooder Manor Holiday Homes
Three and Four star self-catering
- 0136 4621 391
- www.woodermanor.com

OTHER ACCOMMODATION

BEAWORTHY, Devon
Blagdon Farm Country Holidays
Ashwater, Beaworthy EX21 5DF
- 01409 211509

Self-catering cottages in the countryside, designed to be useable by disabled people.

BODMIN, Devon
Penrose Burden Cottages
St Breward, near Bodmin PL30 4LZ
- 01208 850277
- enquiries@penroseburden.com
- www.penroseburden.co.uk

Cottages designed for disabled people.

ENGLAND

NATIONAL MARITIME MUSEUM CORNWALL

The museum to have fun in!

Celebrating the sea, boats and Cornwall, this multi award winning Museum not only has 15 galleries, over five floors beautifully illustrating the past, present and future of this island nation but also offers a number of stunning exhibitions.

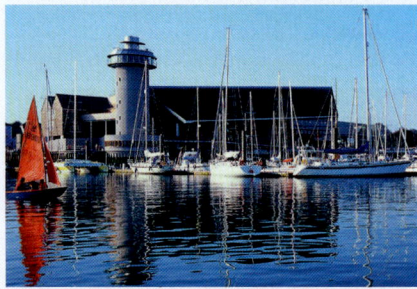

New exhibition

The new blockbuster Search & Rescue exhibition invites you to enter the world of the maritime rescue services where ordinary people lead extraordinary lives, risking their lives to save yours. Experience the drama of a rescue, climb aboard a Sea King helicopter, meet the crews, explore a lifeboat, hit the 'beach' on a quad bike, revisit rescues from the past and discover what it takes to bring you home safely when the worst happens at sea and around our coast.

With hands-on activities every school holiday, talks, lectures, workshops, rotating events and exhibitions, there's so much happening, don't miss your chance for a visit. You'll find more than you might expect.

Opening times

Open daily 10am-5pm, 7 days a week.
Closed Christmas Day & Boxing Day
- T 01326 313388
- F 01326 317878
- E enquiries@nmmc.co.uk

Prices

Adults £11.00
Children (0-5) free, (6-15) £7.60
Senior (60+) £9.00
Family (two adults and up to three children) £31.00.
Groups discounts are available for groups of 10 or more.

Pay once and get in FREE for a full 12 months!

www.nmmc.co.uk

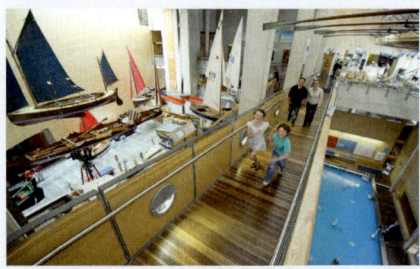
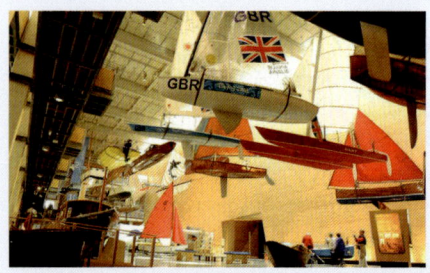

EXMOUTH, Devon
Holiday Homes Trust Caravans
- 020 8433 7290
- scout.holiday.homes@scouts.org.uk
- www.holidayhomestrust.org

Adjacent adapted units in Exmouth, Devon.

IVYBRIDGE, Devon
Hannah's at Ivybridge
Woodland Road, Ivybridge PL21 9HQ
- 01752 892461
- enquiries@discoverhannahs.org

Bungalows designed for wheelchair users.

PAIGNTON, Devon
Holiday Homes Trust Caravan
Hoburne Torbay, Grange Road, Goodrington, Paignton TQ4 7JP
- 020 8433 7290
- scout.holiday.homes@scouts.org.uk
- www.holidayhomestrust.org

Adapted units with views over Torbay.

ST AUSTELL, Cornwall
Holiday Homes Trust Caravans
Pentewan Sands Holiday Park, St Austell PL26 6BT
- 020 8433 7290
- scout.holiday.homes@scouts.org.uk
- www.holidayhomestrust.org

Adjacent adapted units on coastal site.

TEIGNMOUTH, Devon
Cliffden
Dawlish Road, Teignmouth TQ14 8TE
- 01626 770052
- cliffden@visionhotels.co.uk
- www.visionhotels.co.uk

Hotel in large grounds near seafront and town centre for visually impaired people and their companions.

WOOLACOMBE, Devon
Lions Bungalow
Golden Coast Holiday Village, Woolacombe
- 01271 883677

Apply: Mr Taylor, Ilfracombe & District Lions Club, Danesbury, King Street, Combe Martin EX34 0AD

Purpose-built bungalow for wheelchair users and their families.

ENGLAND

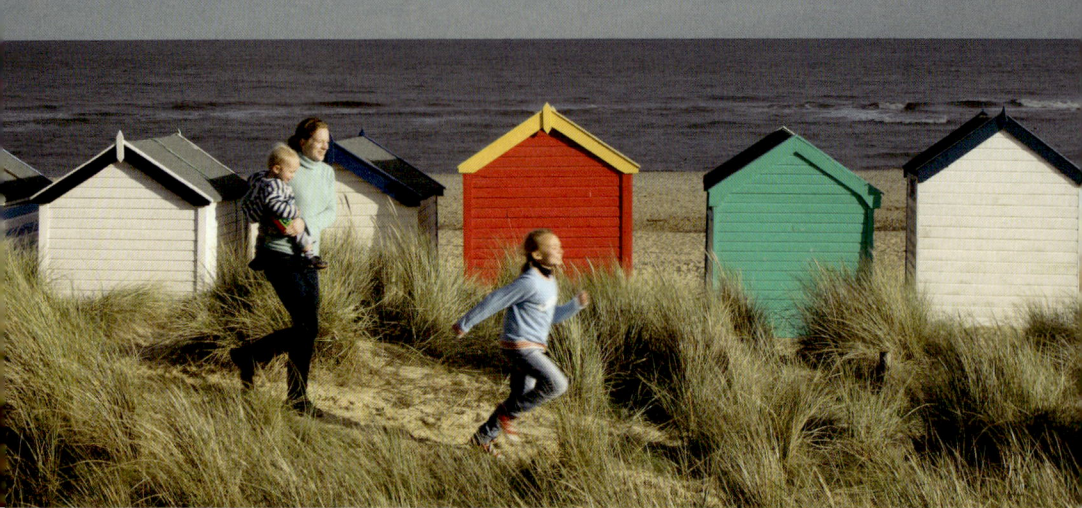

About Eastern England

The East of England region includes Bedfordshire, Cambridgeshire, Essex, Hertfordshire, Norfolk and Suffolk. It stretches from the fringes of London and the Thames Estuary to the Wash and encompasses historic towns, varied countryside and a long coastline.

A string of coastal resorts, most with level promenades, cater for every taste of seaside holiday. Great Yarmouth, Clacton and Southend have a long tradition of providing a range of lively entertainment for their visitors, whether staying in the area or on day trips. Quieter resorts include Hunstanton and Sheringham on the north Norfolk coast, Lowestoft and the old port of Southwold in Suffolk and Frinton in Essex. Harwich and Felixstowe are still important commercial ports as well as resorts.

The region is rich in historic houses and other buildings, including Colchester Castle in England's oldest town, Tilbury Fort, run by English Heritage where

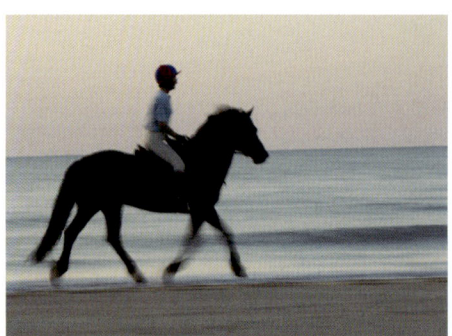

Elizabeth I rallied her troops before the Spanish Armada, Melford Hall in Suffolk and Hatfield House in Hertfordshire. Ancient cathedrals and churches can be visited in Ely, Norwich, Peterborough, Bury St Edmunds and St Albans.

In Cambridge, visitors can join the regular walking tours to see the Colleges and other historic buildings. Norwich, which was once the second largest town in England has the largest collection of medieval buildings and street patterns in the country. Other notable towns in the area include Bedford, Huntingdon, Kings Lynn, Saffron Walden, Sudbury and Woodbridge. The countryside between Ipswich and Colchester was immortalised by painter John Constable.

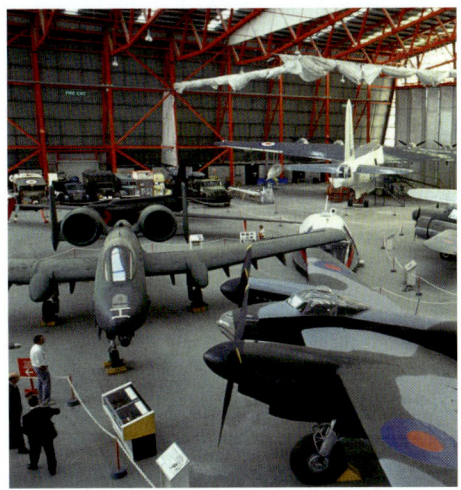

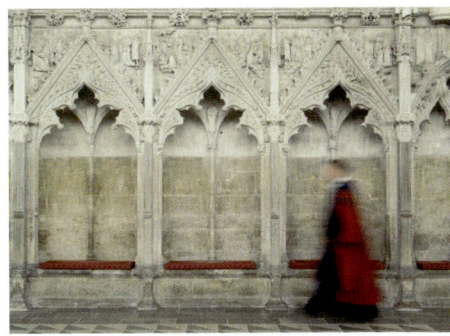

The Norfolk Broads just inland from the coast on the Norfolk/Suffolk border are now a National Park and offer many opportunities for boating, bird watching and enjoying the unique scenery. Other sites of interest to country lovers include the Wildfowl & Wetlands Trust site at Welney near Peterborough, Ferry Meadows Country Park, the National Trust's Wicken Fen near Ely and Needham Lake in Suffolk. Country Parks with facilities for disabled visitors include Sandringham in West Norfolk and Aldenham at Elstree, Hertfordshire.

More formal gardens in the area include the Swiss Garden at Biggleswade in central Bedfordshire, the extensive Gardens of the Rose at St Albans and the University Botanic Garden at Cambridge. Near King's Lynn, Norfolk Lavender is a commercial lavender farm holding the national collection of the plant. Other outdoor attractions include the Museum of East Anglian Life at Stowmarket, Woburn Park in Bedfordshire and the Raptor Foundation near Huntingdon. The North Norfolk Railway, running between Sheringham and Holt has a restored coach equipped for wheelchair users. For an up-to-the-minute shopping experience the region has the Lakeside Shopping Centre at Thurrock.

ENGLAND

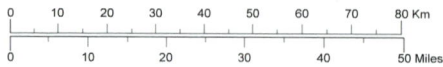

EASTERN ENGLAND

Resources

Tourism

East of England Tourist Board
Visit East Anglia Limited, The Grove, Kenninghall Road, Banham, Norfolk NR16 2HE
- 0333 320 4202
- www.visiteastofengland.com

Official Tourist Board for the east England region.

Information & advice

Disability Essex
Centre for Disability Studies, 34 Rocheway, Rochford, Essex SS4 1DQ
- 0844 412 1770 and 0844 412 1771
- info@disabilityessex.org
- www.disabilityessex.org

Provide holiday information to disabled people in Essex as well as general information on disability.

DIAL
Offer free, impartial and confidential information and advice by telephone to disabled people, their relatives and professionals. Local branches of DIAL change at regular intervals, however, at the time of writing, the following groups were members of DIAL UK and may be able to help visitors in their areas. Please call before travelling to check whether the service and organisation is still available:

DIAL Basildon and South Essex
- 01268 294 400 and 01268 294 401

DIAL Lowestoft and Waveney
- 01502 511 333
   Textphone 01502 405453

DIAL Peterborough
- 01733 265551

DIAL Southend
- 01702 356 033

Disability Advice Service East Suffolk
- 01394 387 070

Disability Cambridgeshire
- 01480 839 192

Disability Information Service Huntingdonshire
- 01480 830 833

The Disability Resource Centre Dunstable
- 01582 470 900
   Textphone 01582 470 968

Hertfordshire Action on Disability
- 01707 324581

Ipswich Disabled Advice Bureau
- 01473 217 313

Norfolk Coalition of Disabled People
- 01508 491210
   Textphone 01508 491 570

POhWER (East of England)
- 0300 456 2370

THINGS TO SEE OR DO

Ferry Meadows Country Park
Country Park at the heart of Nene Park, west of Peterborough. Most paths within the central area are hard surfaced, relatively flat and suitable for push chairs and wheelchairs. All buildings and toilets, including the bird watching hides overlooking the Nature Reserve, are accessible to wheelchair users. Guide dogs and assistance dogs are welcome.
- www.neneparktrust.org.uk

ENGLAND

Visiting Norfolk?

The majority of our buses are now low-floor
Please check with local bus operators for full details

Also coming soon in 2013, RNIB React "talking bus stops" in Norwich City Centre

More details available from:
www.norfolk.gov.uk/travel_and_transport
www.traveline.info

Norfolk County Council at your service

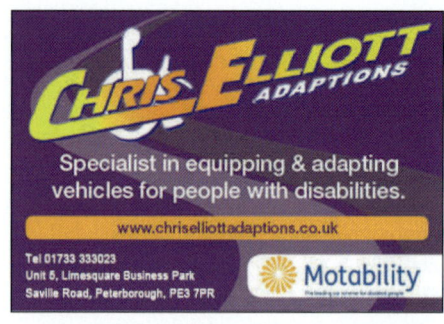

Year round access at Harrold Odell Country Park

Open every day of the year, the park is a haven for wildlife. There is a river, two lakes, meadow and woodland. The 2.5km surfaced route around the large lake is good for wheelchair users. The visitor centre and toilets are wheelchair accessible, the car park has designated spaces for elderly and disabled.

Harrold Odell Country Park is situated between Harrold and Odell villages to the north west of Bedford. Follow the signs from the A6 at Sharnbrook.

T: 01234 720016 W: www.hocp.co.uk

BEDFORD BOROUGH COUNCIL

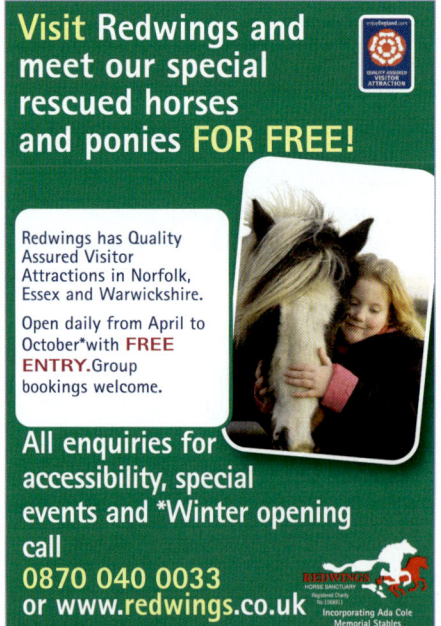

Visit Redwings and meet our special rescued horses and ponies **FOR FREE!**

Redwings has Quality Assured Visitor Attractions in Norfolk, Essex and Warwickshire.

Open daily from April to October*with **FREE ENTRY.** Group bookings welcome.

All enquiries for accessibility, special events and *Winter opening call
0870 040 0033
or **www.redwings.co.uk**

ANGLIA SQUARE
SHOPPING CENTRE

is pleased to support
Disability Rights UK

A GREAT VARIETY OF STORES AND SAFE PARKING

Anglia Square,
Norwich NR3 1DZ

206   HOLIDAYS IN THE BRITISH ISLES

Optua Advice and Advocacy Service
Stowmarket
☎ 01449 672781

West Norfolk DIS
☎ 01553 782558

Equipment hire

SHOPMOBILITY
The National Federation of Shopmobility UK (NFSUK), PO Box 6641, Christchurch BH23 9DQ
☎ 0844 4141 850
✉ Info@shopmobilityuk.org
🌐 www.shopmobilityuk.org
Scheme which lends manual wheelchairs, powered wheelchairs and powered scooters to members of the public with limited mobility to shop and to visit leisure and commercial facilities within the town, city or shopping centre. You can find the nearest Shopmobility scheme to you through their on-line directory. Contact specific Shopmobility Schemes to make equipment bookings or find out more information.

The Disability Resource Centre
Poynters House, Poynters Road, Dunstable LU5 4TP
☎ 01582 470970
✉ equipment@drcbeds.org.uk
    information@drcbeds.org.uk
🌐 www.drcbeds.org.uk
This service allows you to try before you buy. They offer free impartial advice on daily living aids to people of any age with any disability. Drop-in service on Wednesdays – no appointment necessary. They also have wheelchairs for hire and a range of small equipment for sale.

The HAND Partnership
Horning Road, West, Hoveton, Norwich NR12 8QJ
☎ 01603 784 777
🌐 www.thpmobility.org.uk
Wheelchairs and scooters are available to hire for people living in or on holiday in Norfolk. They also carry out scooter repairs.

Hertfordshire Action on Disability
The Woodside Centre, The Commons, Welwyn Garden City AL7 4DD
☎ 01707 384260 (equipment hire)
   01707 375159 (transport)
✉ info@hadnet.org.uk
🌐 www.hadnet.org.uk
Operate a wheelchair hire scheme and an accessible transport service.

Maple Mobility DGT Services
Unit 7, Buckingham Court, Dairy Road, Dukes Park Industrial Estate, Chelmsford CM2 6XW
☎ 01245 451514
🌐 www.maplemobility.co.uk
Manual/powered wheelchairs and scooters are available at weekly rates. Delivery and collection in the Chelmsford area.

Publications

Bedford and District Access Group
☎ 01234 718 565 (for the access officer)
🌐 www.bedford.gov.uk
A range of leaflets giving information on accommodation, places to eat and transport. Produced by the Borough Council in association with Bedford Access Group. Available free from Bedford Tourist Information Centre, Town Hall, St Paul's Square, Bedford MK40 1SJ.
☎ 01234 718 112

ENGLAND

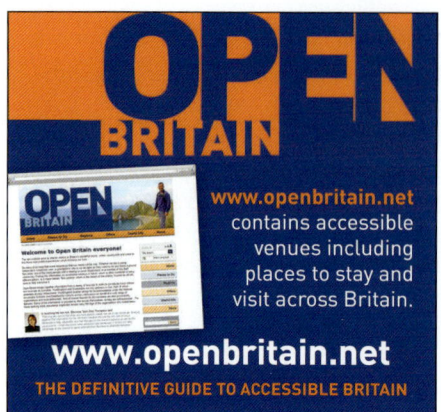

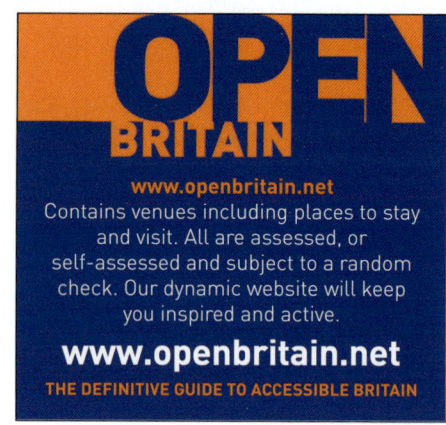

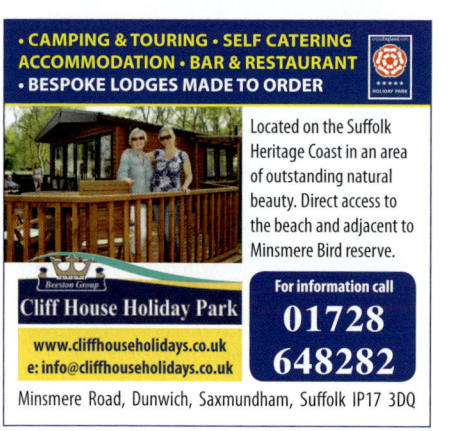

Julian Ellis

Chartered Accountants

Specialising in Small Business Accountancy,

Taxation Services

Paye & VAT Services

15a Bull Plain, Hertford SG14 1DX
Telephone/Fax:
01992 550424

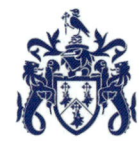

King's Lynn & West Norfolk Council

are pleased to support
Disability Rights UK

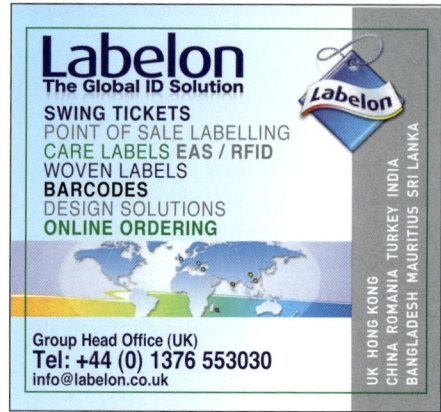

EASTERN ENGLAND

Accessible Holiday Accommodation in East England (Norfolk, Suffolk and Lincolnshire)
Online information sheet about accessible accommodation in Norfolk, Suffolk and Lincolnshire compiled by Disabled Holiday Information (July 2009).
- W www.disabledholidayinformation.org.uk /documents/EastEnglandAccessible Accommodation.pdf

Accommodation

NAS ASSESSED ACCOMMODATION

ALDEBURGH, Suffolk
The Brudenell Hotel
Four star hotel
- T 01728 452071
- E generalmanager@brudenellhotel.co.uk
- W www.brudenellhotel.co.uk

ASHDON, Essex
Hill Farm Holiday Cottages
Three star self-catering
- T 01799 584 881
- E hillfarm-holiday-cottages@hotmail.co.uk
- W www.hillfarmcottages.net

THINGS TO SEE OR DO
Central Beach
Sandy beach in Great Yarmouth between Britannia and Wellington Piers next to Marine Parade. Ramps to the beach are available at several locations. Adapted beach wheelchairs are available for hire free of charge at the Tourist Information Centre located on Marine Parade.
- W www.great-yarmouth.co.uk

AYLMERTON, Norfolk
Roman Camp Inn
Four star inn
- T 01263 838291
- E enquiries@romancampinn.co.uk
- W www.romancampinn.co.uk

BACTON, Norfolk
Primrose Cottage
Three star self-catering
- T 01692 650667
- E holiday@cablegap.co.uk
- W www.ukparks.co.uk/cablegap

Castaways Holiday Park
Three star holiday park
- T 01692 650 436 / 650418
- E castaways.bacton@hotmail.co.uk
- W www.castawaysholidaypark.co.uk

BECCLES, Suffolk
The Lodge
Four star self-catering
- T 0150 2716 428
- E karenrenilson@hotmail.com
- W www.catherinehouse.net

BEESTON, Norfolk
Holmdene Farm
Three star self-catering
- T 01328 701 284
- E holmdenefarm@farmersweekly.net
- W www.northnorfolk.co.uk/holmdenefarm

BLAXHALL, Suffolk
YHA Blaxhall
Three star hostel
- T 0162 9592 686
- E margaretgibson@yha.org.uk
- W www.yha.org.uk

ENGLAND

BOXFORD, Suffolk
Sherbourne Lodge Cottages
Four star self-catering
- 01787 210885
- enquiries@sherbournelodgecottages.co.uk
- www.sherbournelodgecottages.co.uk

BURGH NEXT AYLSHAM, Norfolk
North Farm Cottages
Four star cottages
- 0160 3737 974
- info@northfarm.info
- www.northfarm.info

BURGH ST PETER, Norfolk
Waveney River Centre
Five star holiday park
- 01502 677343
- ruth@waveneyrivercentre.co.uk
- www.waveneyrivercentre.co.uk

CARLTON COLVILLE, Suffolk
Ivy House Country Hotel
Hotel
- 01502 501353
- admin@ivyhousecountryhotel.co.uk
- www.ivyhousecountryhotel.co.uk

CASTLE HEDINGHAM, Essex
The Lodge at Hedingham Castle
Three star cottages
- 01787 460261
- sarah@hedinghamcastle.co.uk
- www.hedinghamcastle.co.uk

CHELMSFORD, Essex
Boswell House Hotel
Two star small hotel
- 0124 528 7587
- boswell118@aol.com
- www.boswellhousehotel.co.uk

CRATFIELD, Suffolk
School Farm Cottages
Four star self-catering
- 01986 798844
- schoolfarmcotts@aol.com
- www.schoolfarmcottages.com

EAST HARLING, Norfolk
Berwick Cottage
Four star self-catering
- 01787 372343
- info@thelinberwicktrust.org.uk
- www.thelinberwicktrust.org.uk

EAST RUNTON, Norfolk
Incleborough House Luxury Self Catering
Five star self-catering
- 0126 3515 939
- enquiries@incleboroughhouse.co.uk
- www.incleboroughhouse.co.uk

EDGEFIELD, Norfolk
Wood Farm Cottages Ltd
Four star self-catering
- 01263 587347
- info@wood-farm.com
- www.wood-farm.com

ELM, Cambridgeshire
The Elm Tree Inn
Four star inn
- 0194 5587 009
- theelmtreeinn@mail.com
- www.elmtree-inn.com

ELY, Cambridgeshire
Little Downham Anchor
Three star hotel
- 01353 699333
- ld.anchor@aol.com
- under construction

EASTERN ENGLAND

FOXLEY WOOD, Norfolk
Moor Farm Stable Cottages
Three and Four star self-catering
- 0136 2688 523
- mail@moorfarmstablecottages.co.uk
- www.moorfarmstablecottages.co.uk

FRITTON, Norfolk
Decoy Barn
Four star guesthouse
- 01493 488222
- karenwilder9@aol.com
- www.decoybarn.co.uk

GREAT BARTON, Suffolk
Wylene
Four star self-catering
- 0135 9271 130
- chriswhitton@aol.com
- wyleneholidayhome.co.uk

GREAT FINBOROUGH, Suffolk
Jack Bridge Cottage @ Jack Bridge Farm
Four star self-catering
- 01449 672177
- pembertons@jackbridgefarm.plus.com
- www.farmstayanglia.co.uk/jackbridge

GREAT SNORING, Norfolk
Vine Park Cottage
Four star farmhouse
- 01328 821016
- rita@vineparkcottagebandb.co.uk
- www.vineparkcottagebandb.co.uk

HAPPISBURGH, Norfolk
Boundary Stables
Four star self-catering
- 01692 650 171
- bookings@boundarystables.co.uk
- boundarystables.co.uk

HAUGHLEY, Suffolk
Red House Farm
Three and Four star self-catering
- 01449 673323
- John@redhousefarmhaughley.co.uk
- www.redhousefarmhaughley.co.uk

HENLEY, Suffolk
Damerons Farm Holidays
Four star self-catering
- 01473 832454
- info@dameronsfarmholidays.co.uk
- www.dameronsfarmholidays.co.uk

HITCHAM, Suffolk
The White Horse Inn
Four star inn
- 0144 9740 981
- lewis@thewhitehorse.wanadoo.co.uk
- www.thewhitehorsehitcham.co.uk

HORNING, Norfolk
Norfolk River Cottages
Four star cottages
- 01692 631581
- carol@norfolkrivercottages.co.uk
- www.norfolkrivercottages.co.uk

Heron Cottage
Five star cottage
- 0778 8 853332
- info@heron-cottage.com
- www.heron-cottage.com

King Line Cottages
Three and Four star self-catering
- 01692 630297
- info@norfolk-broads.co.uk
- www.norfolk-broads.co.uk

HOLIDAYS IN THE BRITISH ISLES

ENGLAND

HUNSTANTON, Norfolk
Foxgloves Cottage
Four star self-catering
- 01485 532 460
- deepdenehouse@btopenworld.com
- www.foxglovescottage.co.uk

Caley Hall Hotel
Three star hotel
- 01485 533486
- mail@caleyhallhotel.co.uk
- www.caleyhallhotel.co.uk

KELLING, Norfolk
The Pheasant Hotel
Two star hotel
- 01263 712201
- enquiries@pheasanthotelnorfolk.co.uk
- www.pheasanthotelnorfolk.co.uk

LITTLE DOWNHAM, Cambridgeshire
Wood Fen Lodge
Four star guesthouse
- 01353 862495
- info@woodfenlodge.co.uk
- www.woodfenlodge.co.uk

LITTLE SNORING, Norfolk
Jex Farm Barn and Stable
Four star self-catering
- 0132 887 8257
- farmerstephen@jexfarm.wanadoo.co.uk
- www.jexfarm.co.uk

MAUTBY, Norfolk
Lower Wood Farm Country Cottages
Four and Five star self-catering
- 0129 7324 63
- jenny.trice@premiercottages.co.uk
- www.lowerwoodfarm.co.uk

METHWOLD, Norfolk
Next Door at Magdalen House
Four star self-catering
- 0136 6727 255
- k.cootes@btconnect.com
- www.magdalenhouse.co.uk

MICKFIELD, Suffolk
Read Hall Cottage
Five star self-catering
- 0144 9711 366
- andy@readhall.co.uk
- www.readhall.co.uk

MIDDLEWOOD GREEN, Suffolk
Leys Farmhouse Annexe
Three star self-catering
- 01449 711 750
- hevtrev@btopenworld.com
- www.leysfarmhouseannexe.co.uk

NAYLAND, Suffolk
Gladwins Farm
Four and Five star self-catering
- 0120 6262 261
- contact@gladwinsfarm.co.uk
- www.gladwinsfarm.co.uk

NORWICH, Norfolk
Prince's Barn
Four star holiday cottages
- 01692 630276
- fbaugh@netcom.co.uk

Spixworth Hall Cottages
Four star self-catering
- 01603 898190
- hallcottages@btinternet.com
- www.hallcottages.co.uk

EASTERN ENGLAND

PAKEFIELD, Suffolk
Pakefield Caravan Park
Four star holiday park
- 01502 561136
- shelley@normanhurst.net
- www.pakefieldpark.co.uk

PULHAM MARKET, Norfolk
The Old Bakery
Five star bed & breakfast
- 01379 676492
- info@theoldbakery.net
- www.theoldbakery.net

REYDON, SOUTHWOLD, Suffolk
Newlands Country House
Four star guest accommodation
- 0150 272 2164
- info@newlandsofsouthwold.co.uk
- www.newlandsofsouthwold.co.uk

SAINT OSYTH, Essex
Lee Wick Farm Holiday Cottages
Four star self-catering
- 01255 823 031
- info@leewickfarm.co.uk
- www.leewickfarm.co.uk

SANDRINGHAM, Norfolk
Park House Hotel
Three star hotel
- 0148 554 3000
- tess.gilder@lcdisability.org
- www.parkhousehotel.org.uk

SANDY, Bedfordshire
Fullers Hill Cottages
Four star cottages
- 01767 651163
- bookings@fullershillcottages.co.uk
- www.fullershillcottages.co.uk

SHERINGHAM, Norfolk
YHA Sheringham
Three star hostel
- 0162 9592 686
- margaretgibson@yha.org.uk
- www.yha.org.uk

Sheringham Cottages
Four star self-catering
- 01263 577560
- trevor.claydon@which.net
- www.sheringhamcottages.com

SHOTLEY, Suffolk
Orwell View Barns
Five star self-catering
- 0147 3788 497
- info@orwellviewbarns.co.uk
- www.orwellviewbarns.co.uk

SIBTON, Suffolk
Park Farm Sibton
Four star self-catering
- 0172 8668 324
- annelawrence28@btinternet.com
- www.sibtonparkfarm.co.uk

SISLAND, Norfolk
Owl Barn at Sisland Tithe Barn
Four star self-catering
- 0150 8520 520
- info@sisland-tithe-barn.co.uk
- www.sisland-tithe-barn.co.uk

SOUTH WALSHAM, Norfolk
Break-O-Day
Self-catering house
- 0149 3728 707
- angela@atebbutt.plus.com

HOLIDAYS IN THE BRITISH ISLES

SWILLAND, Suffolk
Swilland Mill
Five star self-catering
- 0147 3785 122
- jamie@swillandmill.co.uk
- www.swillandmill.com

THORPE-LE-SOKEN, Essex
Lifehouse Spa & Hotel
Four star hotel
- 0125 5863 464
- imogen.b@lifehouse.co.uk
- www.lifehouse.co.uk

TITCHWELL, Norfolk
Titchwell Manor Hotel
Three star hotel
- 01485 210221
- margaret@titchwellmanor.com
- www.titchwellmanor.com

TRIMINGHAM, Norfolk
Woodland Leisure Park
Four star holiday and touring park
- 0126 3579 208
- carole@woodland-park.co.uk
- www.woodland-park.co.uk

WALTHAM CROSS, Hertfordshire
YHA Lee Valley Village
Four star hostel
- 0162 9592 686
- margaretgibson@yha.org.uk
- www.yha.org.uk

WALTON-ON-THE-NAZE, Essex
Bufo Villae Guest House
Four star guest accommodation
- 01255 672644
- bufovillae@btinternet.com
- www.bufovillae.co.uk

WATTISFIELD, Suffolk
Jayes Holiday Cottages
Three star self-catering
- 01359 251255
- info@jayesholidaycottages.co.uk
- www.jayesholidaycottages.co.uk

WATTISHAM, Suffolk
Wattisham Hall Holiday Cottages
Four star self-catering
- 01449 744288
- michellesquirrell212@btinternet.com
- www.wattishamhall.co.uk

WELLS-NEXT-THE-SEA, Norfolk
YHA Wells-next-the-Sea Youth Hostel
Four star hostel
- 0162 9592 686
- margaretgibson@yha.org.uk
- www.yha.org.uk

WENDLING, NR DEREHAM, Norfolk
Greenbanks
Four star guesthouse
- 01362 687742
- enquiries@greenbankshotel.co.uk
- www.greenbankshotel.co.uk

WEST RUDHAM, Norfolk
Oyster House
Four star bed & breakfast
- 01485 528327
- oyster-house@tiscali.co.uk
- www.oysterhouse.co.uk

WEYBOURNE, Norfolk
Home Farm Holiday Cottages
Four star cottages
- 0126 3588 334
- sally.j.middleton@btinternet.com
- www.weybourne-holiday-cottages.co.uk

EASTERN ENGLAND

WISBECH ST MARY, Cambridgeshire
Common Right Barns
Four star self-catering
- T: 0194 541 0424
- E: teresa@commonrightbarns.co.uk
- W: www.commonrightbarns.co.uk

WISSETT, Suffolk
The Old Stables, Wissett Lodge
Four star self-catering
- T: 01986 873173
- E: mail@wissettlodge.co.uk
- W: www.wissettlodge.co.uk

WORTHAM, Suffolk
Ivy House Farm
Four star self-catering
- T: 0129 7324 63
- E: jenny.trice@premiercottages.co.uk
- W: www.ivyhousefarmcottages.co.uk

OTHER ACCOMMODATION

CHIGWELL, Essex
Vitalise Jubilee Lodge
Grange Farm, High Road, Chigwell IG7 6DP
- T: 0303 303 0145
- E: bookings@vitalise.org.uk
- W: www.vitalise.org.uk

Centre on the edge of Epping Forest for breaks for people with disabilities.

CLACTON-ON-SEA, Essex
Groomshill
8 Holland Road, Clacton-on-Sea
Contact: Livability
- T: 08456 584 478
- E: selfcatering@livability.org.uk
- W: www.livability.org.uk

Holiday bungalow adapted for disabled people near town centre and seafront. Sleeps six.

GREAT YARMOUTH, Norfolk
Holiday Homes Trust Caravan
Seashore Holiday Park, North Denes, Great Yarmouth, Norfolk NR30 4HG
- T: 020 8433 7290
- T: scout.holiday.homes@scouts.org.uk
- T: www.holidayhomestrust.org

Adapted unit in Great Yarmouth, Norfolk.

HOLT, Norfolk
Norfolk Country Cottages
The Old Crab Shop, 1 Cross Street, Holt, Norfolk NR25 6HZ
- T: 01603 715 779
- E: info@norfolkcottages.co.uk
- W: www.norfolkcottages.co.uk

A leading provider of self-catering holiday accommodation in Norfolk. Some of their properties are suitable for disabled people.

THINGS TO SEE OR DO

Nancy Oldfield Trust
Outdoor pursuits centre offering disabled and disadvantaged people a day out on the Norfolk Broads. Activities include sailing, canoeing, nature observation, fishing or a leisurely cruise on Barton Broad. A fully accessible, self-catering bungalow for up to 10 people can be booked.
- W: www.nancyoldfield.org.uk

HOVETON, Norfolk
Broomhill
Station Road, Hoveton, near Wroxham
Contact: Livability
- T: 08456 584478
- E: selfcatering@livability.org.uk
- W: www.livability.org.uk

Self-contained flats by Wroxham Broad, owned by Livability, designed for wheelchair users.

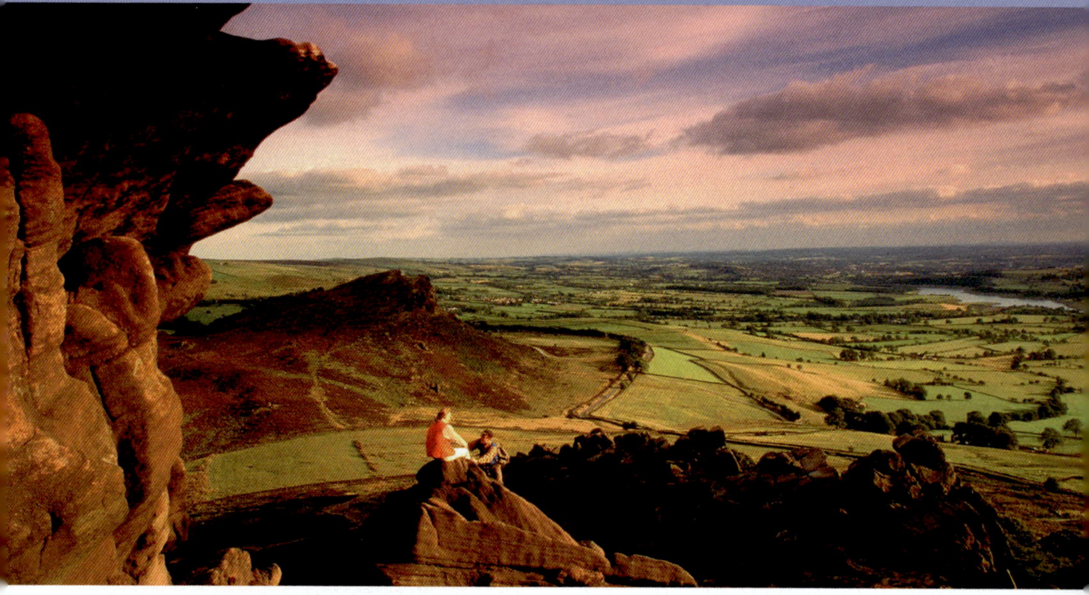

ENGLAND

About the East Midlands

This region, ranging from the wide, flat Fens to the mountainous Peak District, comprises the counties of Derbyshire, Leicestershire, Lincolnshire, Northamptonshire, Nottinghamshire and Rutland.

Around the Lincolnshire coast resorts such as Cleethorpes, Skegness and Mablethorpe provide the opportunity for seaside holidays with a level seafront and much traditional entertainment. Inland there is a choice between staying in historic towns or more rural localities.

Many important historic events took place and myths were formed in the area. You can learn more of Hereward the Wake in the Fens around Crowland or Robin Hood in Nottingham and Sherwood Forest. The Wars of the Roses ended at Bosworth in Leicestershire, where there is a Visitor Centre and Country Park, and the Civil War began at Nottingham Castle, now an art gallery and museum.

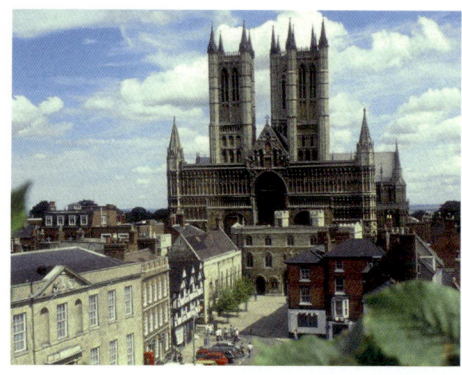

HOLIDAYS IN THE BRITISH ISLES

EAST MIDLANDS

The two largest cities in the region are Leicester and Nottingham. Both provide opportunities to enjoy music, theatre and sporting events and have a variety of attractions depicting the history and industries of the area. Other important towns include Derby, Northampton and Lincoln, with its magnificent Cathedral towering over the surrounding countryside at the top of a steep hill.

Many smaller towns are also worth visiting. At Boston the church tower dominates the surrounding fenland. In nearby Spalding the Springfields Gardens are renowned, as befits a town that is the centre of Britain's major flower growing area. Another town proud of its parks is Buxton where the museum has an exhibition on the surrounding Peak District. The twisted spire on the parish church of Chesterfield is another of the noted landmarks of the region.

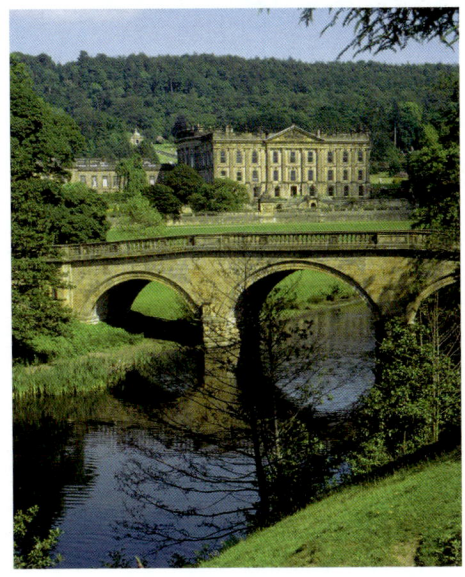

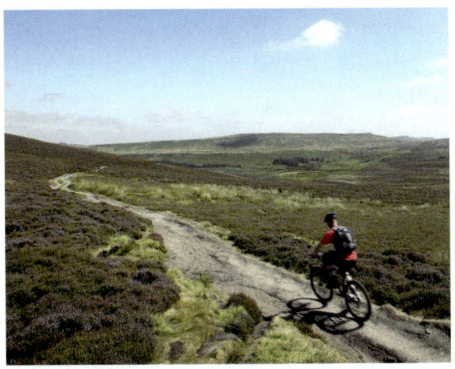

Most of the Peak District National Park is in Derbyshire. Other countryside attractions include accessible trails in Grafton Park and Boughton Park near Kettering, the Saltfleetby National Nature Reserve on the Lincolnshire Coast and the Rufford Country Park in Nottinghamshire. There are opportunities for water sports, birdwatching, fishing and many other activities at Rutland Water. Life on an Edwardian estate can be experienced at Elvaston Country Park near Derby.

The region is home to a number of transport attractions including the Crich Tramways Village in Derbyshire, the Great Central Railway in Nottinghamshire and Leicestershire and the National Space Science Centre at Leicester. Those with literary interests can compare the background of D H Lawrence at the Durban House Heritage Centre at Eastwood with that of Lord Byron at Newstead Abbey only a few miles away in the outskirts of Nottingham.

ENGLAND

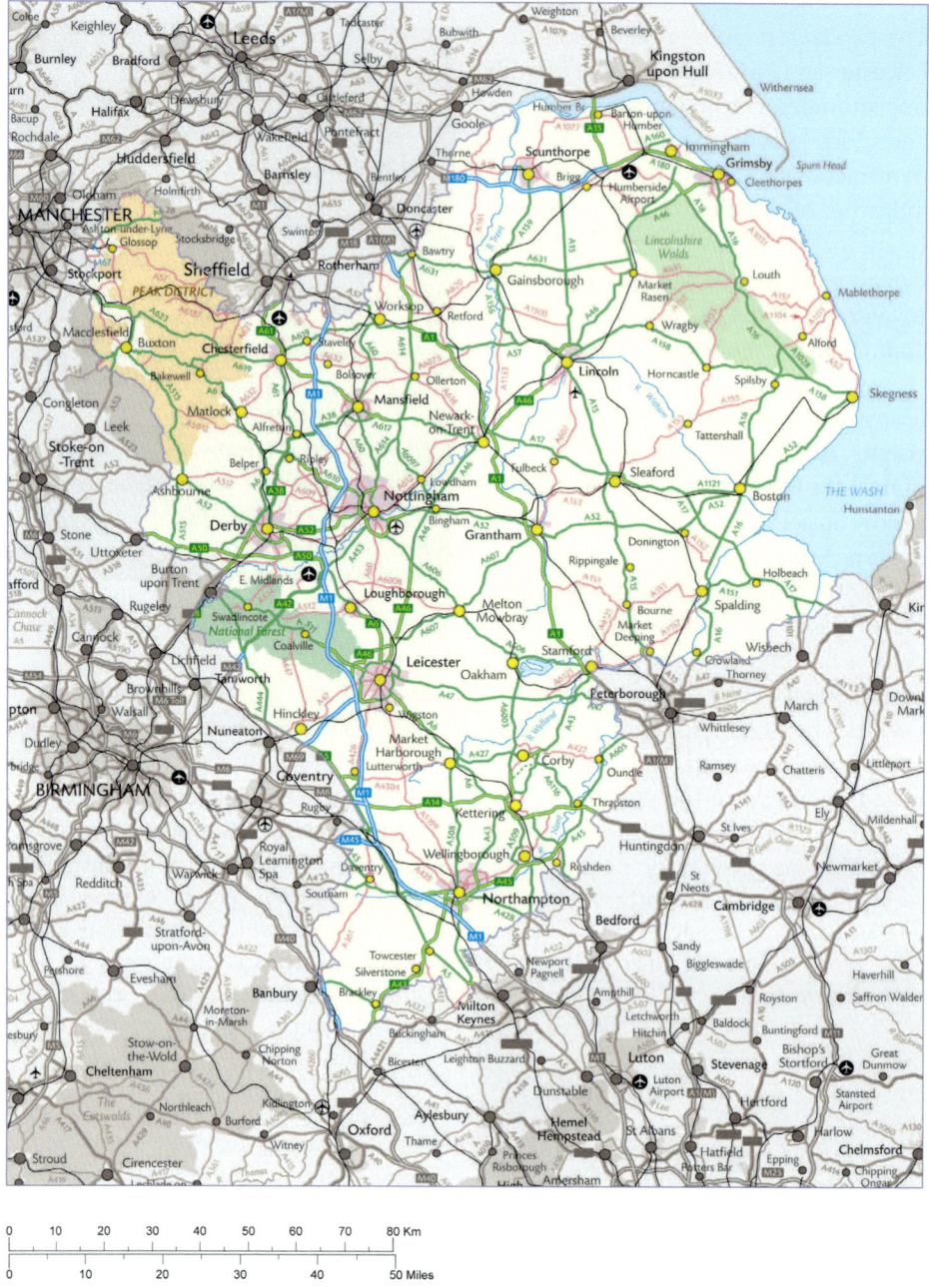

HOLIDAYS IN THE BRITISH ISLES

EAST MIDLANDS

Resources

Tourism

Tourist Information Centres
You can locate details of Tourist Information Centres throughout this region using the destination finder on the VisitEngland website. You will also find destination guides, ideas, events, attractions and accommodation:
- www.visitengland.com/ee/DestinationFinder

Information & advice

Mosaic: shaping disability services
2 Oak Spinney Park, Ratby Lane, Leicester Forest East LE3 3AW
- 0116 2318720
- enquiries@mosaic1898.co.uk
- www.mosaic1898.co.uk

Voluntary organisation providing a range of services to disabled people, their families and carers. They have two accessible self-catering bungalows at Overstrand, North Norfolk. Bookings are always taken on a first come, first served basis. During high season bookings are only taken for one week at a time. At other times you can book for a fortnight.

Disability Lincs Ltd
Ancaster Day Centre, Boundary Street, Lincoln LN5 8NJ
- 01522 870602
- enquiries@disabilitylincs.org.uk
- www.disabilitylincs.org.uk

Enquiries to the administrative officer.

DIAL
Offer free, impartial and confidential information and advice by telephone to disabled people, their relatives and professionals. Local branches of DIAL are constantly changing but at the time of writing, the following groups were members of DIAL UK and may be able to help visitors in their areas. Please call before travelling to check whether the service and organisation is still available:

Brigg Carers' Support Centre
- 01652 650585

DIAL Northants Corby
- 01536 204742

DIAL Northants Daventry
- 01327 701646

Disability Nottinghamshire
- 01623 625891

Leicester CIL
- 0116 222 5005

THINGS TO SEE OR DO

Sherwood Pines White Trail
Near Mansfield, deep within the Sherwood Pine Forest is the White Trail. This takes in some of the oldest trees in the forest and was created with easy access in mind with seating at regular intervals along the way. It covers a distance of approximately one and a half miles. Facilities, which are all wheelchair accessible, include toilets, café, picnic area and, adjacent to the café, a raised board walk play area.
- 01623 822447

HOLIDAYS IN THE BRITISH ISLES

ENGLAND

Access made easy

Loughborough's four star hotel provides you with an enjoyable and relaxing stay

Enjoy England Mobility three award accredited
Ample disabled parking
Accessible bedrooms
Gold standard customer service

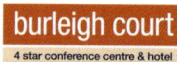
burleigh court
4 star conference centre & hotel

Conferences | Weddings | Accommodation | Spas

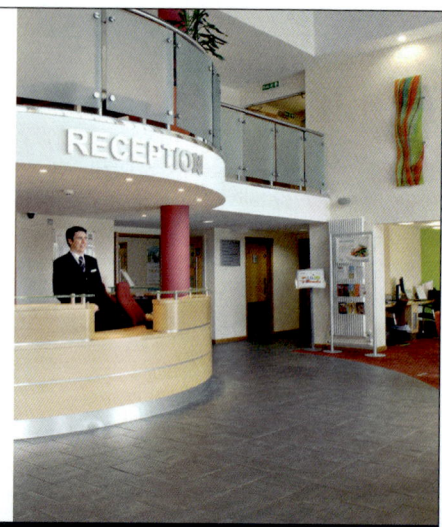

imago @ Loughborough Ltd, Loughborough University, Leicestershire, LE11 3TD
01509 228101 | info@welcometoimago.com | www.welcometoimago.com/weddings

imago your experience, our expertise.

elms farm cottages
stay somewhere special

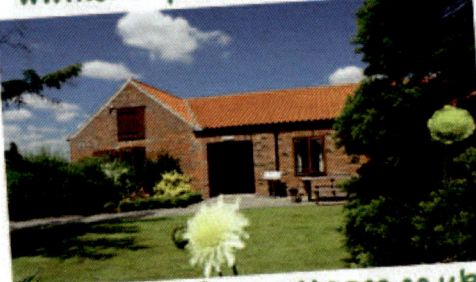

www.elmsfarmcottages.co.uk

Nine award winning holiday cottages, fully equipped and furnished to a high standard, with level access throughout.

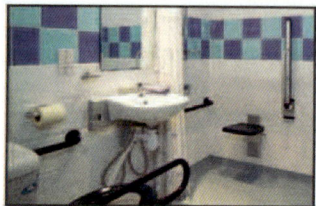

carol@elmsfarmcottages.co.uk

Boston, Lincolnshire
t: 01205 290840 m: 07887 652021

Village pub within 350 metres
2 & 3 bedroomed cottages
Open all year, sleeps 2 - 34

Equipment hire

SHOPMOBILITY
The National Federation of Shopmobility UK (NFSUK), PO Box 6641, Christchurch BH23 9DQ
- 📞 0844 41 41 850
- ✉ info@shopmobilityuk.org
- 🌐 www.shopmobilityuk.org

Scheme which lends manual wheelchairs, powered wheelchairs and powered scooters to members of the public with limited mobility to shop and to visit leisure and commercial facilities within the town, city or shopping centre. You can find the nearest Shopmobility scheme to you through their on-line directory. Contact specific Shopmobility Schemes to make equipment bookings or find out more information.

Scooter Serv
15 Moat Lane, Towcester, Northamptonshire NN12 6AD
- 📞 0845 612 1912
- ✉ service@scooterserv.com
- 🌐 www.scooterserv.com

This company can hire manual and powered wheelchairs and scooters for use on the UK mainland.

Publications

Access for All
- 📞 01629 816200
- ✉ customer.service@peakdistrict.gov.uk

Guides giving information for disabled visitors to the Peak District including car parks, public transport, accessible trails, public toilets and guided walks. Available in print from Peak District National Park, Aldern House, Baslow Road, Bakewell DE45 1AE. The information is also available on:
- 🌐 www.peakdistrict.org

THINGS TO SEE OR DO

Lincolnshire beaches

Sutton-on-Sea has a good car park right beside the sea wall, just a short distance to a long promenade on the sea wall. Ideal for those who find walking difficult, wheelchair users and buggies.

Mablethorpe Beach has toilets with disabled facilities and is reached from the promenade via steps or ramps. Blue Flag Award, Quality Coast Award and Marine Conservation Society recommended.

ENGLAND

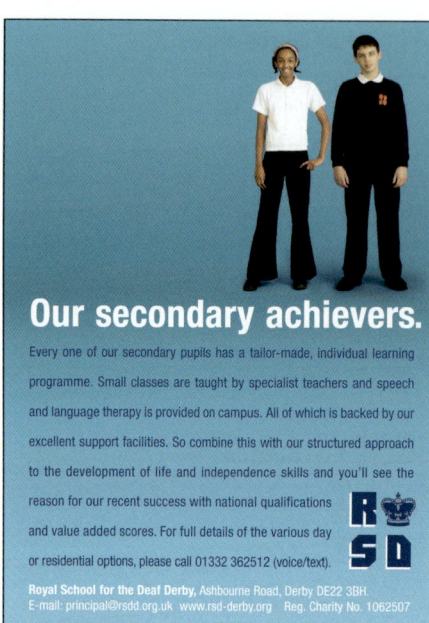

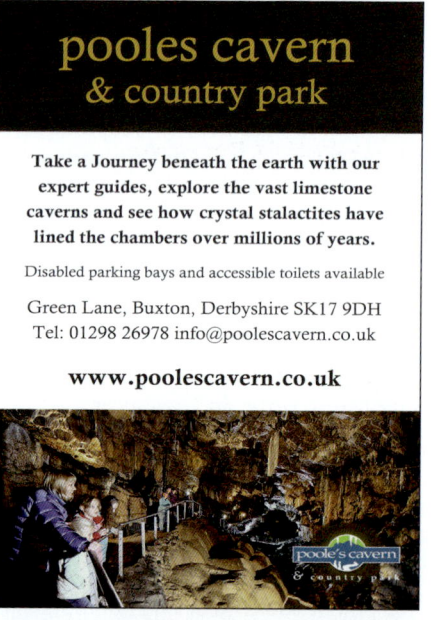

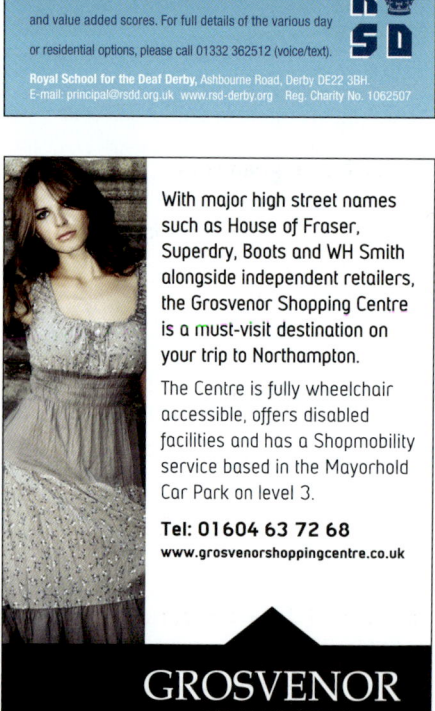

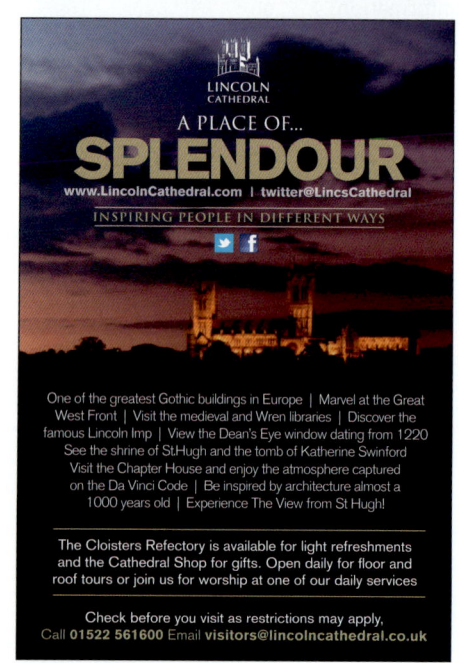

EAST MIDLANDS

Accommodation

NAS ASSESSED ACCOMMODATION

ALDERWASLEY, Derbyshire
Wiggonlea Stable and Fletchers Barn
Four star self-catering
- 01773 852344
- wiggonlea@uwclub.net
- www.wiggonlea.uwclub.net

ALFORD, Lincolnshire
Half Moon Hotel and Restaurant
Three star small hotel
- 0150 7463 477
- halfmoonalford25@aol.com
- www.halfmoonalford.co.uk

ASHBOURNE, Derbyshire
Ravenscliffe Farm Holidays
Four star self-catering
- 07872 315889
- info@ravenscliffefarm.co.uk
- www.ravenscliffefarm.co.uk

Callow Hall Country House Hotel & Restaurant
Four star hotel
- 01629 734474
- idh@eastlodge.com
- www.callowhall.co.uk

ASHBY-CUM-FENBY, Lincolnshire
Hall Farm Hotel & Restaurant
Four star small hotel
- 0147 2220 666
- info@hallfarmhotelandrestaurant.co.uk
- www.hallfarmhotelandrestaurant.co.uk

BAMFORD, Derbyshire
Yorkshire Bridge Inn
Four star self-catering
- 0143 3651 361
- info@yorkshire-bridge.co.uk
- www.yorkshire-bridge.co.uk

Ladybower Apartments
Five star self-catering
- 01433 651361
- enquiries@ladybowerapartments.co.uk
- www.ladybowerapartments.co.uk

BICKER, Lincolnshire
Supreme Inns
Three star hotel
- 0120 5822 804
- sales@supremeinns.co.uk
- www.supremeinns.co.uk

BLYTH, Nottinghamshire
The Courtyard at Hodsock Priory
Five star guest accommodation
- 01909 591204
- lj@hodsockpriory.com
- www.hodsockpriory.com

BLYTON, Lincolnshire
Blyton Ponds
Four star bed & breakfast
- 01427 628240
- blytonponds@msn.com
- www.blytonponds.co.uk

BRASSINGTON, Derbyshire
Hoe Grange Holidays
Four star self-catering
- 0162 9540 262
- info@hoegrangeholidays.co.uk
- www.hoegrangeholidays.co.uk

HOLIDAYS IN THE BRITISH ISLES

ENGLAND

Wishing Disability Rights UK every success

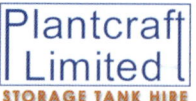

Plantcraft Limited
STORAGE TANK HIRE

Flixborough Industrial Estate
Scunthorpe, North Lincs
DN15 8SJ
Tel: 01724 850224
Fax: 01724 289317

www.plantcraft.co.uk

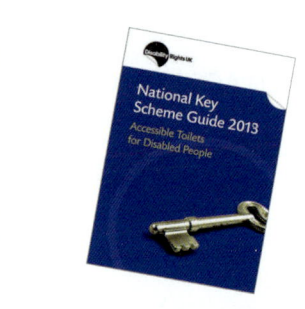

National Key Scheme Guide 2013
Accessible Toilets for Disabled People

Available to order from our online shop
www.disabilityrightsuk.org

THE COTTAGE BY THE POND

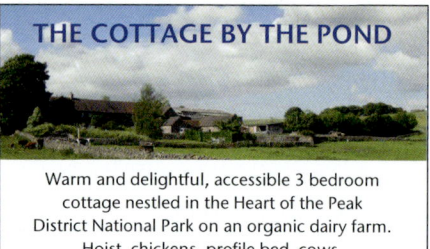

Warm and delightful, accessible 3 bedroom cottage nestled in the Heart of the Peak District National Park on an organic dairy farm. Hoist, chickens, profile bed, cows, wet room, lambs and gorgeous views!

01335 310274
stay@beechenhill.co.uk
www.beechenhill.co.uk

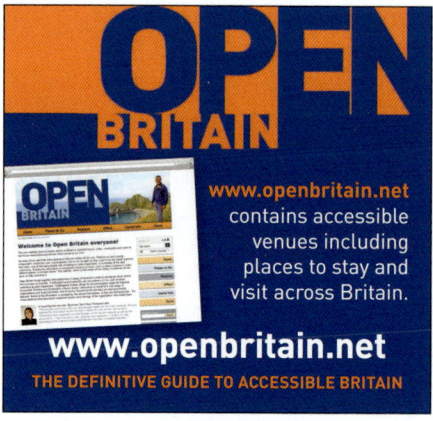

OPEN BRITAIN

www.openbritain.net
contains accessible venues including places to stay and visit across Britain.

www.openbritain.net
THE DEFINITIVE GUIDE TO ACCESSIBLE BRITAIN

Disabled holidays home and away

I am a quadriplegic myself and have adapted this apartment and chalet for myself and others. The chalet is in Mablethorpe, Lincolnshire and is very child/dog/wheelchair friendly.

The apartment is in Rojales, Spain and overlooks a beautiful guitar-shaped pool and is very close to local bars, multi-market and medical centre. The local town is a 15 minute wheel.

Both places have wheel-in shower with chair provided and mobile hoist with electric beds.

Please do not hesitate to contact me for any further details.

www.disabledapartment.com   Mobile: 00447515541300

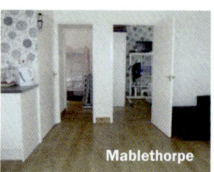
Mablethorpe

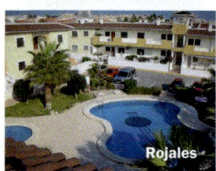
Rojales

HOLIDAYS IN THE BRITISH ISLES

EAST MIDLANDS

BURGH ON BAIN, Lincolnshire
Bainfield Lodge
Four star self-catering
- 0150 7313 540
- dennis.walker1@btinternet.com
- www.bainfieldholidaylodge.co.uk

BUXTON, Derbyshire
Alpine Lodge Guest House
Four star guesthouse
- 0129 8261 55
- jean@jeangreenwaycole.plus.com
- www.alpinelodgebuxton.co.uk

CHURCH BROUGHTON, Derbyshire
Oaklands Country Lodges
Four star self-catering
- 01283 730283
- redfern751@btinternet.com
- www.oaklandscountrylodges.co.uk

CLOPTON, Northamptonshire
Nene Valley Cottages
Five star cottages
- 0129 7324 63
- jenny.trice@premiercottages.co.uk
- www.nenevalleycottages.co.uk

CLUMBER PARK, WORKSOP, Nottinghamshire
Clumber Park Hotel & Spa
Hotel
- 01623 835 333
- jh@clumberparkhotel.com
- www.clumberparkhotel.com

DISEWORTH, Leicestershire
Lady Gate Guest House
Four star guesthouse
- 01332 811565
- enquiries@ladygateguesthouse.co.uk
- www.ladygateguesthouse.co.uk

EARL STERNDALE, Derbyshire
Wheeldon Trees Farm
Four star self-catering
- 0129 7324 63
- jenny.trice@premiercottages.co.uk
- www.wheeldontreesfarm.co.uk

EAST BARKWITH, Lincolnshire
The Grange Holiday Cottages
Four star self-catering
- 01673 858670
- sarahstamp@farmersweekly.net
- www.thegrange-lincolnshire.co.uk

EDWINSTOWE, Nottinghamshire
Forest Lodge Hotel
Hotel
- 0162 3824 443
- audrey@forestlodgehotel.co.uk
- www.forestlodgehotel.co.uk

YHA Sherwood Forest
Four star hostel
- 0162 9592 686
- margaretgibson@yha.org.uk
- www.yha.org.uk

GOULCEBY, LOUTH, Lincolnshire
Bay Tree Cottage
Four star self-catering
- 0150 734 3230
- info@goulcebypost.co.uk
- www.goulcebypost.co.uk

GRAINTHORPE, Lincolnshire
Canal Farm Cottages
Four star self-catering
- 01472 388 825
- r-ma@canalfarmcottages.co.uk
- www.canalfarmcottages.co.uk

ENGLAND

Get Motoring

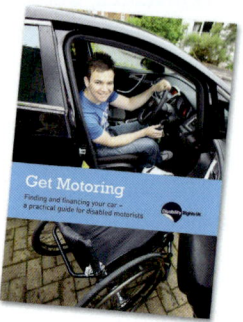

A practical guide for disabled motorists to help find and finance a car. New 2012 edition.

Available to order from our online shop
www.disabilityrightsuk.org

Get Mobile

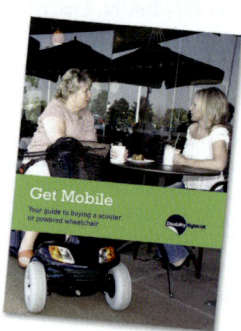

A guide to buying a mobility scooter or powered wheelchair. New 2012 edition.

Available to order from our online shop
www.disabilityrightsuk.org

Supporting
Disability Rights UK

H Kemp & Son Ltd

259 Hallgate
Cottingham
East Riding of Yorkshire
HU16 4BG

Tel: 01482 844 695

Genuine family-run business Established in 1893

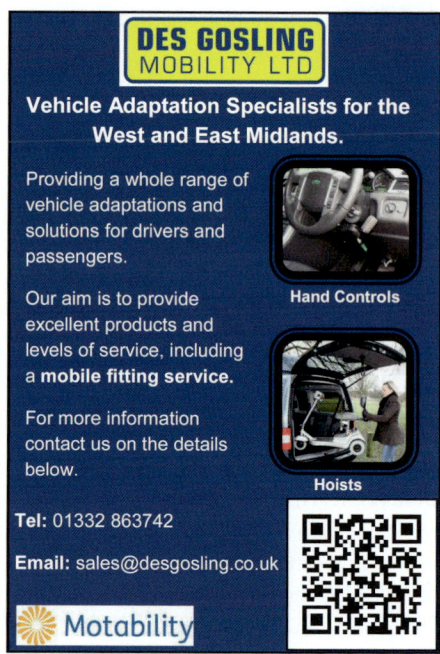

DES GOSLING MOBILITY LTD

Vehicle Adaptation Specialists for the West and East Midlands.

Providing a whole range of vehicle adaptations and solutions for drivers and passengers.

Our aim is to provide excellent products and levels of service, including a **mobile fitting service.**

For more information contact us on the details below.

Tel: 01332 863742

Email: sales@desgosling.co.uk

Hand Controls

Hoists

Motability

EAST MIDLANDS

GUILSBOROUGH, Northamptonshire
Coton Lodge
Five star farmhouse
- T 0160 4740 215
- E jo@cotonlodge.co.uk
- W www.cotonlodge.co.uk

HALLGATES, CROPSTON, Leicestershire
Horseshoe Cottage Farm
Five star bed & breakfast
- T 0116 2350038
- E lindajee@ljee.freeserve.co.uk
- W www.horseshoecottagefarm.com

HAREBY, Lincolnshire
Meridian Retreats
Four star self-catering
- T 01205 870210
- E office@ewbowser.com
- W www.meridianretreats.co.uk

HARPSWELL, Lincolnshire
The Old Stables
Four star self-catering
- T 01427 668 412
- E pam.tatam@gmail.com
- W www.hall-farm.co.uk

HELSEY, NR HOGSTHORPE, Lincolnshire
Helsey House Cottages
Four star self-catering
- T 01754 872 927
- E eaepcs@yahoo.co.uk
- W www.helseycottages.co.uk

HINCKLEY, Leicestershire
Barceló Hinckley Island Hotel
Four star hotel
- T 0870 1688 833
- W www.barcelo-hotels.co.uk

Sketchley Grange Hotel
Hotel
- T 0145 5251 133
- E conference@sketchleygrange.co.uk
- W www.sketchleygrange.co.uk

HUBBERTS BRIDGE, NR BOSTON, Lincolnshire
Elms Farm Cottages
Four and Five star self-catering
- T 01205 290 840
- E carol@elmsfarmcottages.co.uk
- W www.elmsfarmcottages.co.uk

INGOLDMELLS, Lincolnshire
Ingoldale Park
Four star self-catering
- T 01754 872335
- E ingoldalepark@btopenworld.com
- W www.ingoldmells.net

LEICESTER, Leicestershire
Belmont Hotel
Hotel
- T 0116 254 4773
- E info@belmonthotel.co.uk
- W www.belmonthotel.co.uk

Hilton Leicester
Accredited hotel
- T 020 7856 8380
- E john.dixon@hilton.com
- W www.hilton.co.uk

Leicester Marriott Hotel
Hotel
- T 0116 282 0106
- E jo.dempster@marriotthotels.com
- W www.marriott.co.uk

ENGLAND

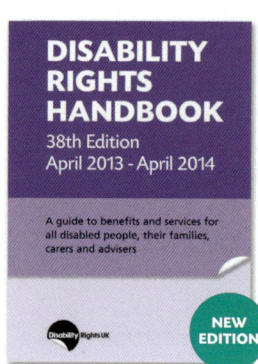

As comprehensive as ever
- How the benefit system works and how to make a claim
- Benefits for people with an illness, injury or disability
- Benefits for carers, young people and children and those looking for work, or in retirement
- Benefits for people injured at work or serving in the Armed Forces
- Challenging benefit decisions
- Getting and paying for care services

New in 2013
For people aged 16-64
- Personal Independence Payment: how to claim, what to do if you are turned down and what happens to people on Disability Living Allowance
- Extra information on Access to Work
- The new sanctions rules for Jobseeker's Allowance and Employment and Support Allowance
- The benefit cap: who will be affected and how it works

For families with disabled children
- Expanded guidance on Disability Living Allowance for children

For people 65 and over:
- Additional information on claiming Attendance Allowance

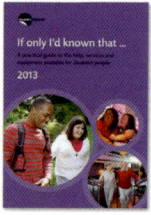

Personal Independence Payment is coming ...

From April 2013, Disability Living Allowance for people aged 16-64 will start to be replaced by a new benefit, the Personal Independence Payment. Over 2 million people will be affected.

The next two years will also see the biggest changes to the benefits system since the introduction of the welfare state. In this period of unprecedented change and benefits cuts, keeping up with the new rules is crucial.

Information and advice you can trust
The new edition of our Disability Rights Handbook, fully updated for 2013, provides in-depth information on the entire benefits system and comprehensive guidance on these critical changes.

The must-buy edition – out May 2013
Disability Rights Handbook 2013-2014 (38th Edition)
£29.99 inc P&P (£15.00 for people claiming benefits)
Order online at www.disabilityrightsuk.org

Stay informed – know your rights
This year's Handbook explains Personal Independence Payment and includes new additional guidance on Disability Living Allowance for children and Attendance Allowance (for people 65 and over) with tactics and tools to help make a successful claim.

It introduces Universal Credit which will replace several income-related benefits and tax credits and is planned to be phased in from April 2013.

All benefits explained in one book
Written in plain English by benefits specialists and legally referenced, it's the only user-friendly benefits guide designed specifically for both claimants and their advisers. It has the answers you need to help ensure the quality of your advice or to claim what you are entitled to.

Keep your Handbook up to date all year
Become a member of Disability Rights UK and we'll keep you up-to-date throughout the year with 'Disability and Welfare Rights Updates' our bi-monthly PDF magazine. 20+ pages of news and page-by-page Handbook updates. Download a free sample copy from our website.

If only I'd known that ...
Our companion guide, 'If only I'd known that a year ago' provides practical advice on accessing the help, services and equipment available for disabled people of all ages. See overleaf for more information.

Order your copy now at www.disabilityrightsuk.org

EAST MIDLANDS

LOUGHBOROUGH, Leicestershire
Imago at Burleigh Court
Four star hotel
- 01509 633 007
- g.hodge@burleigh-court.co.uk
- www.welcometoimago.com

LOUTH, Lincolnshire
Nursery Cottage, The Granary, Millhouse & The Stables
Four star self-catering
- 0150 7358 256
- nurserycottage@hotmail.co.uk
- www.mealsfarm.com

Brackenborough Hall Coach House Holidays
Four and Five star self-catering
- 01507 603 193
- paulandflora@brackenboroughhall.com
- www.brackenboroughhall.com

MARKET HARBOROUGH, Leicestershire
The Angel Hotel & Restaurant
Three star hotel
- 01858 462 702
- d.barton@theangel-hotel.co.uk
- www.theangelhotel.co.uk

MARTIN, Lincolnshire
The Manor House Stables
Four star self-catering
- 01526 378 717
- sherryforbes@hotmail.com
- www.manorhousestables.co.uk

MARTON, Lincolnshire
Black Swan Guest House
Guesthouse
- 01427 718878
- info@blackswanguesthouse.co.uk
- www.blackswanguesthouse.co.uk

MOIRA, Leicestershire
YHA National Forest
Four star hostel
- 0162 9592 686
- margaretgibson@yha.org.uk
- www.yha.org.uk

MOULTON EAUGATE, NR SPALDING, Lincolnshire
Stennetts Farm Cottages
Four star cottages
- 01406 380 408
- info@stennettsfarmcottages.co.uk
- www.stennettsfarmcottages.co.uk

NEWARK, Nottinghamshire
Dairy Cottage
Four star self-catering
- 0194 9850 309
- william-baird@btconnect.com
- www.hallfarmaccommodation.co.uk

NEWHAVEN, Derbyshire
Old House Farm Cottages
Four star self-catering
- 01629 636268
- s.flower1@virgin.net
- www.oldhousefarm.com

NORTH CARLTON, Lincolnshire
Cliff Farm Cottage
Four star self-catering
- 01522 730475
- info@cliff-farm-cottage.co.uk
- www.cliff-farm-cottage.co.uk

NORTH WILLINGHAM, Lincolnshire
The Old Dairy Cottage
Self-catering cottages
- 0167 3838 272
- carole.wright394@btinternet.com
- www.ashfarmbarns.co.uk

OAKHAM, Leicestershire
Lodge Trust Country Park
Three star self-catering
- 01572 768073
- bookings@lodgetrust.org.uk
- www.lodgecountrypark.org.uk

OLD BRAMPTON, Derbyshire
Chestnut Cottage and Willow Cottage
Four star self-catering
- 01246 566159
- patricia_green@btconnect.com

OUNDLE, Northamptonshire
Oundle Cottage Breaks
Three and Four star self-catering
- 01832 275508
- richard@simmondsatoundle.co.uk
- www.oundlecottagebreaks.co.uk

THINGS TO SEE OR DO
Rufford Abbey Country Park
This 150 acre park in Ollerton is one of Nottinghamshire's most popular visitor attractions, containing the remains of a 12th century Cistercian monastery and a later country house. It is a fairly flat site, and most areas of the park are accessible except the upper level of the Abbey ruins. Mobility scooters and wheelchairs can be booked in advance. All facilities, including toilets, are wheelchair accessible. An Access Statement is available online.
- 01623 821338
- www.nottinghamshire.gov.uk enjoying/countryside/countryparks/rufford/

PARTNEY, NR SPILSBY, Lincolnshire
The Red Lion Inn
Four star inn
- 01790 752 271
- enquiries@redlioninnpartney.co.uk
- www.redlioninnpartney.co.uk

SKEGNESS, Lincolnshire
Chatsworth
Three star guest accommodation
- 01754 764177
- lynne@chatsworthhotel.co.uk
- www.chatsworthskegness.co.uk

SOUTH SCARLE, Nottinghamshire
Greystones Guest Accommodation
Four star bed & breakfast
- 01636 893 969
- sheenafowkes@greystonesguests.co.uk
- www.greystonesguests.co.uk

STAINFIELD, Lincolnshire
Rural Roosts
Four star self-catering
- 01526 398 492
- katie@ruralroosts.co.uk
- www.ruralroosts.co.uk

SWADLINCOTE, Derbyshire
Forest Lodges
Three and Four star self-catering
- 0128 356 3483
- debbie@roslistonforestrycentre.co.uk
- www.roslistonforestrycentre.co.uk

SWEPSTONE, Leicestershire
Church View Barn
Three star self-catering
- 0153 0272 481
- wendydavis39@hotmail.com

EAST MIDLANDS

THORGANBY, Lincolnshire
Thorganby Hall Farm Cottages, Little Walk and Marris
Three, Four and Five star self-catering
- 01472 398270
- emma@thorganby.plus.com
- www.thorganbyhall.co.uk

THORPE ST PETER, Lincolnshire
Ings Barn
Self-catering cottages
- 0152 2595 164
- manorbarn13@hotmail.co.uk

THRUSSINGTON, Leicestershire
Walton Thorns Farm Holiday Cottages
Four star self-catering
- 01509 880315
- liz@waltonthorns.co.uk
- www.waltonthorns.co.uk

WOODHALL SPA, Lincolnshire
Bluebell Retreat
Four star cottage
- 0152 6388 341
- gibbs.alison@btinternet.com
- www.bluebellretreatcottage.co.uk

Village Limits Country Pub, Restaurant and Motel
Four star guest accommodation
- 01526 353312
- info@villagelimits.co.uk
- www.villagelimits.co.uk

Petwood Hotel
Three star hotel
- 01526 352411
- Jon@petwood.co.uk
- www.petwood.co.uk

WORKSOP, Nottinghamshire
Browns
Five star bed & breakfast
- 01909 720659
- browns.holbeck@btconnect.com
- www.brownsholbeck.co.uk

WYCOMB, Leicestershire
Stonepits Farm Bed & Breakfast
Four star farmhouse
- 0166 444 4597
- stay@stonepitsfarm.co.uk
- www.stonepittsfarm.co.uk

OTHER ACCOMMODATION

BOSTON, Lincolnshire
Special Needs Activity Centre Lincolnshire
14 Croppers Way, Freiston, Boston PE22 0QT
- 01205 761373
- info@snac.org.uk
- www.snac.org.uk
Special Needs Activity Centre in Lincolnshire.

MILFORD, Derbyshire
The Ebenezer Chapel
Derwent River Bridge, Milford
- 01332 840564
- ann.wayne@derbyshire-holidays.com
- www.derbyshire-holidays.com
Converted former chapel in riverside village of Milford.

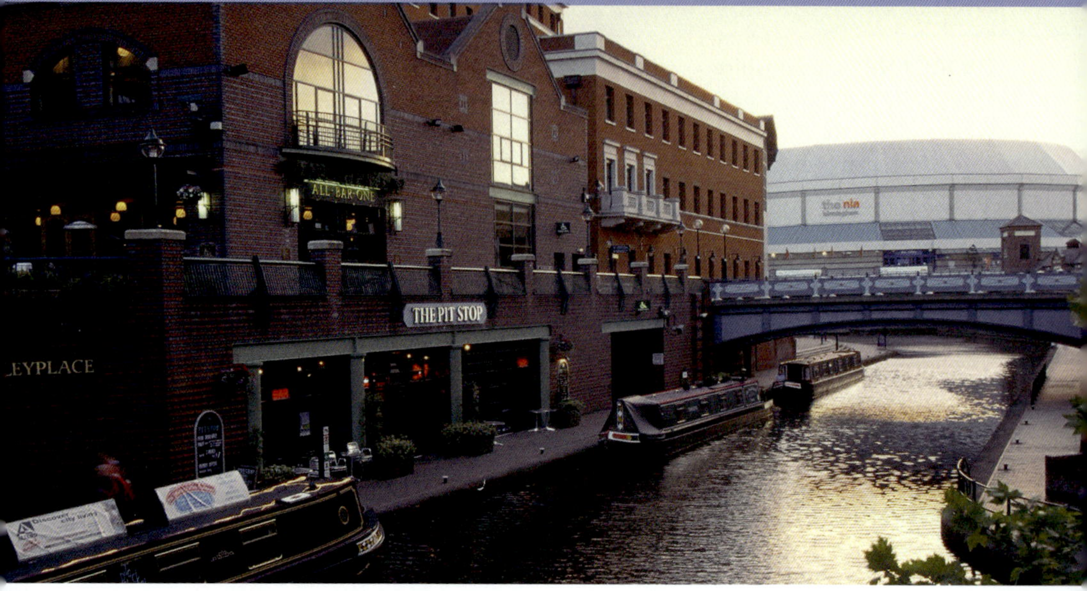

About the West Midlands

The Heart of England region comprises Herefordshire, Shropshire, Staffordshire, Warwickshire, West Midlands and Worcestershire. It is an area that combines a major urban centre, a rich historic and industrial heritage and some of England's most typical and unspoilt countryside.

The rivers Severn and Wye flow through Shropshire, Worcestershire and Herefordshire on the Welsh border.

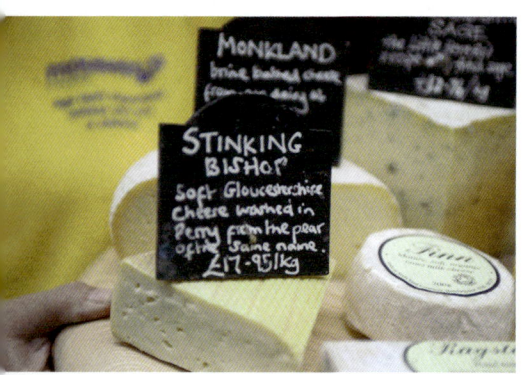

Fruit blossom attracts visitors to the Vale of Evesham in the spring. To the north, Staffordshire shares the Peak District with its neighbouring counties.

Birmingham, the country's second largest city, provides the full range of urban attractions and has more miles of canals than Venice. The Barber Institute of Fine Arts features the work of many of the greatest names in Western art while recent developments in the city centre include the Symphony Hall and a rebuilt shopping area around the

Bullring. There is also a wide range of museums, shops, parks, sporting venues and other activities. Outside the city centre the National Exhibition Centre and Arena hosts a full programme of concerts, exhibitions and other events.

Ironbridge in Shropshire, the birthplace of the Industrial Revolution, is a World Heritage Site supporting a cluster of museums that are largely accessible. The Black Country Living Museum at Dudley is a large open-air site depicting life and industry in the area. The pottery industry can be explored at visitor centres and factory shops in Stoke-on-Trent and Worcester. In Birmingham, a late 19th century jewellery factory has been recreated as the Jewellery Quarter Discovery Centre. The development of the motor industry can be experienced at the Heritage Motor Centre at Gaydon near Warwick and the Coventry Transport Museum.

For other tastes there are museums devoted to beer in Burton-on-Trent and

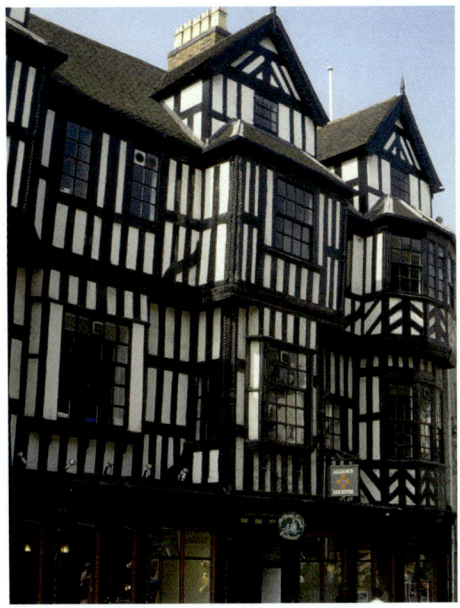

cider in Hereford, Cadbury World in Birmingham and the Ryton Organic Gardens near Coventry.

The literary and artistic heritage of the area is considerable. Pride of place must go to Stratford-upon-Avon, birthplace of William Shakespeare, and home to the fully accessible Shakespeare Centre. The hills of Shropshire and Worcestershire were immortalised by A E Houseman. Other notables include Dr Johnson from Lichfield, George Elliot from Nuneaton and Edward Elgar from Worcester.

At Britain's first major theme park, Alton Towers in Staffordshire, the grounds and many of the attractions are accessible and help can be provided getting onto rides. Dedicated holiday shoppers can visit the Merryhill Centre near Dudley.

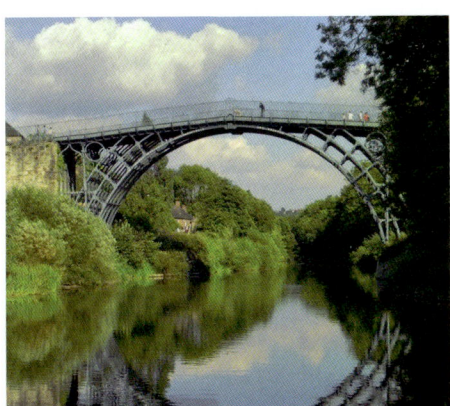

ENGLAND

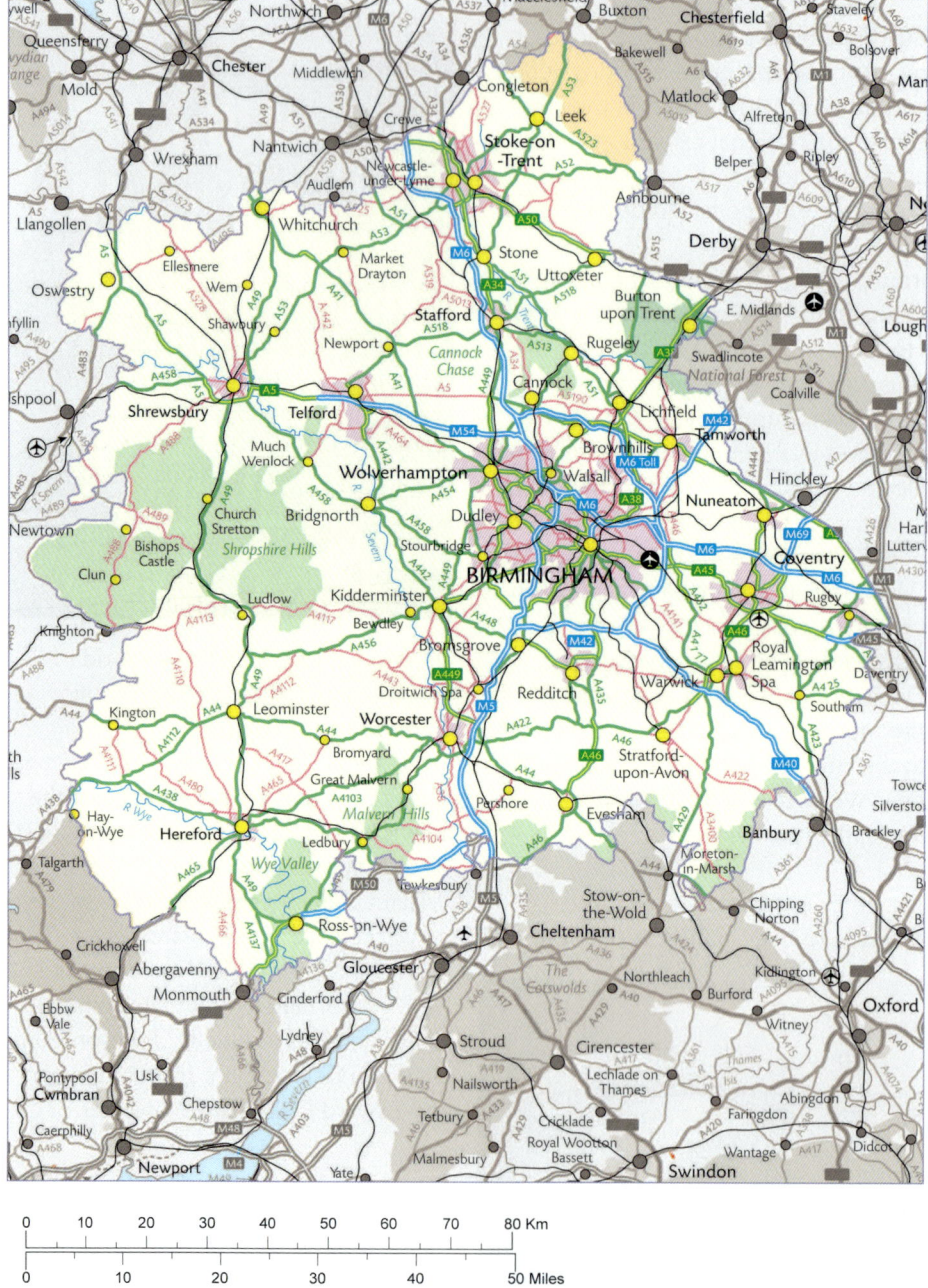

Resources

Tourism

Heart of England Tourist Board
The official tourist board for the 'Heart of England'. Their website includes suggested attractions, places to stay and events.
- Ⓦ www.visitheartofengland.com

Information & advice

DIAL
Offer free, impartial and confidential information and advice by telephone to disabled people, their relatives and professionals. Local branches of DIAL are constantly changing but at the time of writing, the following groups were members of DIAL UK and may be able to help visitors in their areas. Please call before travelling to check whether the service and organisation is still available:

CARES Sandwell
- Ⓣ 0121 558 7003 (also Textphone)

DIAL North Worcestershire
- Ⓣ 01562 60241
- Helpline 0845 200 1072

DIAL Solihull
- Ⓣ 0121 770 0333 (also Textphone)

DIAL South Worcestershire
- Ⓣ 01905 27790
- Textphone 01905 22191

Disability Solutions, Stoke
- Ⓣ 01782 683100
- Textphone 01782 683800

Liseux Trust Birmingham
- Ⓣ 0121 382 6660
- Textphone 0121 350 8182

Walsall DIAL
- Ⓣ 01922 635588

Equipment hire

SHOPMOBILITY
The National Federation of Shopmobility UK (NFSUK), PO Box 6641, Christchurch BH23 9DQ
- Ⓣ 0844 41 41 850
- Ⓔ info@shopmobilityuk.org
- Ⓦ www.shopmobilityuk.org

Scheme which lends manual wheelchairs, powered wheelchairs and powered scooters to members of the public with limited mobility to shop and to visit leisure and commercial facilities within the town, city or shopping centre. You can find the nearest Shopmobility scheme to you through their on-line directory. Contact specific Shopmobility Schemes to make equipment bookings or find out more information.

> **THINGS TO SEE OR DO**
>
> **The Barber Institute of Fine Arts**
> Gallery within the University of Birmingham that regularly organises free tours for deaf visitors with a fully qualified BSL interpreter on Sundays. Outside these dates, groups of 8 or more can book a BSL interpreted, guided gallery tour at a cost of £4 per person. Audio descriptive gallery tours for blind and partially sighted visitors can also be arranged for groups of 8 people or more with fully trained guides, for £4 per person.
> - Ⓣ 0121 414 2261
> - Ⓔ education@barber.org.uk

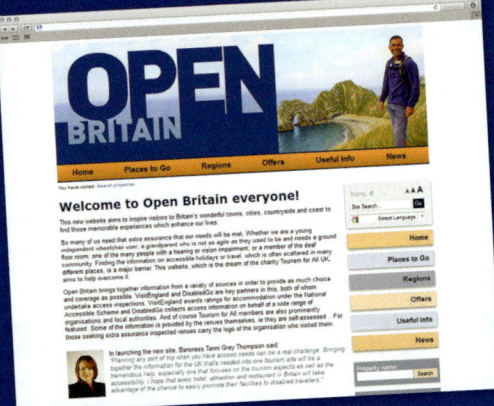

WEST MIDLANDS

Leamington Spa Shopmobility
Shopmobility Unit, Level 4, Royal Priors Car Park, Park St, Leamington Spa CV32 4XT
- 01926 470450
- info@leamingtonshopmobility.org.uk
- www.leamingtonshopmobility.org.uk

Boston Community Transport
The Len Medlock Centre, St Georges Road, Boston PE21 8TY
- Dial A Ride 01205 315934
  Voluntary Car Scheme 01205 315935
  Shopmobility 01205 314936
- transport@southlincscvs.org.uk

As part of a Shopmobility Scheme, scooters and both powered and manual wheelchairs are available for hire for both residents for use elsewhere and people visiting the area. Users have to be members of the scheme for insurance purposes. Vehicles can be delivered, at an additional charge, to addresses within 10 miles of Boston.

Publications

Getting Around Access Guide
- 0121 214 7214
- customerrelations@centro.org.uk
- www.centro.org.uk

A guide to accessible public transport in the West Midlands PTA area. Published each April, it includes information on the accessible Midland Metro light rail service between Birmingham and Wolverhampton and lists local public toilets for disabled people. Available in standard or large print, Braille or on tape or CD from CENTRO Customer Relations, 16 Summer Lane, Birmingham B19 3SD.

Wheelchair User's Guide to Accessible Tourist Attractions & Accommodation for Shropshire
- www.disabledholidayinfo.org.uk

Wheelchair User's Guide to Accessible Countryside Sites & Trails in Shropshire & the Borderlands 2007/8 and *Wheelchair User's Guide to Accessible Activities in & around Shropshire* (both researched by a wheelchair user). Send a A5 addressed envelope with a first class stamp for each title to: Disabled Holiday Information, PO Box 186, Oswestry SY10 1AF.

Online resources

www.stratford-upon-avon.co.uk
Detailed information on access at tourist attractions and other facilities is given on this site.

THINGS TO SEE OR DO

Shakespeare's Houses
The ground floors of Shakespeare's Birthplace, Nash's House, Hall's Croft and Mary Arden's Farm and most of the gardens in Stratford-Upon-Avon are accessible to those with restricted mobility, and toilet facilities for wheelchair users are available.
- www.shakespeare.org.uk

ENGLAND

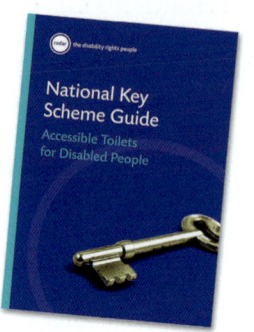

National Key Scheme Guide

Updated every year, this guide lists the location of 9,000 NKS toilets around the UK. It shows opening times, provider name and whether the toilet is unisex.

Available to order from our online shop
www.disabilityrightsuk.org

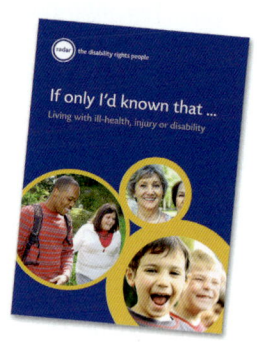

If Only I'd Known That ...

An information-packed guide to services, welfare rights, facilities and support for anyone with a disability or health condition, this guide includes resources for all ages from childhood to later years.

Available to order from our online shop
www.disabilityrightsuk.org

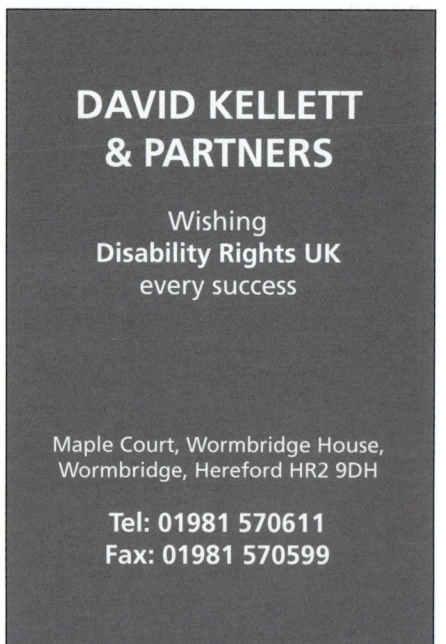

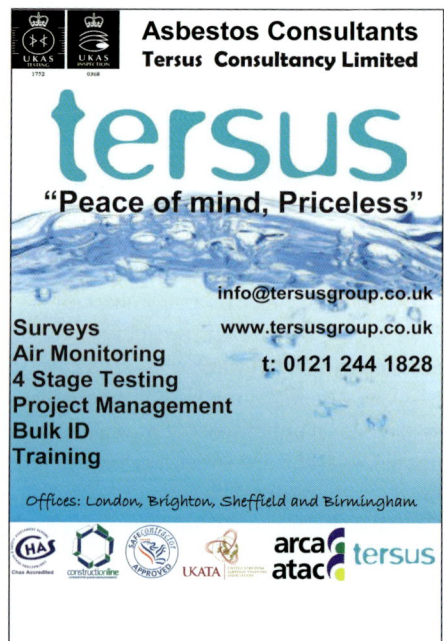

WEST MIDLANDS

Accommodation

NAS ASSESSED ACCOMMODATION

BAGNALL, Staffordshire
Cordwainer Cottage
Three star self-catering
- 0178 2302 575
- enquiries@cordwainercottage.co.uk
- www.cordwainercottage.co.uk

BIRMINGHAM, West Midlands
SACO Livingbase
Four star serviced apartments
- 0845 1220 405
- janejones@sacoapartments.co.uk
- www.sacoapartments.co.uk

BRIDGENORTH, Shropshire
The Malthouse
Four star self-catering
- 0175 062 218
- janetkr@ker-russell.me.uk
- www.cottages4you.co.uk

BROMYARD, Herefordshire
Durstone Cottage
Three star self-catering
- 0188 5400 221
- sarah.mulroy@btconnect.com
- www.durstonefarm.co.uk

COALPORT, Shropshire
YHA Coalport
Three star hostel
- 0162 9592 686
- margaretgibson@yha.org.uk
- www.yha.org.uk

DIDDLEBURY, Shropshire
Goosefoot Barn Cottages
Four star self-catering
- 01584 861326
- info@goosefootbarn.co.uk
- www.goosefootbarn.co.uk

DILHORNE, Staffordshire
Little Summerhill Cottages
Four star self-catering
- 0178 2550 967
- info@holidaycottagesstaffordshire.com
- www.holidaycottagesstaffordshire.com

EATON-UNDER-HEYWOOD, Shropshire
Eaton Manor
Four and Five star self-catering
- 0129 7324 63
- jenny.trice@premiercottages.co.uk
- www.eatonmanor.co.uk

GRAFTON, Herefordshire
Anvil Cottage, Apple Bough and Cider Press
Four star self-catering
- 01432 268689
- jennielayton@ereal.net
- www.graftonvilla.co.uk

HEREFORD, Herefordshire
Poston Mill Park
Four star self-catering
- 01981 550225
- info@poston-mill.co.uk
- www.postonmillholidays.co.uk

HINDLIP, Worcestershire
The Manor Coach House
Four star guest accommodation
- 01905 456457
- info@manorcoachhouse.co.uk
- www.manorcoachhouse.co.uk

ENGLAND

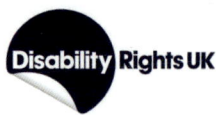

Visit our online shop
For products and books that open doors to independent living.

www.disabilityrightsuk.org

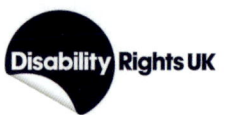

Make a donation
Support our work with a one-off or regular donation.

www.disabilityrightsuk.org

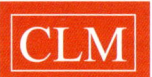

Currall Lewis and Martin
Construction Limited
are happy to support
the work of Disability Rights UK

www.clmconstruction.co.uk

D & HB Associates Ltd

Is pleased to support
Disability Rights UK

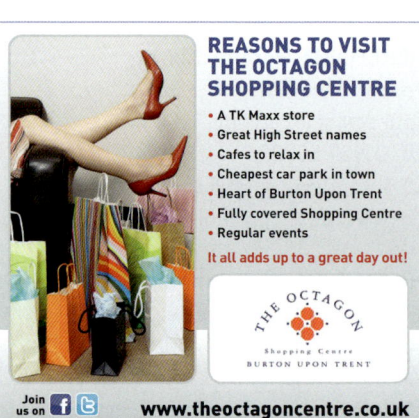

VULCO SPRING
& PRESSWORK CO. LTD
EVESHAM ROAD, ASTWOOD BANK,
REDDITCH, WORCESTERSHIRE, B96 6DU
TEL. (01527) 892447
www.vulcosprings.com

SPRINGS, WIRE FORMS, PRESSINGS, SPANNERS, CONTACTS, BRACKETS AND CLIPS, ASSEMBLIES, MULTIFORMS AND TRADITONAL, TOOL MAKING TO YOUR REQUIREMENTS

WEST MIDLANDS

ILAM, Staffordshire
Beechenhill Cottage and The Cottage by the Pond
Four star self-catering
- 01335 310274
- stay@beechenhill.co.uk
- www.beechenhill.co.uk

The Orchards
Four star self-catering
- 01538 308205
- rushley.farm@btopenworld.com

YHA Ilam Hall
Four star hostel
- 0162 9592 686
- margaretgibson@yha.org.uk
- www.yha.org.uk

KINETON, Warwickshire
Long Ground Barn
Five star self-catering
- 01926 641829
- carolyn@heartofthecountryholidays.co.uk
- www.heartofthecountryholidays.co.uk

KNIGHTCOTE, Warwickshire
Knightcote Farm Cottages
Five star self-catering
- 0129 7324 63
- jenny.trice@premiercottages.co.uk
- www.farmcottages.com

LEDBURY, Herefordshire
The Old Kennels Farm
Three and Four star self-catering
- 01531 635024
- info@oldkennelsfarm.co.uk
- www.oldkennelsfarm.co.uk

LEOMINSTER, Herefordshire
The Wain House
Four star self-catering
- 0198 1580 442
- info@tkfarm.co.uk
- www.trippenkennettfarm.co.uk

YHA Leominster
Four star hostel
- 0162 9592 686
- margaretgibson@yha.org.uk
- www.yha.org.uk

LIGHTHORNE, Warwickshire
Church Hill Farm B&B
Four star bed & breakfast
- 01926 651251
- sue@churchhillfarm.co.uk
- www.churchhillfarm.co.uk

LUDLOW, Shropshire
Ludlow Mascall Centre
Three star hotel
- 01584 873882
- marketing@ludlowmascallcentre.co.uk
- www.ludlowmascallcentre.co.uk

Mocktree Barns Holiday Cottages
Three star self-catering
- 01547 540441
- mocktreebarns@care4free.net
- www.mocktreeholidays.co.uk

MALVERN, Herefordshire
Hidelow House Cottages
Four and Five star self-catering
- 01886 884547
- stay@hidelow.co.uk
- www.hidelow.co.uk

ENGLISH

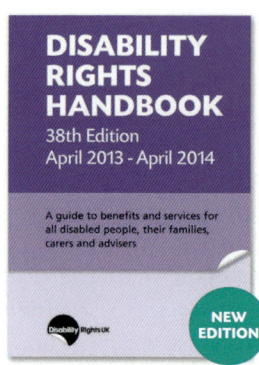

As comprehensive as ever
- How the benefit system works and how to make a claim
- Benefits for people with an illness, injury or disability
- Benefits for carers, young people and children and those looking for work, or in retirement
- Benefits for people injured at work or serving in the Armed Forces
- Challenging benefit decisions
- Getting and paying for care services

New in 2013
For people aged 16-64
- Personal Independence Payment: how to claim, what to do if you are turned down and what happens to people on Disability Living Allowance
- Extra information on Access to Work
- The new sanctions rules for Jobseeker's Allowance and Employment and Support Allowance
- The benefit cap: who will be affected and how it works

For families with disabled children
- Expanded guidance on Disability Living Allowance for children

For people 65 and over:
- Additional information on claiming Attendance Allowance

Personal Independence Payment is coming ...

From April 2013, Disability Living Allowance for people aged 16-64 will start to be replaced by a new benefit, the Personal Independence Payment. Over 2 million people will be affected.

The next two years will also see the biggest changes to the benefits system since the introduction of the welfare state. In this period of unprecedented change and benefits cuts, keeping up with the new rules is crucial.

Information and advice you can trust
The new edition of our Disability Rights Handbook, fully updated for 2013, provides in-depth information on the entire benefits system and comprehensive guidance on these critical changes.

The must-buy edition – out May 2013
Disability Rights Handbook 2013-2014 (38th Edition)
£29.99 inc P&P (£15.00 for people claiming benefits)
Order online at www.disabilityrightsuk.org

Stay informed – know your rights
This year's Handbook explains Personal Independence Payment and includes new additional guidance on Disability Living Allowance for children and Attendance Allowance (for people 65 and over) with tactics and tools to help make a successful claim.

It introduces Universal Credit which will replace several income-related benefits and tax credits and is planned to be phased in from April 2013.

All benefits explained in one book
Written in plain English by benefits specialists and legally referenced, it's the only user-friendly benefits guide designed specifically for both claimants and their advisers. It has the answers you need to help ensure the quality of your advice or to claim what you are entitled to.

Keep your Handbook up to date all year
Become a member of Disability Rights UK and we'll keep you up-to-date throughout the year with 'Disability and Welfare Rights Updates' our bi-monthly PDF magazine. 20+ pages of news and page-by-page Handbook updates. Download a free sample copy from our website.

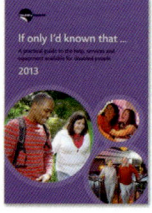

If only I'd known that ...
Our companion guide, 'If only I'd known that a year ago' provides practical advice on accessing the help, services and equipment available for disabled people of all ages. See overleaf for more information.

Order your copy now at www.disabilityrightsuk.org

WEST MIDLANDS

MICHAELCHURCH ESCLEY, Herefordshire
Holt Farm
Four star self-catering
- 0174 7828 170
- enq@hideaways.co.uk
- www.holtfarmholidays.com

ROSS-ON-WYE, Herefordshire
Trevase Granary
Five star self-catering
- 01989 730210
- pursey.trevase@btconnect.com
- www.trevasecottages.co.uk

Flanesford Priory
Three and Five star self-catering
- 01989 770157
- info@flanesfordpriory.co.uk
- www.flanesfordpriory.co.uk

Tump Farm
Three star self-catering
- 01600 891029
- clinwilcharmaine@hotmail.com
- www.wyedeantourism.co.uk

SHREWSBURY, Shropshire
Lyth Hill House
Five star bed & breakfast
- 0174 3874 660
- bnb@lythhillhouse.com
- www.lythhillhouse.com

STANSHOPE, Staffordshire
Church Farm Cottage & Ancestral Barn
Four and Five star self-catering
- 01335 310243
- enquiries@dovedalecottages.co.uk
- www.dovedalecottages.co.uk

TRETIRE, Herefordshire
Penblaith Barn
Five star self-catering
- 0198 9730 210
- stay@trevasecottages.co.uk
- www.trevasecottages.co.uk

WHITCHURCH, Herefordshire
Portland House Guest House
guest accommodation
- 01600 890757
- info@portlandguesthouse.co.uk
- www.portlandguesthouse.co.uk

WROXETER, NR SHREWSBURY, Shropshire
Wroxeter Hotel
Three star country house hotel
- 01743 761256
- info@thewroxeterhotel.co.uk
- www.thewroxeterhotel.co.uk

OTHER ACCOMMODATION

ROSS-ON-WYE, Herefordshire
Merton House Hotel
Edde Cross Street, Ross-on-Wye HR9 7BZ
- 01989 563252
- merton.house@clara.co.uk
- www.mertonhouse.org

Hotel in own grounds specially adapted for disabled and elderly guests.

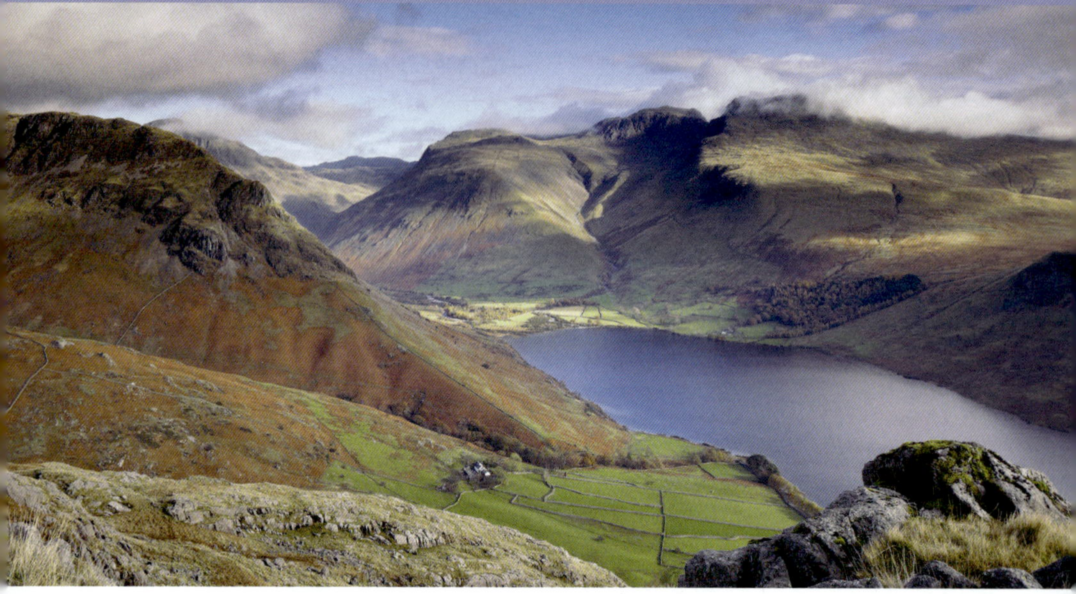

ENGLAND

About North West England

The North West region of England is a wide and varied place – Cheshire, Cumbria, Greater Manchester, Lancashire and Merseyside all feature including the spectacular Lake District National Park. Whether you are looking for urban or rural scenery, the North West can offer whatever you need for a relaxing break or a full-on adventure holiday.

The North West is a region of contrast ranging from the modern cities of Manchester and Liverpool to the Roman and medieval heritage of Chester to the rolling hills of Lancashire and the stunning scenery of the Lake District.

The leading seaside resort in the North is Blackpool with miles of redeveloped level promenade, piers, entertainments and, of course, the famous Blackpool Tower and Pleasure Beach, at which many rides can be enjoyed by disabled visitors.

Former European City of Culture, Liverpool boasts a wide array of visitor opportunities including the redeveloped

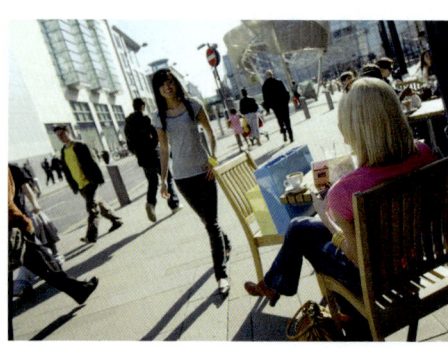

HOLIDAYS IN THE BRITISH ISLES

NORTH WEST ENGLAND

Albert Dock Centre which houses a variety of shops, restaurants, museums and galleries including Tate Liverpool, the International Slavery Museum and the Beatles Museum. Other attractions include the Walker Art Gallery, Liverpool One shopping centre and Mersey Ferries.

A short distance away is Manchester offering top class theatre, music and sport with a wide range of shops and restaurants. In the redeveloped Castlefields area you can visit the Museum of Science & Industry housed in the world's first passenger railway station. Away from the city centre, waterside developments include The Lowry and Imperial War Museum North at Salford Quays and the Trafford Centre for out-of-town shopping. You can also visit Manchester United football ground and take an accessible tour.

Historic towns of the region include Carlisle, Lancaster and Chester where the original city walls surround picturesque shopping streets and the cathedral. Advice on accessible sight-seeing routes can be obtained from the Tourist Information Centre. There is also no shortage of historic houses in the region, most notably Chatsworth House in Cheshire, one of the UK's largest stately homes.

Parks and gardens in the area include Liverpool University's Botanic gardens at Ness on the Wirral, the Topiary Gardens at Levens Hall in the Lake District and Tatton Park near Knutsford in Cheshire. The Forest of Bowland in Lancashire, an Area of Outstanding Natural Beauty is well worth a visit – hire an all-terrain wheelchair buggy to explore. If wildlife is your thing you can choose from attractions including Chester Zoo and the Wildfowl & Wetlands Trust's Martin Mere near Ormskirk. In the Lake District a number of scenic paths have been developed for disabled people including the National Trust's Friars Crag Walk beside Derwentwater and the Ridding Wood Sculpture Trail in Grizedale Forest.

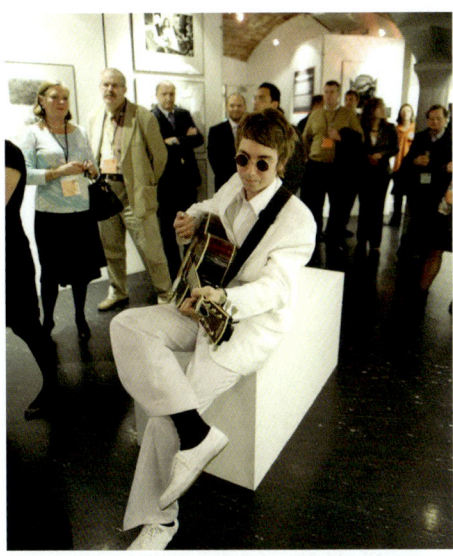

Throughout the area are displays of the local industrial heritage. The silk industry is explored at Macclesfield and the craft of glassmaking is on display at The World of Glass in St Helens. Small Pennine mill towns can be visited by the restored, award-winning East Lancashire Railway.

ENGLAND

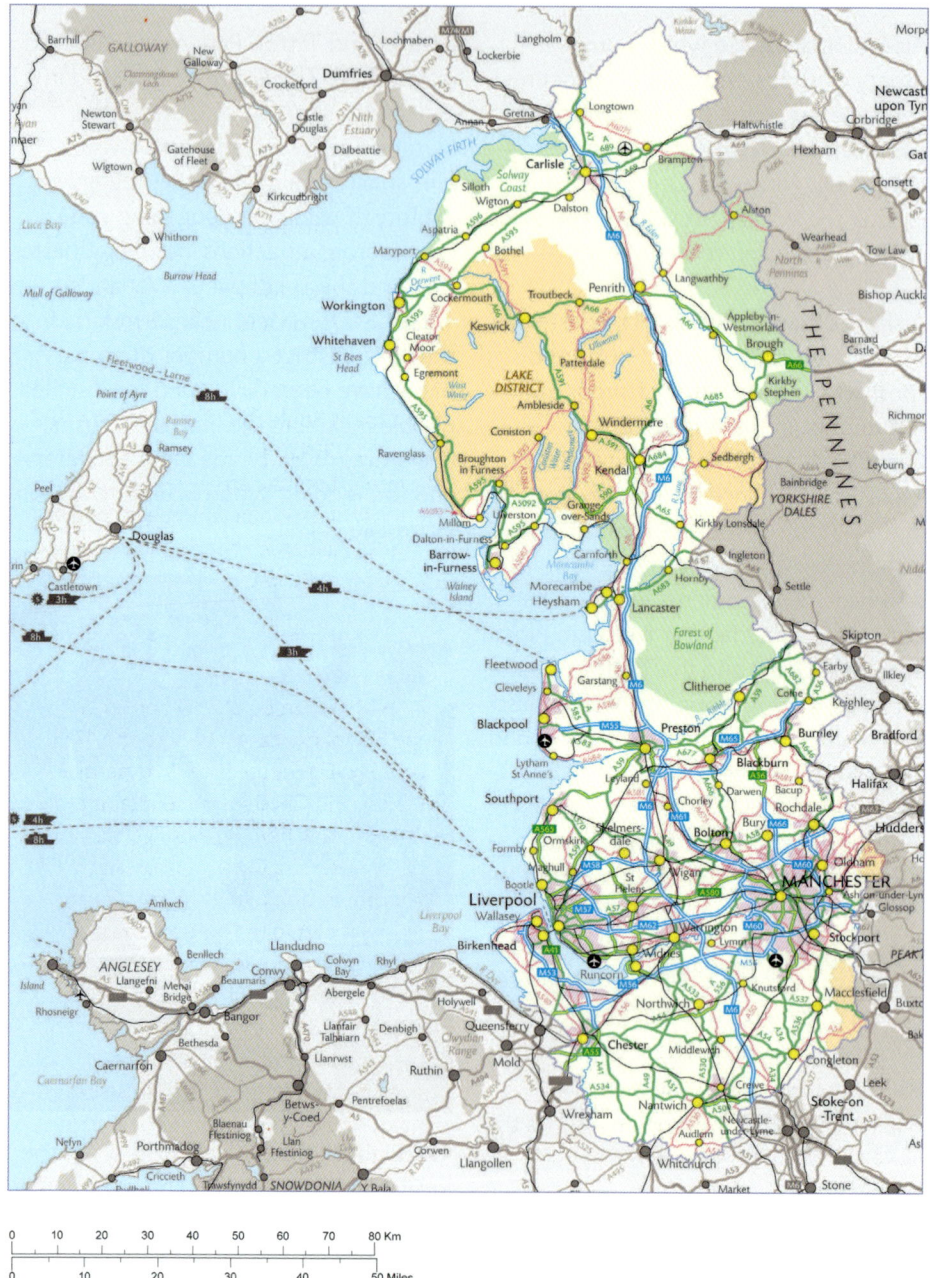

HOLIDAYS IN THE BRITISH ISLES

Resources
Tourism

The North West of England does not have a single regional tourism organisation. Instead you should contact the relevant organisation below.

Visit Chester & Cheshire
Chester Railway Station, 1st Floor, West Wing Offices, Station Road, Chester CH1 3NT
- T: 0845 647 7868
- W: www.visitchester.com

Provide general information on Chester and Cheshire.

Cumbria Tourism
Windermere Road, Staveley, Cumbria LA8 9PL
- T: 01539 822222
- E: info@golakes.co.uk
- W: www.golakes.co.uk

Provide general information and a number of free publications about the county.

Lancashire & Blackpool Tourist Board
Farington House, Lancashire Enterprise Business Park, Centurion Way, Leyland, PR26 6TW
- T: 01772 426450
- E: info@visitlancashire.com
- W: www.visitlancashire.com

Provide general information on the area to visitors.

Visit Manchester
Manchester Visitor Information Centre, 45-50 Piccadilly Plaza, Portland Street M1 4BT
- T: 0871 222 8223
- E: touristinformation@visitmanchester.com
- W: www.visitmanchester.com

Offers a selection of general tourist information on Manchester and its accommodation and attractions.

Blackpool Pleasure Beach
525 Ocean Boulevard, Blackpool FY4 1EZ
- T: 0871 2221234
- E: info@bpbltd.com
- W: www.blackpoolpleasurebeach.com

Various facilities for disabled are available at the Pleasure Beach.

THINGS TO SEE OR DO

Chatsworth House

One of the largest stately homes in the UK, partly dating back to the 17th century. The house is set in expansive parkland in Cheshire and contains a unique collection of paintings, furniture, Old Master drawings, neoclassical sculptures, books and other artifacts. There is a lift in the house, allowing fully inclusive access to the entire visitor route for visitors with restricted mobility. There is good access to the garden, farmyard, shops and restaurants. Electric scooters can be borrowed. Disabled parking and toilets on site.

- W: www.chatsworth.org

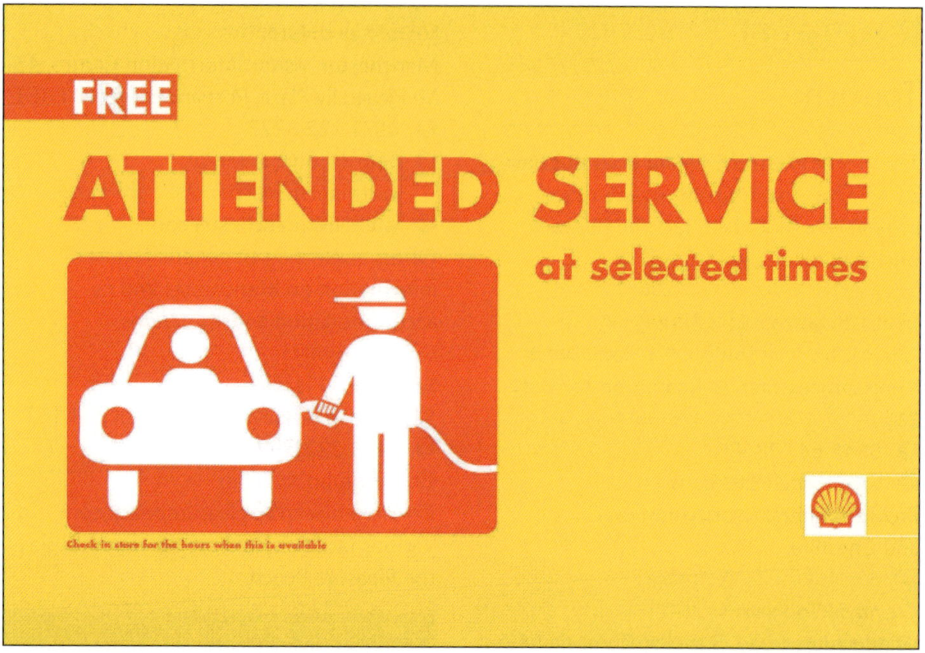

ENGLAND

FREE ATTENDED SERVICE
at selected times

Check in store for the hours when this is available

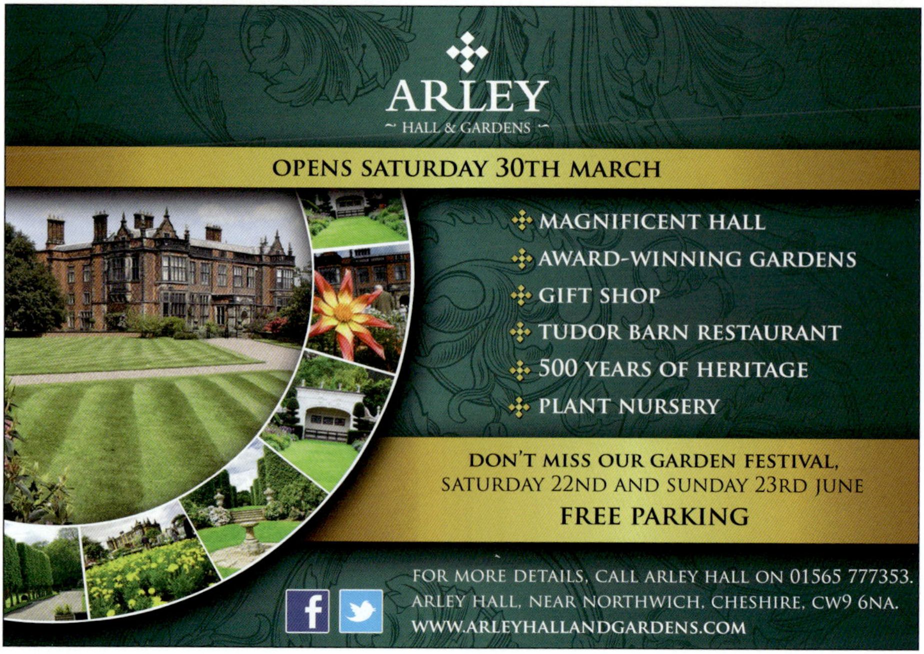

ARLEY
HALL & GARDENS

OPENS SATURDAY 30TH MARCH

- MAGNIFICENT HALL
- AWARD-WINNING GARDENS
- GIFT SHOP
- TUDOR BARN RESTAURANT
- 500 YEARS OF HERITAGE
- PLANT NURSERY

DON'T MISS OUR GARDEN FESTIVAL,
SATURDAY 22ND AND SUNDAY 23RD JUNE
FREE PARKING

FOR MORE DETAILS, CALL ARLEY HALL ON 01565 777353.
ARLEY HALL, NEAR NORTHWICH. CHESHIRE. CW9 6NA.
WWW.ARLEYHALLANDGARDENS.COM

NORTH WEST ENGLAND

Information & advice

Disabled Living
Burrows House, 10 Priestley Road, Wardley Industrial Estate, Worsley, Manchester M28 2LY
- ☎ 0161 607 8200
- ✉ info@disabledliving.co.uk
- 🌐 www.disabledliving.co.uk

Charity which provides impartial information about equipment and services for disabled adults, children, older people and the professionals who support them.

Disability Stockport
23 High Street, Stockport SK1 1EG
- ☎ 0161 480 7248
- ✉ email@disabilitystockport.org.uk
- 🌐 www.disabilitystockport.org.uk

Offer an information service to disabled people in Stockport.

Cheshire Centre for Independent Living
Oakwood Lane, Barnton, Cheshire CW8 4HE
- ☎ 01606 872760
- ✉ office@cheshirecil.org
- 🌐 www.chestercil.org

User-led group of information providers in Cheshire providing information, training, information, practical help, direct payments and advocacy to assist disabled people throughout Cheshire.

DIAL
Offer free, impartial and confidential information and advice by telephone to disabled people, their relatives and professionals. Local branches of DIAL are constantly changing but at the time of writing, the following groups were members of DIAL UK and may be able to help visitors in their areas.

Please call before travelling to check whether the service and organisation is still available:

Access Lancashire
- ☎ 01772 621633

DIAL House Chester
- ☎ 01244 4345655
  Textphone 01244 342472

Disability Equality (NW) Ltd
- ☎ 01772 558863

Macclesfield DIB
- ☎ 01625 501759

Paveways, Wigan
- ☎ 01942 519909

Vale Royal Disability Services
- ☎ 01606 888400

Park Tours & Travel
The Mountain Goat Office, Victoria Street, Windermere, Cumbria LA23 1AD
- ☎ 015394 45161
- 🌐 www.mountain-goat.com

Offer full and half-day tours in the Lake District using mini-buses with experienced drivers. Facilities for wheelchair users, with folding wheelchairs, who can mount steps and walk a few steps can be provided with prior notice.

> **THINGS TO SEE OR DO**
>
> ### Coniston Boating Centre
> Boat centre on Coniston Water in the Lake District. Hires electric motor boats with a moveable ramp, accommodating up to three wheelchair users. The top speed is six mph. Suitable for wheelchair anglers.
> - 🌐 www.conistonboatingcentre.co.uk
> - ☎ 01539 441 366

Lancashire Outdoor Education
Contact us to get out more!
Borwick Hall
A unique Manor house dating back to the 14th century surrounded by beautiful and open countryside.
Easy access to Morecambe bay, an area of outstanding natural beauty and the Lake District National Park.
Tel: 01524 732508 Email: borwickhall@lancashire.gov.uk
Borwick, Carnforth, LA6 1JU
Hothersall Lodge
A purpose built centre surrounded by seven acres of beautiful grounds. Situated in a secluded and picturesque corner of the Ribble Valley with beautiful surrounding countryside, close to Ribchester.
The Centre is particularly suited to providing inclusive adventurous activities for additional needs visitors.
Tel: 01254 878422 Email: hothersall.lodge@lancashire.gov.uk
Hothersall, Longridge, Preston, PR3 2XB
Tower Wood
A beautiful Edwardian house set in twelve acres of lawns and woodland on the shore of Lake Windermere.
Located in the Lake District National Park with easy access to all the lakes and mountains in this unique area.
Tel: 015395 31519 Email: tower.wood@lancashire.gov.uk
Windermere, Cumbria, LA23 3PL
Whitehough
Offers a range of traditional timber lodges in a beautiful setting for an outdoor adventure experience.
Beneath Pendle Hill, with easy access to the Yorkshire Dales National Park and the Trough of Bowland.
Tel: 01282 615688 Email: whitehough.admin@lancashire.gov.uk
Barley New Road, Nr. Burnley, BB12 9LF
Lancashire County Council
www.lancashire.gov.uk/education/outdoor

radar the disability rights people
Doing Transport Differently
How to access public transport – a guide for everyone with lived experience of disability or health conditions
Doing Transport Differently
This guide includes information and travellers' tales to help and inspire people with lived experience of disability or health conditions to use public transport.
Available to order from our online shop
www.disabilityrightsuk.org

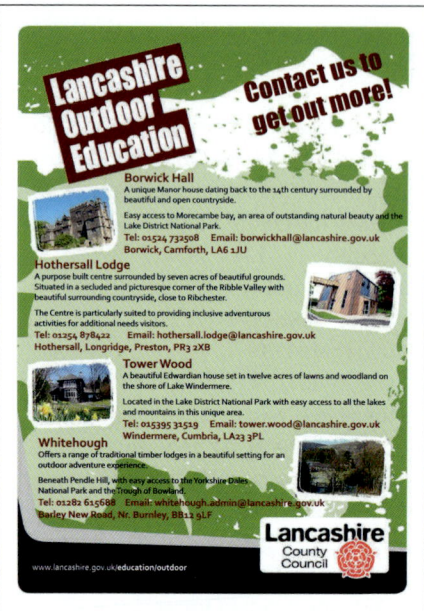

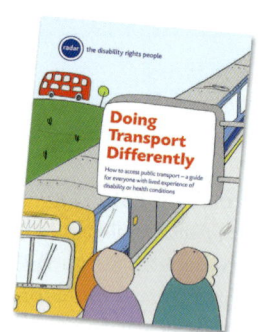

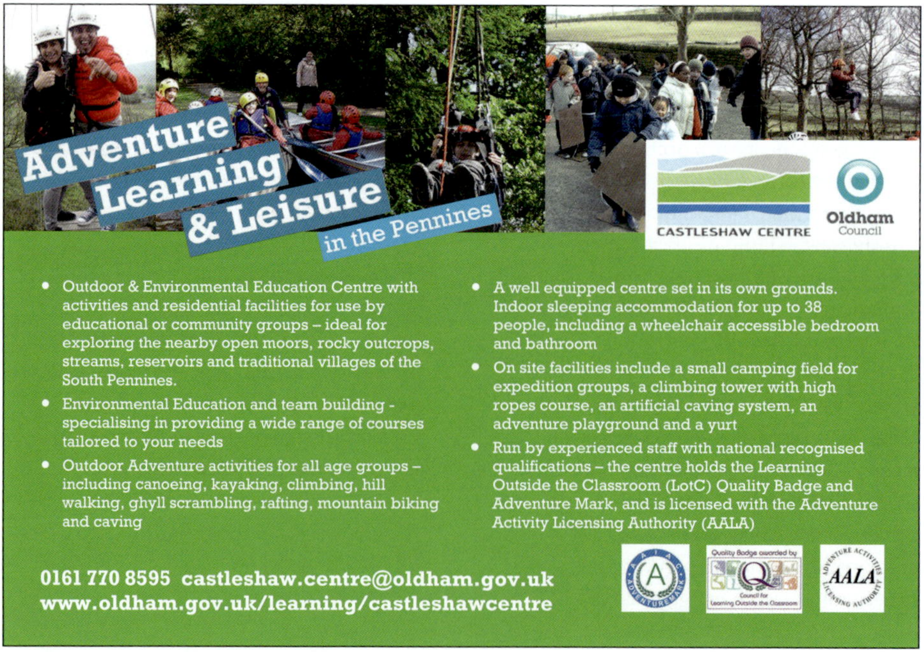

Adventure Learning & Leisure in the Pennines
CASTLESHAW CENTRE
Oldham Council
• Outdoor & Environmental Education Centre with activities and residential facilities for use by educational or community groups – ideal for exploring the nearby open moors, rocky outcrops, streams, reservoirs and traditional villages of the South Pennines.
• Environmental Education and team building - specialising in providing a wide range of courses tailored to your needs
• Outdoor Adventure activities for all age groups – including canoeing, kayaking, climbing, hill walking, ghyll scrambling, rafting, mountain biking and caving
• A well equipped centre set in its own grounds. Indoor sleeping accommodation for up to 38 people, including a wheelchair accessible bedroom and bathroom
• On site facilities include a small camping field for expedition groups, a climbing tower with high ropes course, an artificial caving system, an adventure playground and a yurt
• Run by experienced staff with national recognised qualifications – the centre holds the Learning Outside the Classroom (LotC) Quality Badge and Adventure Mark, and is licensed with the Adventure Activity Licensing Authority (AALA)
0161 770 8595 castleshaw.centre@oldham.gov.uk
www.oldham.gov.uk/learning/castleshawcentre
Quality Badge awarded by Council for Learning Outside the Classroom
AALA

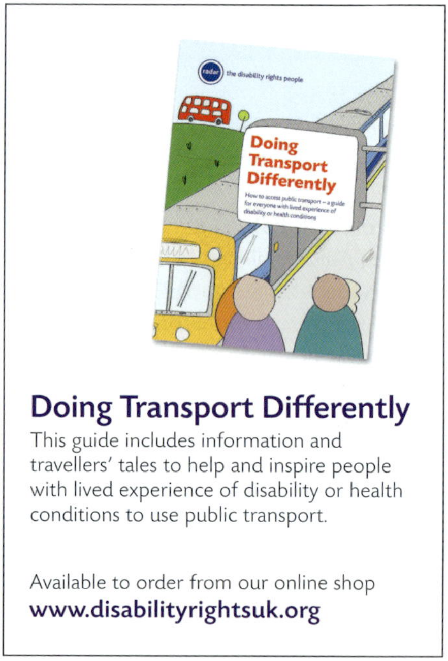

Equipment hire

SHOPMOBILITY

The National Federation of Shopmobility UK (NFSUK), PO Box 6641, Christchurch BH23 9DQ
- ☎ 0844 41 41 850
- ✉ info@shopmobilityuk.org
- 🌐 www.shopmobilityuk.org

Scheme which lends manual wheelchairs, powered wheelchairs and powered scooters to members of the public with limited mobility to shop and to visit leisure and commercial facilities within the town, city or shopping centre. You can find the nearest Shopmobility scheme to you through their on-line directory. Contact specific Shopmobility Schemes to make equipment bookings or find out more information.

Age UK Bolton

72-74 Ashburner Street, Bolton BL1 1TN
- ☎ 01204 382411
- ✉ postmaster@ageukbolton.org.uk
- 🌐 www.ageuk.org.uk/bolton

Manual wheelchairs supplied for periods of up to three weeks to Bolton residents and people over 50 visiting the area.

Blackpool Wheelchair Hire

183 Lytham Road, Blackpool FY1 6EU
- ☎ 01253 408453
- 🌐 www.blackpoolwheelchairs.co.uk

Manual and electric wheelchairs and scooters are available for hire on daily or weekly rates. Delivery to hotels in the area can be arranged.

Blackpool Shopmobility

52 Clifton Street, Blackpool FY1 1JP
- ☎ 01253 476451

Hire manual wheelchairs and scooters for use around Blackpool. Operate a door-to-door community transport service for outings in the area. Radar keys available.

The Helpful Hand

6 Chester Road, Macclesfield SK11 8DG
- ☎ 01625 424438
- 🌐 www.thehelpfulhand.co.uk

Manual and powered wheelchairs, scooters and a range of electric beds, chairs, stairlifts, commodes and incontinence equipment are available for sale and hire.

THINGS TO SEE OR DO

Forest of Bowland Tramper Trails

This area of Lancashire is designated an Area of Outstanding Natural Beauty (AONB). A Tramper is a specially designed four-wheel drive all-terrain electric buggy, which can be used off road and even on rough ground, mud and grass. Tramper Trails are designated paths for less mobile visitors along trails with fantastic views, wildlife rich hedgerows and through tranquil woodlands and parklands. All are graded using the Disabled Ramblers 1 to 5 categories. Trampers are available for hire across the area, they can be booked in advance and delivered to the start point of a particular Tramper trail.
- 🌐 www.forestofbowland.com/access-for-all

ENGLAND

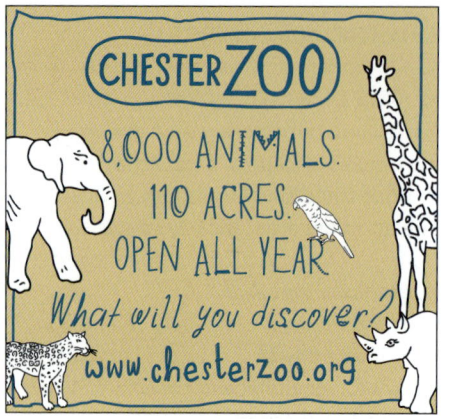

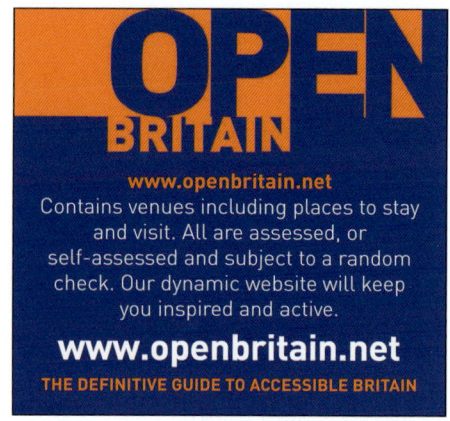

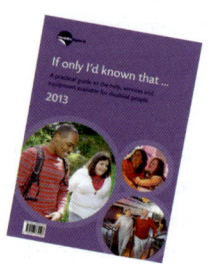

Available to order from our online shop
www.disabilityrightsuk.org

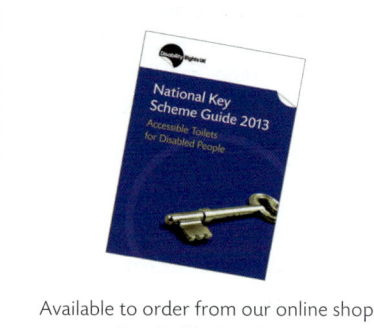

Available to order from our online shop
www.disabilityrightsuk.org

Drybeck Farm, Eden Valley

Traditional Mongolian Yurts and a gypsy caravan – equipped with a loving attention to your comfort.

Close to the Lake District, we are situated in an unspoilt, little-known area of outstanding beauty, in a stunning setting on the banks of the River Eden.

There are two steps up into our yurts and three into our toilets. Please contact us to discuss your needs and how we might meet them at Drybeck.

Phone: 0785 452 3012   www.drybeckfarm.co.uk

A unique back to nature holiday without compromising on luxury and comfort

- One mile from Armathwaite village with two pubs for eating out, village stores and a station on the famous Carlisle-Settle railway
- Within close reach of the historic city of Carlisle
- Ideally situated for walking cycling and fishing
- Enjoy our wood fired hot tub overlooking the River Eden
- Enjoy traditional ethically sourced produce straight from the fields, vegetable plot and orchard
- Children welcome to help feed the farm animals
- Dogs welcome

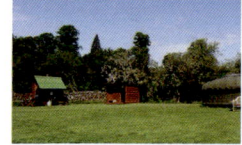
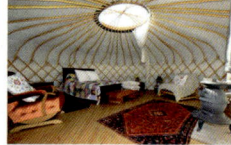

NORTH WEST ENGLAND

Fred Walton Mobility Products
308 Mosley Common Road, Worsley, Manchester M28 1DA
- 0808 108 5678
- www.fredwalton.co.uk

Sell a wide range of equipment and hire manual wheelchairs at weekly rates. Delivery throughout the country.

The Wheelchair Centre
229 Droylsden Road, Audenshaw, Manchester M34 5ZT
- 0161 370 2661/5949
- invalidaids@btconnect.com
- www.thewheelchaircentre.co.uk

Manual wheelchairs are available for hire on daily or weekly basis and lightweight scooters available by the week.

Publications

The Access Guide to Blackpool
Published by Blackpool Tourism. Available from Jubilee Tourist Information Centre, Festival House, Promenade, Blackpool FY1 1AP
- 01253 478222
- tourism@blackpool.gov.uk
- www.visitblackpool.com

Accessible Travel on Merseyside
- 0151 227 5181

Information on public transport services for disabled people in the Merseyside PTA area is available, and updated, on www.merseytravel.gov.uk. Copies in alternative formats can be obtained from Merseytravel, PO Box 1976, Liverpool L69 3HN.

Online resources

Accessible Lake District
- www.nationalparks.gov.uk/visiting/outdooractivities/accessforall/accessible-lakedistrict.htm

Site describes a series of 39 routes, suitable for people with limited mobility, throughout the Lake District.

Accessible countryside for Everyone
- www.accessiblecountryside.org.uk/northwest/cheshire

Contains information on disabled access and wheelchair walks across the countryside and green spaces of Cheshire.

Miles Without Stiles
- www.lake-district.gov.uk

An on-line guide to 41 routes in the Lake District National Park that are considered accessible for people with limited mobility. They are classified into three standards of surface and gradient as well as the distance and other features of the area. Comprehensive information on parking and toilets is also given in the 'Accessible for all' section of their website. There is also a link to a list of shorter paths and approaches to viewpoints that may be accessible to wheelchair users.

ENGLAND

Accommodation

NAS ASSESSED ACCOMMODATION

ACTON BRIDGE, Cheshire
Wall Hill Farm Guest House
Five star guest house
- 0160 685 2654
- info@wallhillfarmguesthouse.co.uk
- www.wallhillfarmguesthouse.co.uk

AINSDALE, SOUTHPORT, Merseyside
Willowbank Holiday Home and Touring Park
Five star holiday & touring park
- 01704 571566
- info@willowbankcp.co.uk
- www.willowbankcp.co.uk

ALSTON, LONGRIDGE, Lancashire
Proven House
Four star self-catering
- 01772 782653
- kenglish56@hotmail.co.uk
- www.theprovenhouse.co.uk

ALTRINCHAM, Greater Manchester
Best Western Cresta Court Hotel
Three star hotel
- 0161 927 7272
- reservations@cresta-court.co.uk
- www.cresta-court.co.uk

AMBLESIDE, Cumbria
Rothay Manor
Three star hotel
- 015394 30892
- hotel@rothaymanor.co.uk
- www.rothaymanor.co.uk

ARNSIDE, Cumbria
YHA Arnside
Three star hostel
- 0162 9592 686
- margaretgibson@yha.org.uk
- www.yha.org.uk

ASHTON WITH STODDAY, Lancashire
Ashton Hall Cottages
Four star self-catering
- 0152 4751 325
- ashtonhallcottages@googlemail.com
- www.ashtonhallcottages.co.uk

BASSENTHWAITE, Cumbria
Sandhills Farm
Four star farmhouse
- 0176 877 6307
- helen.langcake974@btinternet.com
- www.sandhillsfarm.co.uk

BLACKFORD, CARLISLE, Cumbria
Mount Farm B&B
Four star bed & breakfast
- 01228 674 641
- judith.wilson11@btinternet.com
- www.mount-farm.co.uk

BLACKPOOL, Lancashire
Big Blue Hotel
Four star hotel
- 01253 400045
- martin.jackson@bigbluehotel.com
- www.bigbluehotel.com

Ashley Victoria
Four star guest accommodation
- 0125 3348 787
- admin@blackpoolfamilyaccommodation.com
- www.blackpoolfamilyaccommodation.com

NORTH WEST ENGLAND

The Address
Three star guest accommodation
- 01253 624238
- stay@theaddressblackpool.co.uk
- www.theaddressblackpool.co.uk

The Willow Tree House
Two star guest house
- 0125 331 8613
- thebristol.guesthouse@gmail.com
- www.willowtreehouseblackpool.co.uk

Holmsdale
Three star guest house
- 01253 621008
- office@holmsdalehotel-blackpool.com
- www.holmsdalehotel-blackpool.com

The Berkeley
Three and Four star self-catering
- 01253 351244
- info@selfcatering.tv

The Lawton
Three star guest accommodation
- 01253 753471
- thelawtonhotel@gmail.com
- www.thelawtonhotel.co.uk

Coast Apartments
Four star self-catering
- 01253 351377
- enquiries@coastapartments.co.uk
- www.coastapartments.co.uk

Beachwood Guest House
Three star guest accommodation
- 01253 401951
- beachwoodguesthouse30@gmail.com
- www.beachwoodhotel.co.uk

The Beach House
Five star self-catering
- 0125 335 2699
- info@thebeachhouseblackpool.co.uk
- www.thebeachhouseblackpool.co.uk

BLEASDALE, Lancashire
Bleasdale Cottages
Four star self-catering
- 01995 61343
- info@bleasdalecottages.co.uk
- www.bleasdalecottages.co.uk

BLITTERLEES, SILLOTH, Cumbria
Rose Cottage
Four star self-catering
- 0122 8599 950
- sheena@cumbrian-cottages.co.uk
- www.cumbrian-cottages.co.uk

BOSLEY, Cheshire
Strawberry Duck Cottage
Three star self-catering
- 01260 223591
- emonthemove@hotmail.com
- www.strawberryduckcottage.co.uk

BOWNESS ON SOLWAY, Cumbria
The Old Chapel
Three star bed & breakfast
- 01697 351126
- oldchapelbowness@hotmail.com
- www.oldchapelbowness@hotmail.com

BURSCOUGH, Lancashire
Martin Lane Farmhouse Holiday Cottages
Four and five star self-catering
- 0170 489 3527
- cottages@btinternet.com
- www.martinlanefarmhouse.btinternet.co.uk

HOLIDAYS IN THE BRITISH ISLES

ENGLAND

CARLISLE, Cumbria
Old Brewery Residences
Three star self-catering
- 01228 597352
- deec@impacthousing.org.uk
- www.impacthousing.org.uk

CASTLE CARROCK, BRAMPTON, Cumbria
Tottergill Farm Cottages
Four and Five star self-catering
- 0129 7324 63
- jenny.trice@premiercottages.co.uk
- www.tottergill.co.uk

CATLOWDY, LONGTOWN, Cumbria
Bessiestown Farm Country Guesthouse
Five star guest accommodation
- 01228 577219
- info@bessiestown.co.uk
- www.bessiestown.co.uk

CATON, Lancashire
4 The Croft (Ground floor apartment)
Four star self-catering
- 01524 770725
- suebrierly@hotmail.com
- www.holiday-rentals.com/10721

CHESTER, Cheshire
The Chester Abode Limited
Four star hotel
- 0124 4347 000
- gmchester@abodehotels.co.uk
- abodehotels.co.uk/chester

Brookside Hotel
Three star small hostel
- 0124 4381 943
- mariongilfoyle@btinternet.com
- www.brookside-hotel.co.uk

CONGLETON, Cheshire
Sandhole Farm
Four star guest accommodation
- 01260 224419
- veronica@sandholefarm.co.uk
- www.sandholefarm.co.uk

Ladderstile Retreat
Five star farmhouse
- 0126 0223 338
- rose@ladderstileretreat.co.uk
- www.ladderstileretreat.co.uk

CROOK, Cumbria
Lake District Disabled Holidays
Four star self-catering
- 015394 47421
- www.lakedistrictdisabledholidays.co.uk

DOWNHOLLAND, Lancashire
Cross Farm Cottages
Four star self-catering
- 0151 5261 576
- ns.harrison@virgin.net
- crossfarmholidaycottages.co.uk

EDGWORTH, Lancashire
Meadowcroft Barn B&B
Five star farmhouse
- 0120 4853 270
- meadowcroftbarn@btinternet.com
- www.meadowcroftbarn.co.uk

NORTH WEST ENGLAND

Clough Head Farm
Four star self-catering
- 01254 704758
- ethelhoughton@hotmail.co.uk
- www.cloughheadfarm.co.uk

FRODSHAM, Cheshire

Lady Heyes Caravan Park
Four star self-catering
- 0192 8788 557
- nicole@ladyheyespark.com
- www.ladyheyespark.com

GARSTANG, Lancashire

Barnacre Cottages
Five star self-catering
- 0129 7324 63
- jenny.trice@premiercottages.co.uk
- www.barnacre-cottages.co.uk

GRANGE OVER SANDS, Cumbria

Netherwood Hotel
Three star hotel
- 015395 32552
- chris@netherwood-hotel.co.uk
- www.netherwood-hotel.co.uk

GRASMERE, Cumbria

Rothay Lodge & Rothay Lodge Apartment
Four star self-catering
- 0115 923 2618
- enquiries@rothay-lodge.co.uk
- www.rothay-lodge.co.uk

GREAT STRICKLAND, Cumbria

Strickland Manor
Five star self-catering
- 0122 8599 950
- sheena@cumbrian-cottages.co.uk
- www.cumbrian-cottages.co.uk

ISEL, COCKERMOUTH, Cumbria

Linskeldfield Tarn Holiday Cottages
Four star self-catering
- 0190 0822 136
- info@linskeldfield.co.uk
- www.linskeldfield.co.uk

KIRKOSWALD, Cumbria

Howscales
Four star self-catering
- 01768 898666
- liz@howscales.co.uk
- www.howscales.co.uk

LANGHO, Lancashire

Best Western Mytton Fold Hotel and Golf Complex
Three star hotel
- 0125 424 0662
- barbara@myttonfold.co.uk
- www.myttonfold.co.uk

LIVERPOOL, Merseyside

YHA Liverpool
Four star hostel
- 0162 9592 686
- margaretgibson@yha.org.uk
- www.yha.org.uk

Ibis Hotel
Hotel
- 0151 7069 800
- www.ibishotel.com

LONGTHWAITHE, BORROWDALE, Cumbria

YHA Borrowdale
Four star hostel
- 0162 9592 686
- margaretgibson@yha.org.uk
- www.yha.org.uk

ENGLAND

LORTON, COCKERMOUTH, Cumbria
Southwaite Green
Five star self-catering
- 0190 0821 055
- info@southwaitegreen.co.uk
- www.southwaitegreen.co.uk

LYTHAM ST ANNES, Lancashire
The Langdales Hotel
Three star hotel
- 0125 3721 342
- info@langdaleshotel.co.uk
- www.langdaleshotel.co.uk

Avondale
Four star self-catering
- 0125 378 9190
- alvinperkins2@totalise.co.uk

MACCLESFIELD, Cheshire
Kerridge End Holiday Cottages
Five star self-catering
- 0129 7324 63
- jenny.trice@premiercottages.co.uk
- www.kerridgeendholidaycottages.co.uk

MANCHESTER, Greater Manchester
The Midland – Manchester
Four star hotel
- 0161 236 3333
- PBayliss@qhotels.co.uk
- www.qhotels.co.uk

Bewleys Hotel, Manchester Airport
Hotel
- 0161 498 03 33
- manchesterairport@bewleyshotels.com
- www.bewleyshotels.com

Hilton Manchester Deansgate
Accredited hotel
- 020 7856 8380
- sales.manchester@hilton.com
- www.hilton.co.uk/manchesterdeansgate

Lancashire County Cricket Club & Old Trafford Lodge
Three star guest accommodation
- 0161 874 3333
- lodge@lccc.co.uk
- www.lccc.co.uk

YHA Manchester
Four star hostel
- 0162 9592 686
- margaretgibson@yha.org.uk
- www.yha.org.uk

MORECAMBE, Lancashire
Eden Vale Luxury Holiday Flats
Three star self-catering
- 01524 412550
- jicoombs@talktalk.net
- www.edenvalemorecambe.co.uk

MUNGRISDALE, Cumbria
Bannerdale
Self-catering
- 0176 8779 678
- enquiries@nearhowe.co.uk
- www.nearhowe.co.uk

NEWTON-IN-BOWLAND, Lancashire
Stonefold Holiday Cottage
Four star self-catering
- 07966 582834
- www.stonefoldholidaycottage.co.uk

NORTH WEST ENGLAND

PULFORD, Cheshire
Grosvenor Pulford Hotel and Spa
Four star hotel
- 01244 570560
- sue@nelsonnorthwest.co.uk
- www.grosvenorpulfordhotel.co.uk

QUERNMORE, LANCASTER, Lancashire
Knotts Farm Holiday Cottages
Four star self-catering
- 01524 63749
- stay@knottsfarm.co.uk
- www.knottsfarm.co.uk

REDMAIN, NEAR COCKERMOUTH, Cumbria
Redmain Hall Farm
Four star self-catering
- 0122 8599 950
- sheena@cumbrian-cottages.co.uk
- www.cumbrian-cottages.co.uk

RIBCHESTER, Lancashire
Riverside Barn Bed & Breakfast
Five star guest accommodation
- 0125 4878 095 / 0125 4721 000
- sarah.brotherton@btconnect.com
- www.riversidebarn.co.uk

ROCHDALE, Lancashire
Fernhill B&B
Three star bed & breakfast
- 0170 6355 671
- info@fernhillbreaks.co.uk
- www.fernhillbreaks.co.uk

SALFORD, Greater Manchester
The Lowry Hotel
Hotel
- 0161 827 4082
- rpatel@roccofortehotel.com
- www.roccofortehotels.com

SCALES, Cumbria
Scales Farm Country Guest House
Four star guest house
- 01768 779660
- scales@scalesfarm.com
- www.scalesfarm.com

SCORTON, Lancashire
Cleveley Mere Boutique Lodges
Four and five star self-catering
- 0152 479 3644
- enquiries@cleveleymere.com
- www.cleveleymere.com

SEBERGHAM, Cumbria
Monkhouse Hill Cottages
Four and Five star self-catering
- 016974 76254
- cottages@monkhousehill.com
- www.monkhousehill.co.uk

SEDBERGH, Cumbria
Hebblethwaite Hall Farm
Four star self-catering
- 015396 20094
- info@hebblethwaitehallfarm.co.uk
- www.hebblethwaitehallfarm.co.uk

SOUTHPORT, Merseyside
Sandy Brook Farm
Three star self-catering
- 01704 880337
- sandybrookfarm@gmail.com

ST BEES, Cumbria
Springbank Farm Lodges
Four star self-catering
- 01946 822 375
- stevewoodman@talk21.com
- www.springbanklodges.co.uk

ENGLAND

STAVELEY, Cumbria
Avondale
Three star self-catering
- ☎ 015394 45713
- ✉ enquiries@avondale.uk.net
- 🌐 www.avondale.uk.net

THURSTONFIELD, Cumbria
The Tranquil Otter
Five star self-catering
- ☎ 01228 576 661
- ✉ info@thetranquilotter.co.uk
- 🌐 www.thetranquilotter.co.uk

WEST KIRBY, Merseyside
Herons Well
Five star self-catering
- ☎ 0151 6251401
- ✉ stay@heronswell.co.uk
- 🌐 www.heronswell.co.uk

WHINFELL, KENDAL, Cumbria
Top Thorn Farm
Three star self-catering
- ☎ 0153 9824 252
- ✉ info.barnes@btconnect.com

WINDERMERE, Cumbria
Linthwaite House Hotel
Four star country house hotel
- ☎ 015394 88600
- ✉ Andrew@linthwaite.com
- 🌐 www.linthwaite.com

Hawksmoor Guest House
Four star guest house
- ☎ 0153 9442 110
- ✉ enquiries@hawksmoor.com
- 🌐 www.hawksmoor.com

OTHER ACCOMMODATION

AMBLESIDE, Cumbria
Nationwide Bungalow
Borrans Road, Ambleside, Cumbria LA22 0EN
- ☎ 08456 584478
- ✉ info@livability.org.uk
- 🌐 www.livability.org.uk

Holiday bungalow specially adapted for disabled people close to Lake Windermere.

BLACKPOOL, Lancashire
Century Hotel
406 North Promenade, Blackpool FY1 2LB
- ☎ 01253 354598
- 🌐 www.centuryhotel.co.uk

Family owned hotel on the seafront in Blackpool.

Elizabeth Frankland Moore Home
539 Lytham Road, Blackpool FY4 1RA
- ☎ 01253 343313
- ✉ headquarters@blesma.org
- 🌐 www.blesma.org

BLESMA nursing and residential care home for ex-service men and women on southern edge of town.

BOWNESS-ON-WINDERMERE, Cumbria
Windermere Manor
Rayrigg Road, Windermere LA23 1ES
- ☎ 0845 603 0051
- ✉ windermere.manor@actionforblindpeople.org.uk
- 🌐 www.visionhotels.co.uk

Hotel with adaptations and facilities for visually impaired people and their families and friends.

NORTH WEST ENGLAND

BROUGHTON-IN-FURNESS, Cumbria
The Kepplewray Centre
Broughton-in-Furness LA20 6HE
- 01229 716936
- web1@kepplewray.org.uk
- www.kepplewray.org.uk

Activity Centre in southern Lake District also open to people not taking part in organised programmes.

LYTHAM ST ANNES, Lancashire
St Annes Hotel
69-71 South Promenade, St Annes on Sea FY8 1LZ
- 01253 713108
- www.st-annes-hotel.com

Hotel on seafront designed for disabled guests in Lancashire.

NANTWICH, Cheshire
The Wingate Centre
Wrenbury Hall Drive, Wrenbury, Nantwich CW5 8ES
- 01270 780456
- www.wingatecentre.co.uk

Group accommodation for children and adults owned by Wingate Special Children's Trust in rural area.

SOUTHPORT, Merseyside
Salfordian Hotel
37 Park Crescent, Southport PR9 9LT
- 01704 538810
- salfordian@salford.gov.uk
- www.salford.gov.uk/salfordian

Hotel owned by a charity in own grounds.

Vitalise Sandpipers
Fairway, Southport PR9 0AL
- 0303 303 0145
- bookings@vitalise.org.uk
- www.vitalise.org.uk

Centre on shore of Marine Lake, a mile from town centre. Purpose-built for breaks for disabled people.

ENGLAND

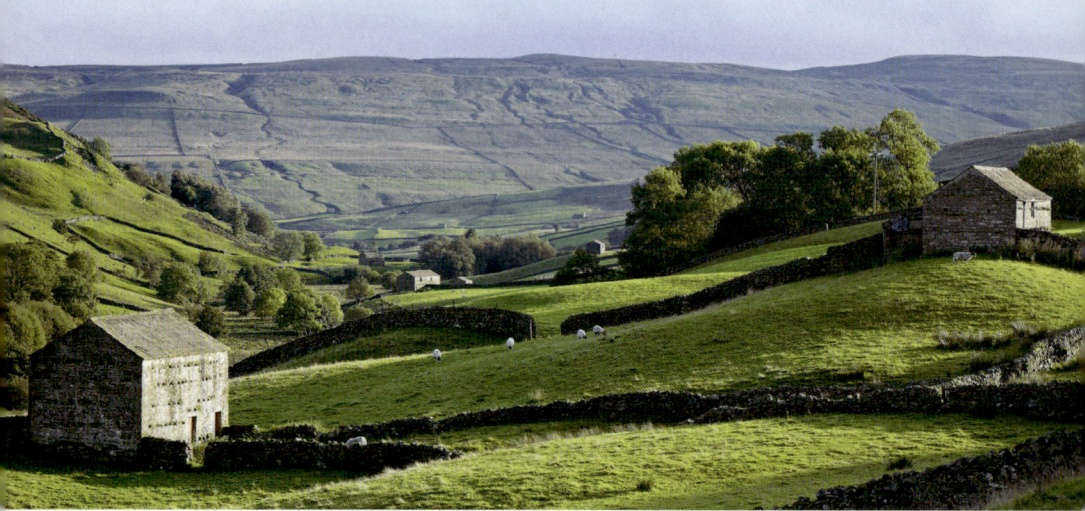

About Yorkshire

The broad acres of England's largest county stretch from the River Tees to the Humber, from the top of the Pennines to the North Sea. Within its borders are attractions for all types of holiday or short break including an increasing number of accessible accommodation and attractions.

The Yorkshire Dales are justifiably famous with deep valleys criss-crossed with limestone dry walls. Contrasting are the wild heather and bracken moors and hump-backed peaks such as Ingleborough and Whernside. One of the best ways to see the Dales is to take a ride on the Settle to Carlisle Railway, an unforgettable journey through some fine landscapes.

The other National Park, the North Yorkshire Moors, is quieter; England's largest expanse of heather moorland.

Where the moors meet the sea are some of Britain's highest cliffs, rich in fossils from the Jurassic times. Little

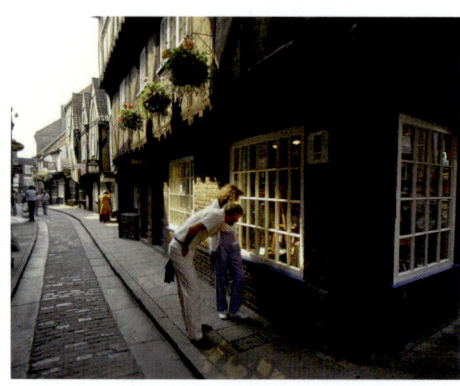

YORKSHIRE

fishing villages lay in gaps between the cliffs: Robin Hoods Bay, Staithes and Runswick Bay. Whitby is amongst them: still a working fishing port, with the smell of kipper smoking, in the shadow of the cliff top abbey.

Further down the coast is Scarborough. Two fine bays separated by a castle-topped headland and amusement arcades compete with cockle stalls – hire an all-terrain wheelchair and explore the South Bay. Nearby are Bempton cliffs; owned by the RSPB, that have some of the richest colonies of seabirds in England; make sure you go when the puffins are at home!

Yorkshire's first golden age was in the middle ages, when Cistercian monks built splendid monasteries. Most impressive is Fountains Abbey, just north of Ripon. In the 18th century its grounds were landscaped, with lakes, woods and hidden temples.

Also in this region is York; home to an impressive cathedral and a complete circle of 13th century walls. Within the walls you can find narrow streets of half-timbered houses and interesting shops. Just North of York you can explore Castle Howard, one of Britain's grandest stately homes.

Should York be a little crowded for your taste, Beverley to the south west is a smaller and much quieter version. It too has a Minster and its other church, St

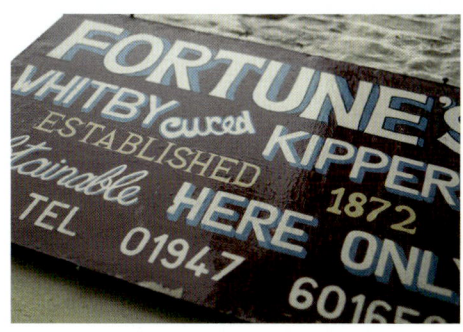

Mary's, has a 13th Century carving of a rabbit, believed to be Lewis Carroll's inspiration for the white rabbit in Alice in Wonderland.

The Southern part of Yorkshire was the heart of the industrial revolution. You will find cobbled streets and some of the countries grandest Victorian architecture. Not only in the big cities of Leeds and Bradford, but in smaller towns like Todmorden and Hebden Bridge. The cities now sport more than their fair share of galleries and museums, often filled with art treasures from local lads and lasses made good: Henry Moore at Leeds, Barbara Hepworth at Wakefield and David Hockney at Saltaire.

If you prefer gloomy and moody, head for Haworth, home to the Bronte sisters. You can get there by steam train on the Keighley and Worth Valley Railway. You can still feel the presence of the three writers in the dark vicarage where they lived with their father and wayward brother, or on the wild moors where they played as children and made up their first tales.

ENGLAND

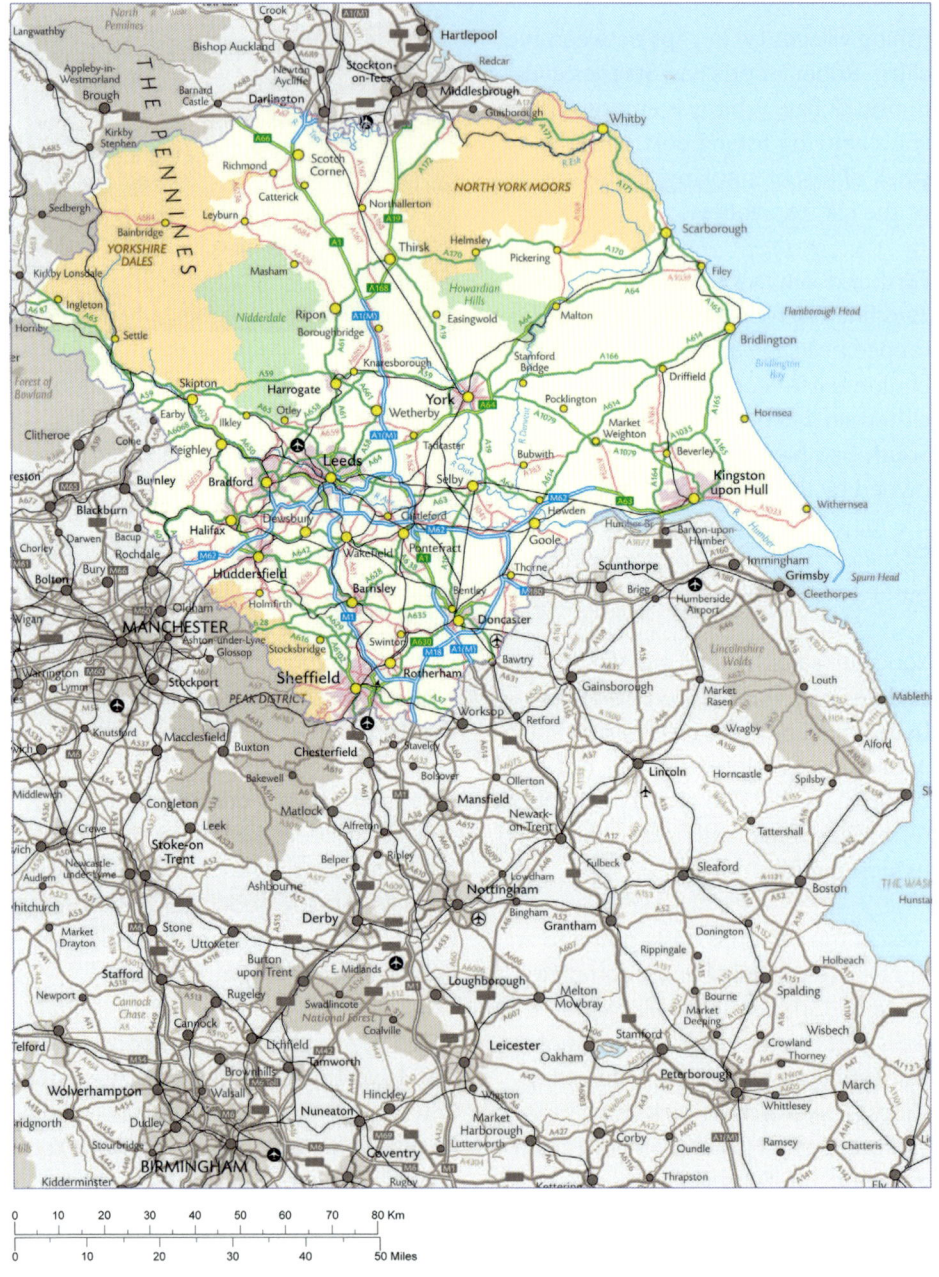

Resources

Tourism

Welcome to Yorkshire
Dry Sand Foundry, Foundry Square, Holbeck, Leeds LS11 5D
- ☎ 01904 707961
- ✉ info@yorkshire.com
- 🌐 www.yorkshire.com

Information & advice

DIAL
Offer free, impartial and confidential information and advice by telephone to disabled people, their relatives and professionals. Local branches of DIAL are constantly changing but at the time of writing, the following groups were members of DIAL UK and may be able to help visitors in their areas. Please call before travelling to check whether the service and organisation is still available:

Bradnet
- ☎ 01274 224444

Disability Advice Bradford
- ☎ 01274 594173
  Textphone 01274 530951

DIAL Doncaster
- ☎ 01302 327800
  Textphone 01302 768297

DIAL Wakefield
- ☎ 01977 723933/4
  Textphone 01977 724081

Scarborough DAG
- ☎ 01723 379397 (also Textphone)

Equipment hire

SHOPMOBILITY
The National Federation of Shopmobility UK (NFSUK), PO Box 6641, Christchurch BH23 9DQ
- ☎ 0844 41 41 850
- ✉ info@shopmobilityuk.org
- 🌐 www.shopmobilityuk.org

Scheme which lends manual wheelchairs, powered wheelchairs and powered scooters to members of the public with limited mobility to shop and to visit leisure and commercial facilities within the town, city or shopping centre. You can find the nearest Shopmobility scheme to you through their on-line directory. Contact specific Shopmobility Schemes to make equipment bookings or find out more information.

THINGS TO SEE OR DO

Castle Howard
Designed by Sir John Vanbrugh at the beginning of the 18th century, Castle Howard is one of the grandest stately homes in Britain, surrounded by extensive grounds and North Yorkshire countryside. All the rooms are accessible by wheelchair, with the exception of the High South area and Chapel. A lift is located just inside the House entrance to carry wheelchairs to the principal floor. Paths throughout the grounds are ramped for easy access and a land-train runs between the Ticket Office, House Entrance and Adventure Playground.
- 🌐 www.castlehoward.co.uk

ENGLAND

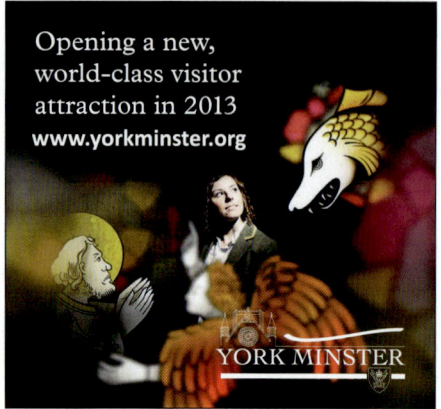

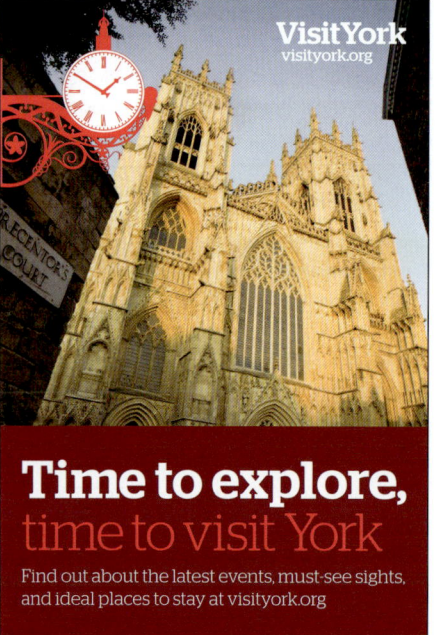

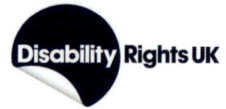

Visit our online shop

For products and books that open doors to independent living.

www.disabilityrightsuk.org

Ratcliffe Disabled Holidays
Run by disabled owner & wife
Ceiling hoists electric hi/lo beds
Wheel-in showers 4 destinations
10 Years Dedicated Service
for Care-Free Holidays
Great facilities-Plenty of space
TOP LOCATIONS & VIEWS
Lake District, East and West Coasts
Sea-front positions
HOUSE FLATS LARGE CARAVANS

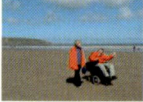 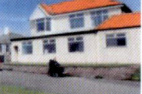

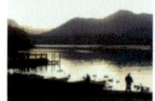 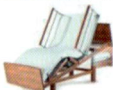

www.theukweb.com/disabledholidays
Phone Allan or Jan 01274 588142

YORKSHIRE

Bayliss Mobility Ltd
Enterprise Complex, Walmgate, York YO1 9TT
- 01904 611516
- info@livingindependent.co.uk
- www.livingindependent.co.uk

Provide second hand, but not a wide choice of wheelchairs for hire as well as selling a wide range of mobility and other equipment.

Skipton & Craven Action for Disability
46/48 Newmarket Street, Skipton BD23 2JB
- 01756 701005
- info@scad.eclipse.co.uk
- www.scad.org.uk

Operate a hire service for manual wheelchairs, an accessible minibus service and have a specially adapted canal boat for day trips. Available for groups.

Whitby & District Disablement Action Group
Church House Centre, Flowergate, Whitby YO21 3BA
- 01947 821001
- whitbydag@btconnect.com
- www.whitbydag.org.uk

Offer a wheelchair hire scheme and have manual wheelchair and scooters. Deposits and hire charges payable in advance. All-terrain wheelchairs are available to hire for use on Whitby beach.

Online resources

www.yorkshire.com/disabled-go
Hosts a wide range of information in the 'DisabledGo' and 'accessible yorkshire' sections.

The North York Moors National Park Authority
- www.moors.uk.net
- 01439 772700

Produced by the North York Moors National Park Authority, this website has a good list of easy-going walking routes, to be found under their 'Accessible Trails' section on the site, as well as a comprehensive 'Access for All' guide on accommodation, toilets and attractions.

> **THINGS TO SEE OR DO**
>
> **South Bay**
> An all-terrain Landeez wheelchair can be hired to enable disabled children and young people to enjoy closer contact with the sand and sea. It can be used on sand, rocks and snow, and is available at The Spa in Scarborough's South Bay. A small deposit is required. Anyone wishing to hire it should contact Briercliffe Children's Centre, Scarborough, on
> - 01609 798700 or 01609 798701

ENGLAND

Accommodation

NAS ASSESSED ACCOMMODATION

BALIFF BRIDGE, West Yorkshire
The Lodge at Birkby Hall
Four star bed & breakfast
- 01484 400 321
- Thelodge@birkbyhall.co.uk
- www.birkbyhall.co.uk

BOROUGHBRIDGE, North Yorkshire
Buckden Pike Loft
Five star self-catering
- 0142 3523 333
- catharine@harrogateholidays.co.uk
- www.harrogateholidays.co.uk

BRIDLINGTON, East Yorkshire
Providence Place
Four star guest house
- 01262 603 840
- enquiries@providenceplace.info
- www.providenceplace.info

Pride-N-Joy
Three star self-catering
- 0122 6390 000
- peter@pride-n-joy.co.uk
- www.pride-n-joy.co.uk

Marina Holiday Apartments
Two and Three star self-catering
- 0148 2629 063
- marinaholidays@hotmail.co.uk

BROUGH, East Yorkshire
Rudstone Walk Country Accommodation
Four star guest accommodation
- 0143 0422 230
- office@rudstone-walk.co.uk
- www.rudstone-walk.co.uk

BUCKDEN, North Yorkshire
9 Dalegarth and Heron Ghyll
Four star self-catering
- 01756 760877
- info@dalegarth.co.uk
- www.dalegarth.co.uk

EASINGWOLD, North Yorkshire
Thornton Lodge Farm
Four star farmhouse
- 01347 821306
- enquiries@thorntonlodgefarm.co.uk
- www.thorntonlodgefarm.co.uk

EBBERSTON, North Yorkshire
Cow Pasture Cottage & Swallowtail Cottage
Three and four star self-catering
- 01723 859285
- brendagreen@yorkshireancestors.com
- www.studleyhousefarm.co.uk

ELLERBY, North Yorkshire
The Ellerby
Four star inn
- 01947 840342
- dra12@live.co.uk
- www.ellerbyhotel.co.uk

YORKSHIRE

FLAMBOROUGH, East Yorkshire
Flamborough Rock Cottages
Three star self-catering
- 0126 2605 957
- jannicegeraghty@hotmail.co.uk
- www.flamboroughrockcottages.co.uk

HARWOOD DALE, North Yorkshire
The Grainary
Four star guest accommodation
- 0172 3870 026
- grainary@btopenworld.com
- www.grainary.co.uk

HELMSLEY, North Yorkshire
YHA Helmsley
Four star hostel
- 0162 9592 686
- margaretgibson@yha.org.uk
- www.yha.org.uk/hostel/helmsley

HIGH CATTON, STAMFORD BRIDGE, North Yorkshire
The Courtyard & Ruxpin Cottage
Four and five star self-catering
- 01759 371 374
- foster-s@sky.com
- www.highcattongrange.co.uk

ILKLEY, West Yorkshire
Ilkley Moor Cottages and Apartments at Westwood Lodge
Four and Five star self-catering
- 0129 7324 63
- jenny.trice@premiercottages.co.uk
- www.westwoodlodge.co.uk

KELFIELD, North Yorkshire
The Dovecote Barns York
Five star self-catering
- 01757 248 331
- info@dovecotebarnsyork.co.uk
- www.dovecotebarnsyork.co.uk

KIRKBYMOORSIDE, North Yorkshire
Partridge Cottage
Four star self-catering
- 01751 430500
- jeff.lee@dispensingdoctor.org
- www.lowhaggfarm.com

LEEDS, West Yorkshire
Weetwood Hall
Four star hotel
- 0113 2306000
- peter.chubb@weetwood.co.uk
- www.weetwood.co.uk

Storm Jameson Court, Charles Morris Hall
Accommodation within University of Leeds
- 0113 343 6085
- j.hynes@adm.leeds.ac.uk
- www.meetinleeds.co.uk

LOCKTON, North Yorkshire
YHA Lockton
Four star hostel
- 0162 9592 686
- margaretgibson@yha.org.uk
- www.yha.org.uk

MIDDLETON, West Yorkshire
The Hawthornes Lodges
Four star self-catering
- 0175 1474 755
- info@thehawthornes.co.uk
- www.thehawthornes.co.uk

HOLIDAYS IN THE BRITISH ISLES

ENGLAND

NEWTON-ON-RAWCLIFFE, North Yorkshire

Sunset Cottage
Four star self-catering
- 01751 472172
- bookings@boonhill.co.uk
- www.boonhill.co.uk

Mel House Cottages
Four star self-catering
- 01751 475396
- holiday@letsholiday.com
- www.letsholiday.com

NORTHALLERTON, North Yorkshire

Lovesome Hill Farm
Four star farmhouse
- 01609 772311
- lovesomehillfarm@btinternet.com
- www.lovesomehillfarm.co.uk

PICKERING, North Yorkshire

Eastgate Cottages
Four and five star self-catering
- 0175 1476 653
- helen.eddon@eastgatecottages.co.uk
- www.northyorkshirecottages.co.uk

Keld Head Farm Cottages
Four star self-catering
- 0129 7324 63
- jenny.trice@premiercottages.co.uk
- www.keldheadcottages.com

PONTEFRACT, West Yorkshire

Tower House Executive Guest House
Five star guest house
- 01977 699988
- towerhouse.guesthouse@virgin.net
- www.towerhouseguesthouse.com

Mel House Cottages
Newton-on-Rawcliffe, Pickering, North Yorkshire YO18 8QA
- 01751 475396
- www.letsholiday.com
- holiday@letsholiday.com
- Contact John & Penny Wicks

Four comfortable well-equipped, four star properties with indoor pool, spa and sauna. Located in attractive 'level' village in the North York Moors National Park (pub, duck pond and children's play area nearby) 4 miles from the market town of Pickering. Ideal for access to the Moors, Cropton & Dalby forests, East Yorkshire coast, the City of York and a nostalgic ride on the North York Moors Steam Railway. Accompanied, children, dogs and horses welcome! You won't be disappointed!

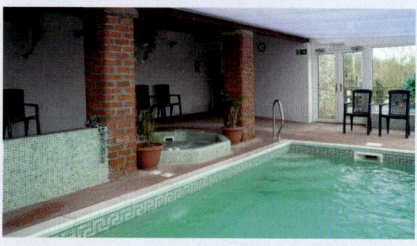

'Mallard' is 'wheelchair accessible' (NAS accredited Level 'M3 Assisted')

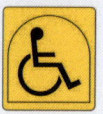
'Swift' is 'wheelchair accessible' (NAS accredited Level 'M3 independent')

'Owl' is suitable for people with mobility impairment (NAS accredited Level 'M1').

YORKSHIRE

PRESTON, HULL, East Yorkshire
Little Weghill Farm
Four star farmhouse
- 0148 2897 650
- info@littleweghillfarm.co.uk
- www.littleweghillfarm.co.uk

SANDSEND, North Yorkshire
Sandsend Bay Cottages
Four star self-catering
- 01947 893231
- info@sandsendbaycottages.co.uk
- www.sandsendbaycottages.co.uk

SAWDON, North Yorkshire
Basin Howe Farm Cottages
Four star self-catering
- 0172 3850 180
- info@basinhowefarm.co.uk
- www.basinhowefarm.co.uk

SCARBOROUGH, North Yorkshire
Scarborough Travel and Holiday Lodge
Three star guest accommodation
- 0172 3363 537
- helen.dean@hotel-group.co.uk
- www.scarborough-lodge.co.uk

Inglenook Guest House
Five star guest house
- 0172 3369 454
- inglenookguesthouse@live.co.uk
- www.inglenookscarborough.co.uk

SEWERBY, East Yorkshire
Field House Farm Cottages
Four and Five star self-catering
- 01262 674932
- john.foster@fieldhousefarmcottages.co.uk
- www.fieldhousefarmcottages.co.uk

STANNINGTON, South Yorkshire
The Cart Shed
Four star self-catering
- 0114 2302 122
- moorwoodequine@googlemail.com
- www.cottage.moorwoodequine.co.uk

STAPE, North Yorkshire
Rawcliffe House Farm
Four star self-catering
- 01751 473292
- stay@rawcliffehousefarm.co.uk
- www.rawcliffehousefarm.co.uk

SUMMERBRIDGE, North Yorkshire
Helme Pasture
Four star self-catering
- 01423 780279
- info@helmepasture.co.uk
- www.helmepasture.co.uk

SWINTON, MALTON, North Yorkshire
Walnut Garth
Four star self-catering
- 01653 691293
- cas@walnutgarth.co.uk
- www.walnutgarth.co.uk

THE BAY, FILEY, North Yorkshire
Bempton Holiday Villa
Four star self-catering
- 0172 3588 042
- thebay@wilfward.org.uk
- www.bemptonholidayvilla.co.uk

THORPE BASSETT, North Yorkshire
The Old Post Office
Four star self-catering
- 01944 758047
- ssimpsoncottages@aol.com
- www.ssimpsoncottages.co.uk

ENGLAND

WAINSTALLS, West Yorkshire
The Crossroads Inn
Four star inn
- ☎ 01422 248151
- ✉ info@thecrossroadsinn.co.uk
- 🌐 www.thecrossroadsinn.co.uk

WHITBY, North Yorkshire
YHA Whitby
Four star hostel
- ☎ 0162 9592 686
- ✉ margaretgibson@yha.org.uk
- 🌐 www.yha.org.uk

Captain Cook's Haven
Three and Four star self-catering
- ☎ 01947 893573
- 🌐 www.hoseasons.co.uk

Whitby Holiday Park
Four star holiday and touring park
- ☎ 01947 602664
- ✉ shelley@normanhurst.net
- 🌐 www.whitbypark.co.uk

> **THINGS TO SEE OR DO**
>
> **Aysgarth Falls**
> Set within the Yorkshire Dales National Park, Aysgarth Falls is a series of cascading falls separated into three forces. The Trail to nearby Freeholders' Wood is a level footpath with great views of the Middle Falls. All gates are accessible and there are seating areas along the route. A further route can be followed along a mud track through the woodland. The National Park Centre café nearby is wheelchair accessible. There are public toilets, including NKS toilets, at the National Park Centre.

WRELTON, North Yorkshire
Beech Farm Cottages
Four and five star self-catering
- ☎ 01751 476612
- ✉ holiday@beechfarm.com
- 🌐 www.beechfarm.com

YAPHAM, East Yorkshire
Wolds View Holiday Cottages
Four and Five star self-catering
- ☎ 01759 302172
- 🌐 www.woldsviewcottages.co.uk

YORK, North Yorkshire
Best Western Monkbar Hotel
Three star hotel
- ☎ 01904 638086
- ✉ gm@monkbarhotel.co.uk
- 🌐 www.monkbarhotel.co.uk

Pound Cottage, Copper Cottage & Crown Cottage
Four star self-catering
- ☎ 01757 248203
- ✉ info@southnewlandsfarm.co.uk
- 🌐 www.southnewlandsfarm.co.uk

OTHER ACCOMMODATION

BEAMSLEY, North Yorkshire
The Beamsley Project
Harrogate Road, Hazlewood, Skipton BD23 6JA
- ☎ 01756 710255
- ✉ info@beamsleyproject.org
- 🌐 www.beamsleyproject.org

Holiday centre in Yorkshire Dales for groups of disabled people and their companions.

YORKSHIRE

BEVERLEY, East Yorkshire

Rudstone Walk Country Cottages
South Cave, Brough, East Yorkshire HU15 2AH
- 01430 422230
- admin@rudstone-walk.co.uk
- www.rudstone-walk.co.uk

Cottages designed for disabled people overlooking The Wolds and Humber.

SKIPSEA, East Yorkshire

Holiday Homes Trust Caravan
Low Skirlington Leisure Park, Skipsea YO25 8SY
Holiday Homes Trust
- scout.holiday.homes@scouts.org.uk
- www.holidayhomestrust.org

Unit on family owned site near Driffield.

YORK, North Yorkshire

Woodlands Respite Care Centre
120 Thief Lane, Hull Road, York YO10 3HU
- 01904 430600
- woodlands@christchurchgroup.co.uk
- http://christchurchgroup.co.uk/facilities/york

Purpose-built centre to meet the needs of people with multiple sclerosis. Located in own grounds to the east of the city of York.

THIRSK, North Yorkshire

Linden Tree
Carlton Road, Carlton Miniott, Thirsk, North Yorkshire YO7 4LX
- 01845 523765
- ptearall@btinternet.com
- www.visitlindentree.co.uk

We offer family run holiday cottages and bed & breakfast accommodation in an ideal location for exploring the Yorkshire Dales and the North Yorkshire Moors, with opportunities for walks and fishing nearby. Our bed & breakfast accommodation is on ground level, and we offer wide doors and a shower room fitted for wheelchair access. Start your day with a hearty traditional breakfast, with continental and vegetarian options available on request. York, Harrogate and Teeside are easily accessible. A warm welcome awaits you at Linden Tree.

ENGLAND

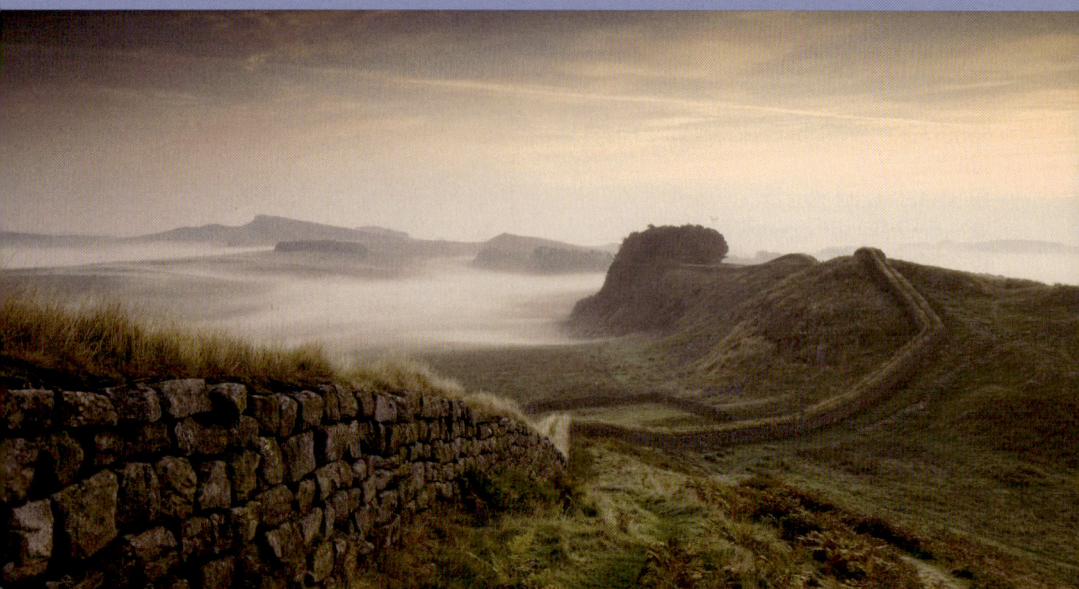

About North East England

The North East region covers the area between the Tees Valley and the Scottish border including County Durham, Northumberland and Tyne and Wear. Within its boundaries are the natural wild areas of the northern Pennines, the dramatic Northumberland Coast, the Tyne valley and the extensive Northumberland National Park.

Much of Britain's history was moulded in this Region. Hadrian's Wall, now a World Heritage Site, was for centuries the northern boundary of the Roman Empire. The Wall and its associated areas can be explored at many sites and via the accessible Hadrian's Wall Country Bus. Britain's early Christian heritage is represented by Lindisfarne Priory on Holy Island near Berwick-upon-Tweed and in this region you can also visit the majestic Durham Cathedral and the historic Bede's World Anglo-Saxon museum at Jarrow. Evidence of the turbulent Middle Ages can be seen at castles such as Bamburgh and Barnard which houses the Bowes Museum, the North's greatest collection of fine and decorative art.

With its extensive coastline, the area has a long seafaring tradition. Captain Cook was born near Middlesbrough where his life and achievements are depicted at the Captain Cook Birthplace Museum. A replica of his ship, 'Endeavour' can be

NORTH EAST ENGLAND

seen at Stockton-on-Tees and an 1800's quayside has been reconstructed at Hartlepool.

The Industrial Revolution brought pioneering developments in mining, engineering, shipbuilding and other heavy industry to the region as depicted at the Discovery Museum in Newcastle. The world's first public railway ran between Stockton and Darlington and the railway heritage is widely displayed including at Locomotion, the National Railway Museum's centre at Shildon in County Durham.

As to the present and future, one of the country's most prominent works of art, the Angel of the North, greets travellers approaching Gateshead where, on the southern bank of the Tyne, the Baltic Centre for Contemporary Art and the

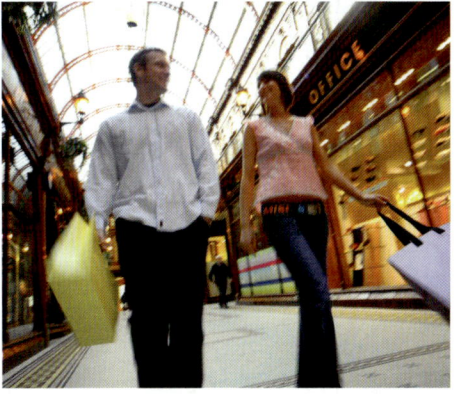

Sage Music Performance Centre were built to mark the Millennium. Across the river in the lively regional capital of Newcastle upon Tyne, another Millennium project, the Life Science Centre focuses on the science of genetics. Holiday shoppers can choose between Newcastle's city centre shops around Eldon Square or the out-of-town MetroCentre in Gateshead.

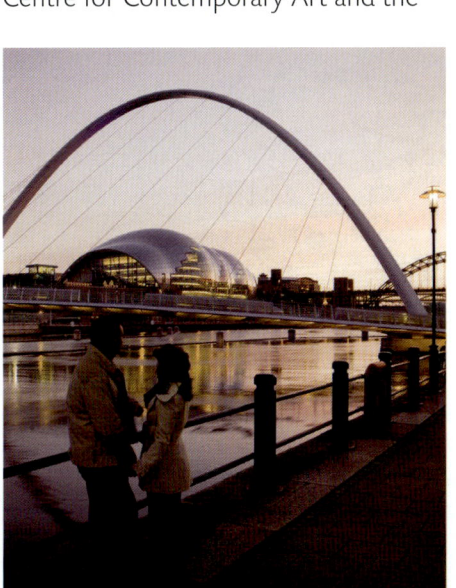

There are many opportunities for countryside recreation and outdoor activities in the region. Kielder Forest, Europe's largest man-made woodland, has a visitor centre at Kielder Castle and a wide range of water sports are available on Kielder Water as well as trips on an accessible cruiser. The Wildfowl & Wetlands Trust has a centre at Washington near Sunderland. At Alnwick in Northumberland, the Gardens of the Castle have been recreated – try the accessible treetop walkway. The Castle itself has frequently appeared on large and small screens, most notably in the first two Harry Potter films.

ENGLAND

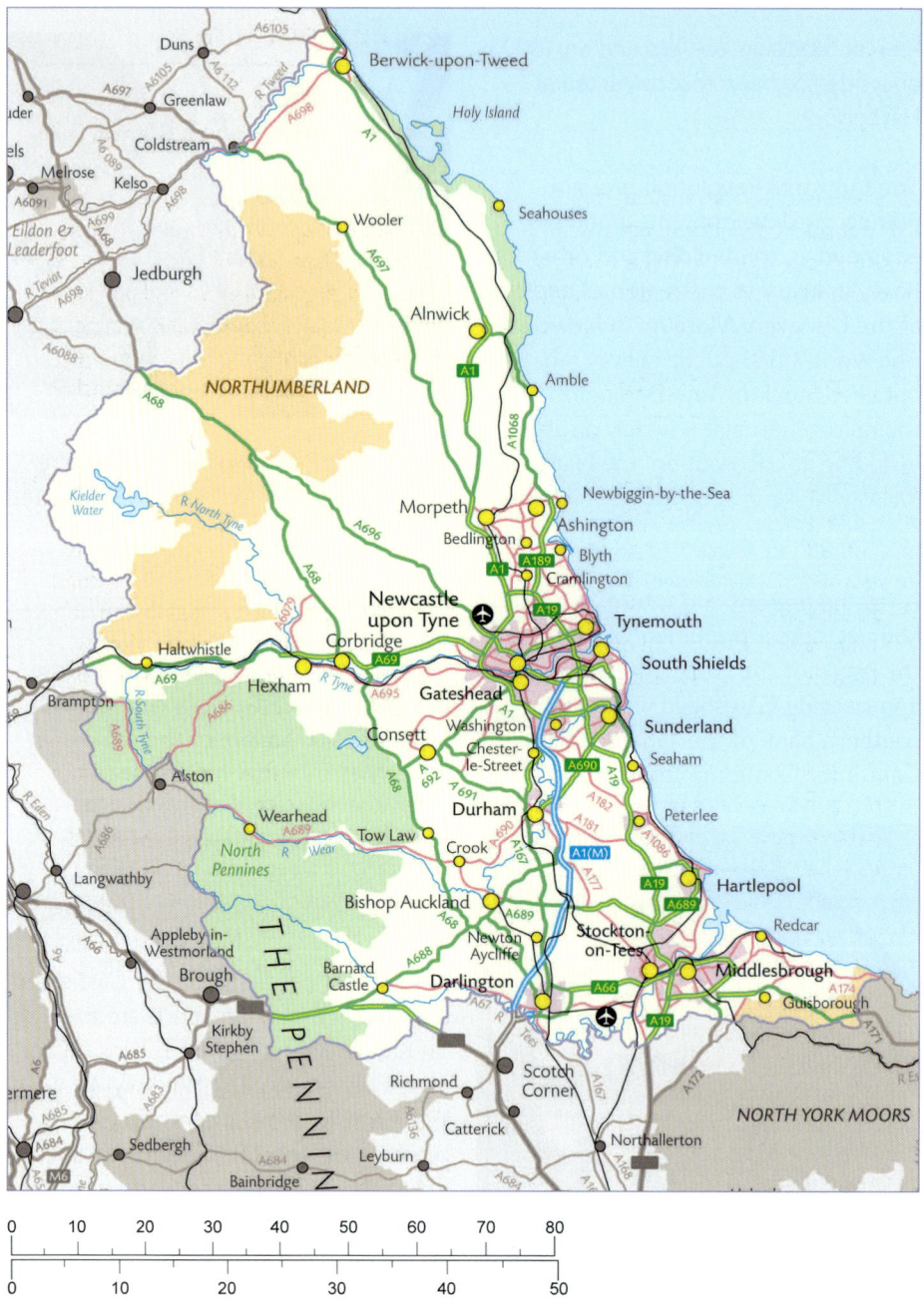

Resources

Tourism

North East England Tourism
- www.visitnortheastengland.com

This website hosts links to numerous tourist offices in the North East and general information on what to do when visiting.

Information & advice

Disability North
The Dene Centre, Castles Farm Road, Newcastle upon Tyne NE3 1PH
- 0191 284 0480
- reception@disabilitynorth.org.uk
- disabilitynorth.org.uk

The Information Service can offer advice on holiday accessible holiday accommodation.

DIAL
Offer free, impartial and confidential information and advice by telephone to disabled people, their relatives and professionals. Local branches of DIAL are constantly changing but at the time of writing, the following groups were members of DIAL UK and may be able to help visitors in their areas. Please call before travelling to check whether the service and organisation is still available:

BLISS-Ability, South Shields
- 0191 427 1666 (also Textphone)

Darlington Association on Disability
- 01325 489999

Equipment hire

Adapt-ABILITY
Sanderson Street, Coxhoe, Durham DH6 4DF
- 0800 0925092
- info@adapt-ability.co.uk
- www.adapt-ability.co.uk

This company has manual and powered wheelchairs and scooters and a range of other equipment for hire from the above address and also from a branch in Hartlepool.

THINGS TO SEE OR DO

Durham Cathedral

In November 2012, a revamped part of the Cathedral was officially opened, improving disabled access to one of the UK's greatest historic landmark buildings significantly. The launch of the Undercroft Foyer and new shop brings visitor amenities together in one location. The steps into the area have been re-modeled, making space for a new platform lift resulting in shorter distances to negotiate for disabled visitors. Baroness Tanni Grey-Thompson called the new area "an open, welcoming and absolutely stunning space" (*The Northern Echo*).

SHOPMOBILITY
The National Federation of Shopmobility UK (NFSUK), PO Box 6641, Christchurch BH23 9DQ
- 0844 4141 850
- Info@shopmobilityuk.org
- www.shopmobilityuk.org

ENGLAND

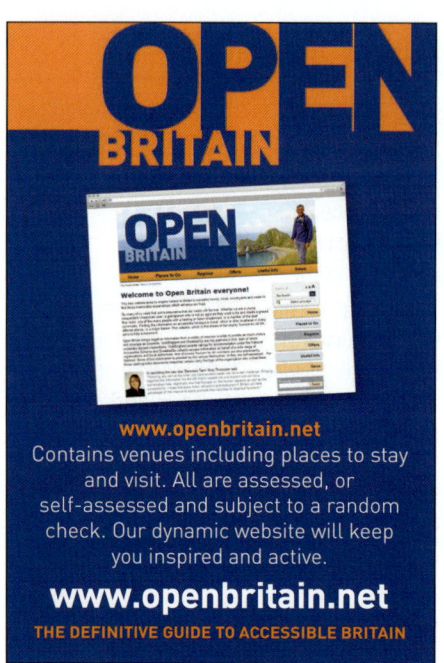

www.openbritain.net

Contains venues including places to stay and visit. All are assessed, or self-assessed and subject to a random check. Our dynamic website will keep you inspired and active.

www.openbritain.net

THE DEFINITIVE GUIDE TO ACCESSIBLE BRITAIN

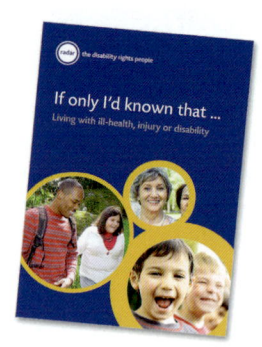

If Only I'd Known That ...

An information-packed guide to services, welfare rights, facilities and support for anyone with a disability or health condition, this guide includes resources for all ages from childhood to later years.

Available to order from our online shop
www.disabilityrightsuk.org

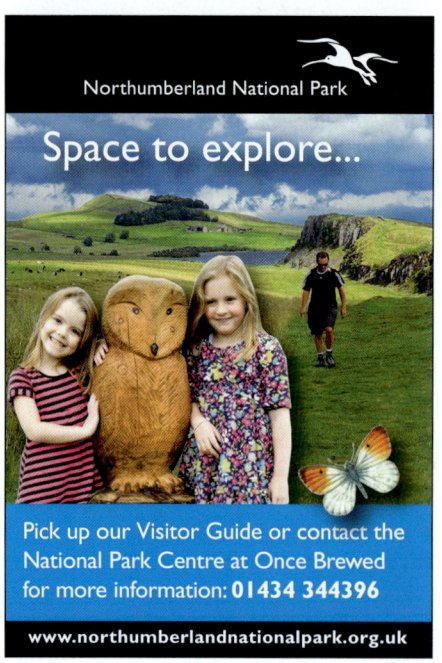

Northumberland National Park

Space to explore...

Pick up our Visitor Guide or contact the National Park Centre at Once Brewed for more information: 01434 344396

www.northumberlandnationalpark.org.uk

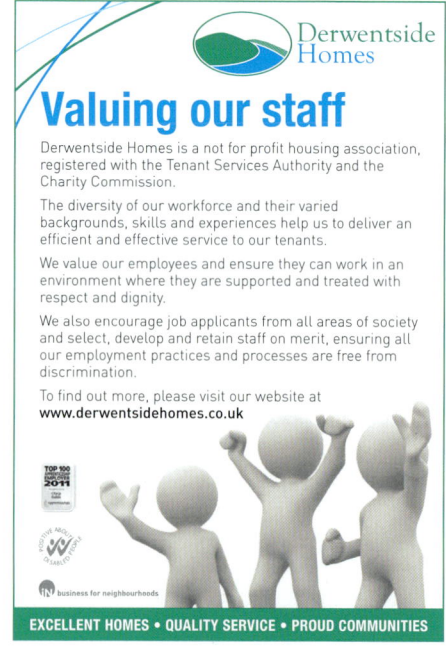

Derwentside Homes

Valuing our staff

Derwentside Homes is a not for profit housing association, registered with the Tenant Services Authority and the Charity Commission.

The diversity of our workforce and their varied backgrounds, skills and experiences help us to deliver an efficient and effective service to our tenants.

We value our employees and ensure they can work in an environment where they are supported and treated with respect and dignity.

We also encourage job applicants from all areas of society and select, develop and retain staff on merit, ensuring all our employment practices and processes are free from discrimination.

To find out more, please visit our website at
www.derwentsidehomes.co.uk

EXCELLENT HOMES • QUALITY SERVICE • PROUD COMMUNITIES

NORTH EAST ENGLAND

Scheme which lends manual wheelchairs, powered wheelchairs and powered scooters to members of the public with limited mobility to shop and to visit leisure and commercial facilities within the town, city or shopping centre. You can find the nearest Shopmobility scheme to you through their on-line directory. Contact specific Shopmobility Schemes to make equipment bookings or find out more information.

THINGS TO SEE OR DO

Hadrian's Wall Country Bus
Northumberland
The award-winning Hadrian's Wall Country Bus AD122 runs from Newcastle Central Station to Carlisle with connecting services to Bowness-on-Solway. Low-floor buses can take wheelchairs. There is a more frequent service to the main Roman sites in the central section. English National Concessionary Travel Scheme passes can be used on the AD122. The service operates between Good Friday and the end of October. For timetables contact:
- 0143 322002
- www.hadrians-wall.org

Publications

County Durham Access Directory
- 0191 383 5383

A booklet published regularly, giving information for people with disabilities about transport services in the county. Available in print, Braille or on tape by post from Passenger Transport, Durham County Council, Environment & Technical Services, County Hall, Durham DH1 5UQ.

Accommodation

NAS ASSESSED ACCOMMODATION

ALNWICK, Northumberland
Holly Lodge
Five star guest house
- 0166 5602 743
- info@hollylodgealnwick.co.uk
- www.hollylodgealnwick.co.uk

BAMBURGH, Northumberland
Outchester & Ross Farm Cottages
Four and Five star self-catering
- 01668 213228
- jbs@rossfarm.f2s.com
- www.rosscottages.co.uk

BARDON MILL, Northumberland
Coach House B&B
Four star bed & breakfast
- 01434 344 779
- mail@bardonmillcoachhouse.co.uk
- www.bardonmillcoachhouse.co.uk

Old High Shield
Four star self-catering
- 0143 434 4791
- highshield@btinternet.com
- www.highshield.co.uk

BEAL, BERWICK-UPON-TWEED, Northumberland
Fenham Farm, Coastal Bed & Breakfast
Four star guest accommodation
- 0128 9381 245
- gillcurry@hotmail.com
- www.fenhamfarm.co.uk

ENGLAND

BELFORD, Northumberland
Elwick Farm Cottages
Four star self-catering
- 01668 213259
- w.r.reay@talk21.com
- www.elwickcottages.co.uk

BELLINGHAM, Northumberland
Brownrigg Lodges
Three star self-catering
- 01434 220 272
- mac.kent@virgin.net
- www.brownrigg-lodges.com

BERWICK-UPON-TWEED, Northumberland
Meadow Hill Guest House
Four star guest house
- 01289 306235
- christineabart@aol.com
- www.meadow-hill.co.uk

West Ord Holiday Cottages
Three and four star self-catering
- 01289 386631
- stay@westord.co.uk
- www.westord.co.uk

Skylark Cottage
Four star self-catering
- 01228 599 950
- sheena@cumbrian-cottages.co.uk
- www.northumbrian-cottages.info

BINGFIELD, Northumberland
The Hytte
Five star self-catering
- 01434 672321
- srgregory@thehytte.com
- www.thehytte.com

BOWES, Durham
Mellwaters Barn
Four star self-catering
- 01833 628181
- mellwatersbarn@aol.com
- www.mellwatersbarn.co.uk

BUTTERKNOWLE, Durham
Little Owl Lodge
Four star self-catering
- 0138 8710 749
- yvonne@alpacas-easthowle.co.uk
- www.alpacas-easthowle.co.uk

CHATHILL, NORTHUMBERLAND, Northumberland
Doxford Hall Hotel & Spa
Four star country house hotel
- 0166 5589 700
- david.hunter@doxfordhall.com
- www.doxfordhall.com

Doxford Cottages
Five star self-catering
- 01665 589 393
- alun@doxfordcottages.co.uk
- www.doxfordcottages.co.uk

COCKFIELD, BISHOP AUCKLAND, Durham
Swallows Nest
Four star self-catering
- 01388 718251
- info@farmholidaysuk.com
- www.farmholidaysuk.com

NORTH EAST ENGLAND

CORNHILL ON TWEED, Northumberland
The Collingwood Arms Hotel
Three star hotel
- 01890 882424
- enquiries@collingwoodarms.com
- www.collingwoodarms.com

CORNRIGGS, COWSHILL, Durham
Cornriggs Cottages
Five star self-catering
- 0169 7746 777
- enquiries@northumbria-byways.com
- www.northumbria-byways.com

CRAMLINGTON, Northumberland
Burradon Farm Cottages and Houses
Four and Five star self-catering
- 0191 447 4616
- judy@burradonfarm.co.uk
- www.burradonfarm.co.uk

CRASTER, Northumberland
Craster Pine Lodges
Four star self-catering
- 01665 576286
- info@crasterholidays.co.uk
- www.crasterpinelodges.co.uk

DARLINGTON, Durham
River Cottage
Five star self-catering
- 01325 730 059
- sarahrutter@me.com
- www.rivercottagegainford.co.uk

EDLINGHAM, Northumberland
Lumbylaw Cottages
Four star self-catering
- 0166 5574 277
- holidays@lumbylaw.co.uk
- www.lumbylaw.co.uk

GAINFORD, Durham
East Greystone Farm Cottages
Four and five star self-catering
- 01325 730236
- sue@holidayfarmcottages.co.uk
- www.holidayfarmcottages.co.uk

GATESHEAD QUAYS, Tyne-and-Wear
Jurys Inn Newcastle Gateshead Quays
Three star hotel
- 0191 401 6800
- suzanne_cannon@jurysinns.com
- www.jurysinns.com

HAYDON BRIDGE, Northumberland
The Old Farmhouse, Grindon Farm
Four star self-catering
- 0143 468 4273
- chris@grindonfarm.co.uk
- www.grindonfarm.co.uk

Shaftoe's
Four star guest house
- 0143 4600 533
- bookings@shaftoes.co.uk
- www.shaftoes.co.uk

Grindon Cartshed
Four star bed & breakfast
- 01434 684273
- cartshed@grindon.force9.co.uk
- www.grindonfarm.co.uk

HIGH HESLEDEN, Durham
The Ship Inn
Four star inn
- 01429 836 453
- sheila@theshipinn.net
- www.theshipinn.net

ENGLAND

INGLETON, Durham
Mill Granary Cottages
Five star self-catering
- T: 0129 7324 63
- E: jenny.trice@premiercottages.co.uk
- W: www.millgranary.co.uk

INGRAM, Northumberland
Cheviot Holiday Cottages
Five star self-catering
- T: 0129 7324 63
- E: jenny.trice@premiercottages.co.uk
- W: www.cheviotholidaycottages.co.uk

KIELDER, Northumberland
Calvert Trust Kielder
Four star self-catering
- T: 01434 250232
- E: tara.martin@calvert-kielder.com
- W: www.calvert-trust.org.uk

Falstone Barns
Five star self-catering
- T: 01434 240251
- E: info@falstonebarns.com
- W: www.falstonebarns.com

KIRKNEWTON, Northumberland
Crookhouse
Four star self-catering
- T: 0129 7324 63
- E: jenny.trice@premiercottages.co.uk
- W: www.crookhouse.co.uk

LAMBLEY, NR BRAMPTON, Northumberland
Clover Hill Cottage
Four star self-catering
- T: 07834 068316
- E: erringtonfarms@live.com
- W: www.cloverhillcumbria.co.uk

LONGHORSLEY, Northumberland
Linden Hall Golf & Country Club
Four star country house hotel
- T: 01670 500000
- E: seamus.coen@macdonald-hotels.co.uk
- W: www.MacdonaldHotels.co.uk/LindenHall

Beacon Hill Farm
Four and five star self-catering
- T: 01670 780900
- E: alun@beaconhill.co.uk
- W: www.beaconhill.co.uk

NEWBROUGH, HEXHAM, Northumberland
Carr Edge Farm
Four star farmhouse
- T: 01434 674788
- E: stay@carredge.co.uk
- W: www.carredge.co.uk

NEWCASTLE UPON TYNE, Tyne & Wear
Hilton Newcastle Gateshead
Accredited hotel
- T: 020 7856 8380
- W: www.hilton.com

Euro Hostel Newcastle
Four star hostel
- T: 08454 900372
- E: newcastle@euro-hostels.co.uk
- W: www.euro-hostels.co.uk

NORTH CHARLTON, Northumberland
The Reading Rooms
Four star self-catering
- T: 01665 600850
- E: enquiries@northumberlandcottages.com
- W: www.northumberlandcottages.com

NORTH EAST ENGLAND

QUEBEC, Durham
Hamsteels Hall Cottages
Four star self-catering
- T 01207 520388
- E june@hamsteelshall.co.uk
- W www.hamsteelshall.co.uk

ROCHESTER, Northumberland
Redesdale Arms
Four star inn
- T 0183 0520 668
- E info@redesdale-hotel.co.uk
- W www.redesdale-hotel.co.uk

SHILBOTTLE, Northumberland
Village Farm
Three, four and five star self-catering
- T 01665 575591
- E crissy@villagefarmcottages.co.uk
- W www.villagefarmcottages.co.uk

SLALEY, NR HEXHAM, Northumberland
The Old Byre (Rye Hill Farm)
Four star self-catering
- T 01434 673259
- E info@ryehillfarm.co.uk
- W www.ryehillfarm.co.uk

SUNNISIDE, NR NEWCASTLE, Tyne & Wear
Hedley Hall Country Cottages
Four star self-catering
- T 0120 7231 835
- E hedleyhall@aol.com
- W www.newcastleselfcatering.co.uk

WARKWORTH, Northumberland
Garden Cottage
Four star self-catering
- T 0191 3883 752
- E info@coquetcottages.co.uk
- W www.coquetcottages.co.uk

WINSTON, Durham
Alwent Mill Cottage
Four star self-catering
- T 01325 730479
- E libby@alwentmill.co.uk
- W www.alwentmillcottage.co.uk

WOOLER, Northumberland
Fenton Hill Farm Cottages
- T 01668 216228
- E stay@fentonhillfarm.co.uk
- W www.fentonhillfarm.co.uk

OTHER ACCOMMODATION

BERWICK-UPON-TWEED, Northumberland
Ord House Country Park
East Ord, Berwick-upon-Tweed TD15 2NS
- T 01289 305288
- E enquiries@ordhouse.co.uk
- W www.ordhouse.co.uk

Park for touring caravans in village near Berwick.

SCOTLAND

> *From stunning natural and historic landscapes, surprising wildlife and delicious food & drink, you can find nature right on your doorstep.*

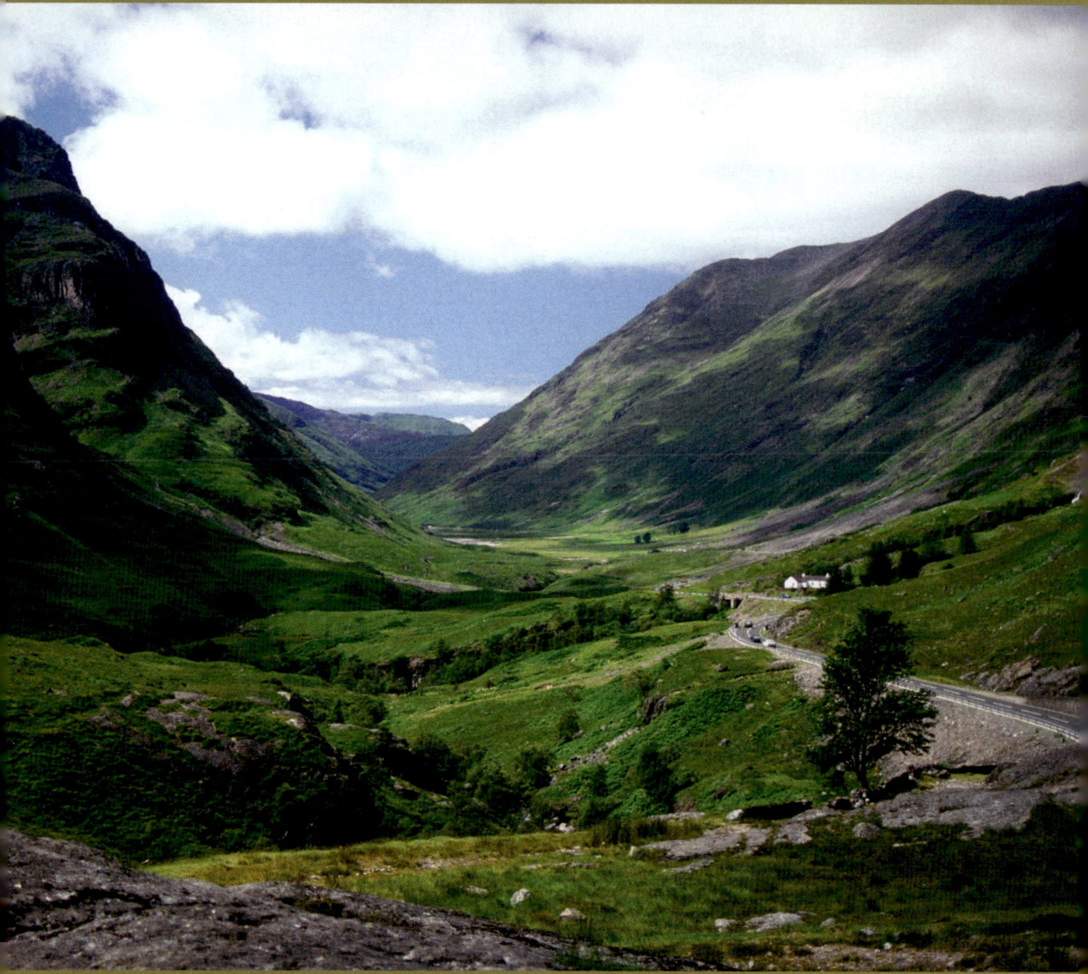

Scotland

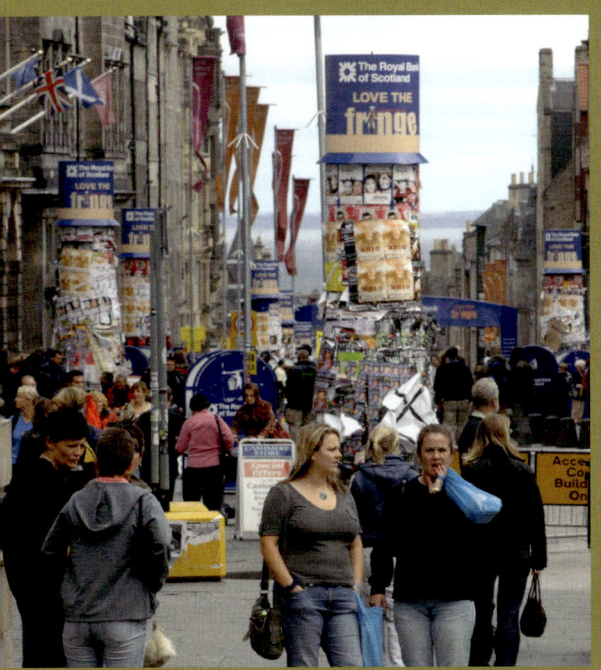
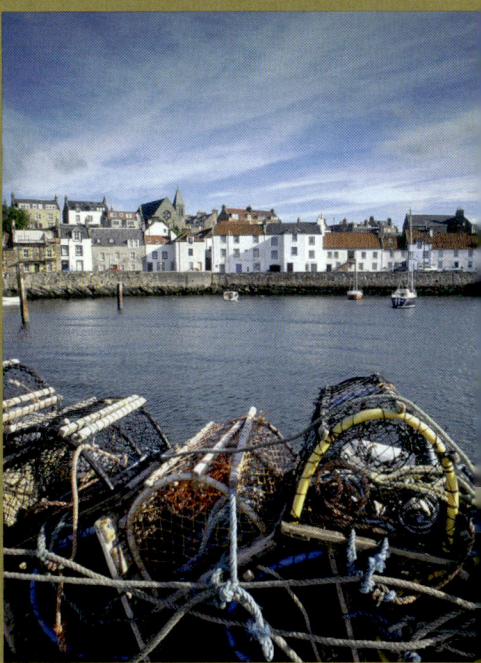
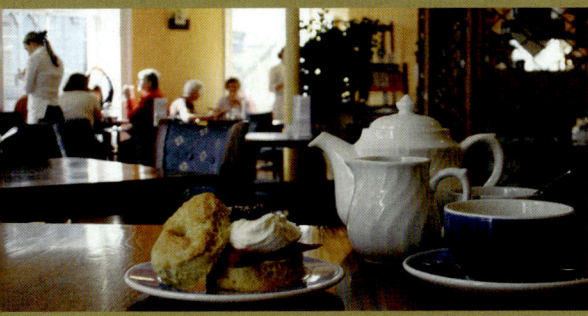

" *Scotland offers an amazing range of landscapes, from gentle rolling hills to breathtaking peaks, rugged coastlines and lochs to sub-tropical gardens.* "

SCOTLAND

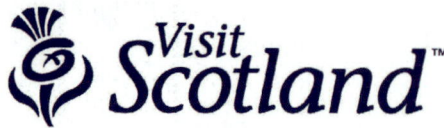

Visit Scotland

As a place to visit for a wonderful holiday, Scotland is hard to beat. We have great places to stay, warm, friendly people, inspiring scenery, superb food and drink, a fascinating culture and history, plus a vast range of things to see and do.

The drama and sheer variety of Scotland's natural features never fails to impress visitors. Though small, the country offers an amazing range of landscapes, from the gentle rolling hills of Dumfries and Galloway to the breath-taking peaks of the Cairngorms, and from the rugged coastlines of the north east to the sub-tropical gardens of Wester Ross. Explore Scotland's lochs and mountains, its interesting geography and its gloriously unpredictable climate.

There are a million ways to fill your holiday in Scotland with many things to see and do. Step onboard an historic boat, take a train ride through a former film set, taste stunning local food or go behind the scenes at whisky distilleries – there are many places to visit in Scotland, whatever your interest. Tourist attractions include charming castles and country houses, fascinating museums and friendly wildlife parks. Unleash your wild side with adventure activities or look out for local wildlife during a quiet stroll or cycle along one of the national cycle routes.

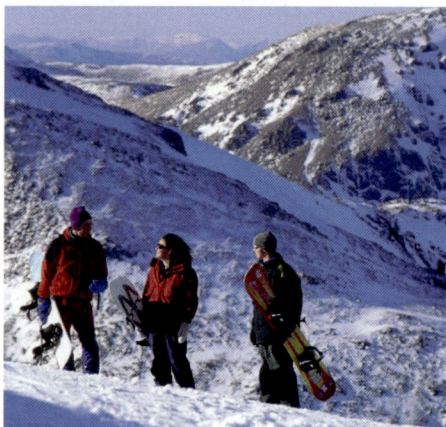

SCOTLAND

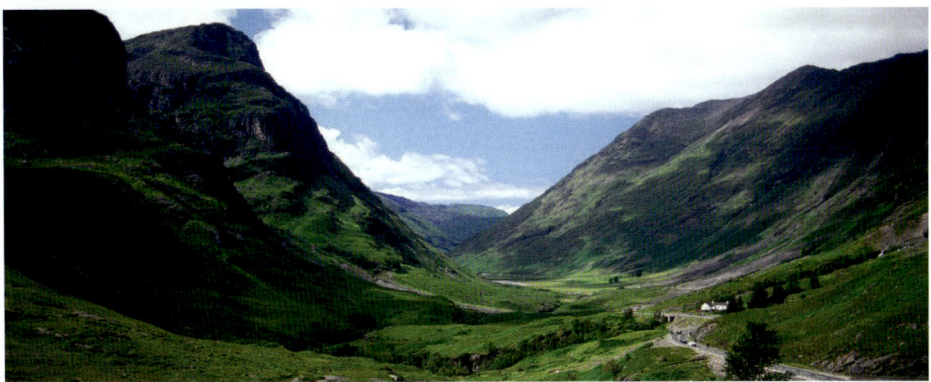

Discover the different historical and cultural elements that can be rightly claimed to be unique to this country.

Year of Natural Scotland 2013

Whatever you want from your holiday, Scotland is waiting to be discovered. We're proud of our beautiful country, proud of our traditions and our history and we look forward to sharing them with you.

2013: Year of Natural Scotland
Come and celebrate Scotland's outstanding natural beauty throughout 2013. From stunning natural and historic landscapes, art inspired by nature, surprising wildlife and delicious food and drink, you can find nature right on your doorstep. Don't miss the chance to experience the great Scottish outdoors for yourself, join in the celebrations with a packed programme of events and discover insider tips from across the country during the Year of Natural Scotland.

Accessible Scotland
If you are planning a holiday in Scotland and have a mobility impairment, then there are a number of ways to choose accommodation and activities that are suitable to your needs. Visit **www.visitscotland.com/guide/where-to-stay/accessible-scotland** and use the links at the foot of the page to check for accommodation that can meet your requirements. Or contact us directly at **info@visitscotland.com** to let VisitScotland advisors not only help find the right place – but also book it for you.

Surprise yourself!

Find out more information about Scotland at:
www.visitscotland.com

SCOTLAND

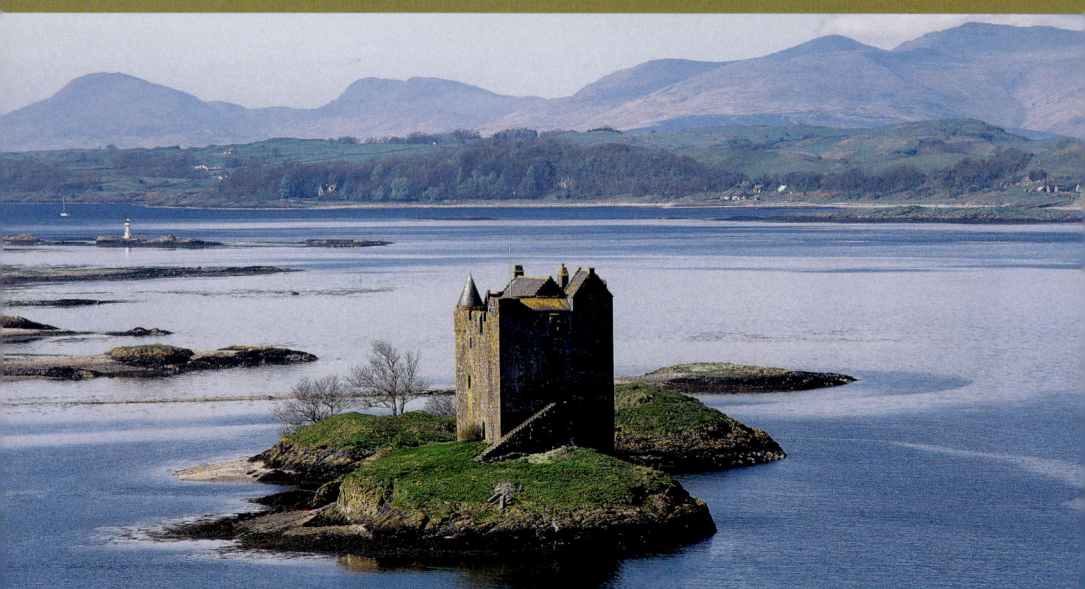

About Scotland

Scotland has something for everyone – dramatic and attractive scenery in the countryside and around the coast, historic towns, a well-established arts scene, seaside resorts, attractions, wilderness areas for solitude and the bustle of major cities.

South east

The historic core of capital city Edinburgh is on the Royal Mile between the Castle and the Palace of Holyroodhouse. Opposite the Palace stands the new home of the Scottish Parliament contrasting with the elegant Georgian terraces in the New Town, north of Princes Street. Attractions include the Museum of Scotland, the National Gallery of Scotland, the Scottish Portrait Gallery, the Scotch Whisky Heritage Centre and Our Dynamic Earth Science Centre (exploring the evolution of our planet). In August the Edinburgh Festival attracts arts lovers to a wide range of events at a variety of venues. To the south, you'll find the small border towns of Peebles, Selkirk and Hawick and small fishing ports such as Eyemouth. Sir Walter Scott's home at Abbotsford near Melrose is closed for restoration until 4 July 2013, but the gardens and a new visitor centre are open.

South west

Glasgow's major growth in the 19th Century has been followed by recent regeneration of the city centre and waterfront. The Riverside houses a museum of transport and travel. On the outskirts, you'll find the Burrell Art Collection at its purpose-built gallery in Pollok Country Park. Other attractions include Greenbank Gardens at Clarkston (National Trust for Scotland), the David Livingstone Centre at Blantyre, Flotterstone (a Countryside Centre in the Pentland Hills) and the Falkirk Wheel, the only revolving boat lift in the world. Further west is the picturesque south-facing coast and countryside of Dumfries and Galloway, and the coastal resorts of Ayr and Largs. Attractions here include The Robert Burns Birthplace Museum at Alloway, Culzean Castle and Country Park near Maybole, Drumlanrig Castle in Dumfriesshire, the World Heritage Site of New Lanark and Viking history centre Vikingar! in Largs.

East

North of the Forth are the major centres of Dundee, Perth and Aberdeen. History devotees can visit the Bannockburn Heritage Centre at Stirling, while country lovers can choose from many sites around the Perthshire towns of Pitlochry or Dunkeld, and the Grampians and visit a whisky distillery. Visitor centres displaying the historic life of the area include the Grampian Transport Museum at Alford, the Aberdeenshire Farming Heritage Centre in Aden Country Park, the Angus Folk Museum and the British Golf Museum at St Andrews in Fife.

Highlands & Islands

Outside Inverness (the main city in this area) is the Culloden Battlefield (National Trust for Scotland). Travelling inland, you reach Loch Ness in the Great Glen (sightings of the monster are not guaranteed!). You'll find dramatic wild countryside and many small towns and villages. The world-famous Inverewe Gardens are at Poolewe in Wester Ross and there are displays of crafts and farming at the Highlands Folk Museum in Kingussie. The Islands have their own attractions. Some, off the west coast can be reached by short ferry trips or, in the case of Skye, by bridge. Highland life 100 years ago is depicted at the Skye Museum of Island Life. Visiting Orkney, Shetland and the Western Isles will need more planning, but all are worth a visit for their distinctive lifestyle and reminders of their prehistoric and Nordic past.

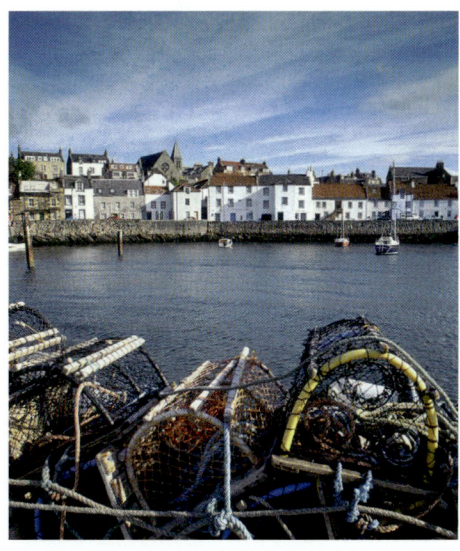

SCOTLAND

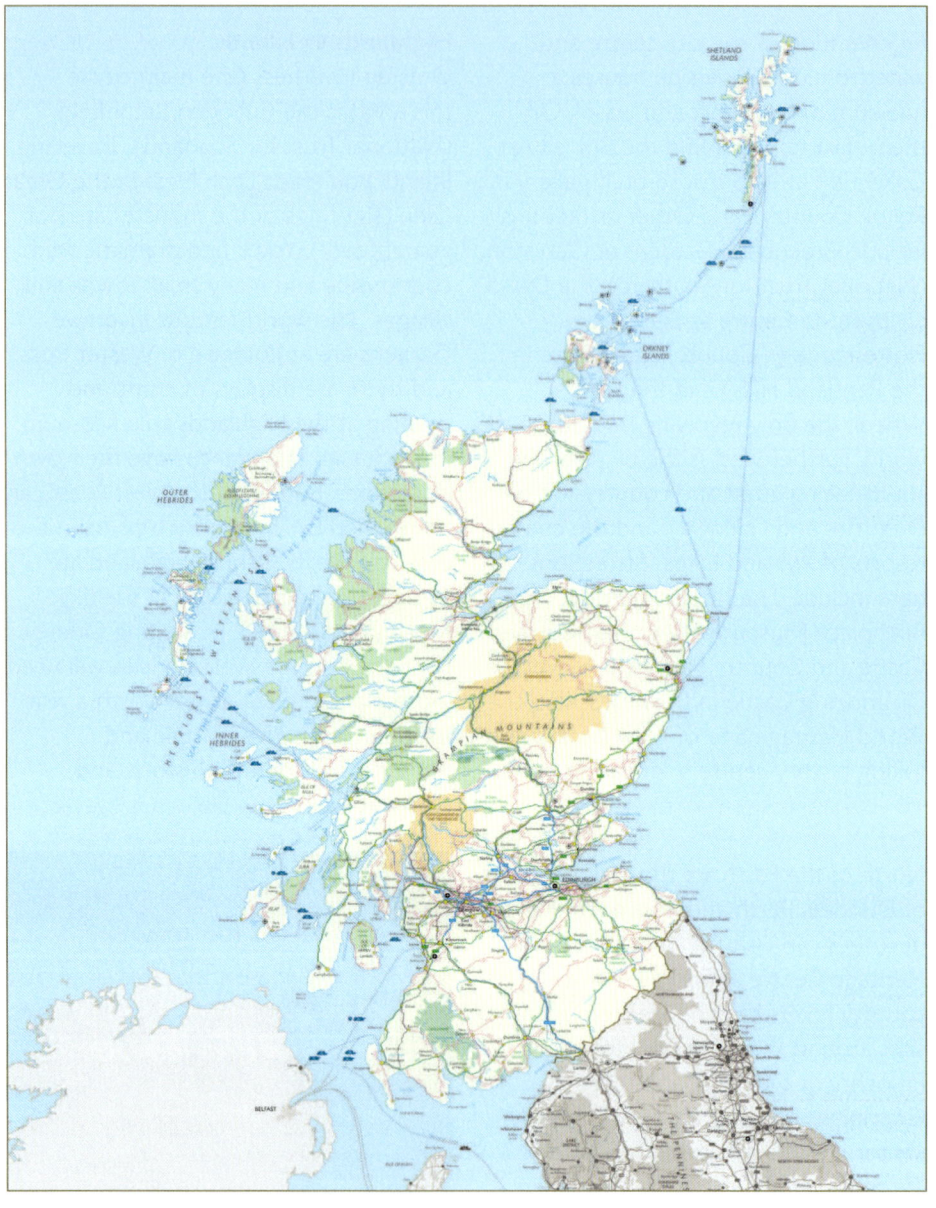

Tourism

VisitScotland
Quality & Standards, Thistle House, Beechwood Park North, Inverness IV2 3ED
- www.visitscotland.com

Operate an Accessibility Scheme for places to stay and attractions that are inspected against specific criteria for three levels of impaired mobility. Search their site for 'Accessible Scotland' to find out more.

Transport

The three largest airports in Scotland are operated by BAA Scotland. For information on the services at each contact:

Aberdeen Airport
- 0844 481 6666
- www.aberdeenairport.com

Edinburgh Airport
- 0844 481 8989
- www.edinburghairport.com

Glasgow Airport
- 0844 481 5555
- www.glasgowairport.com

They share a textphone enquiry number:
- 0844 571 7410

Highlands & Islands Airports Ltd
Head Office, Inverness Airport, Inverness IV2 7JB
- 01667 462445
- info@hial.co.uk
- www.hial.co.uk

Operate 11 airports in northern Scotland providing commercial, tourist and emergency services. Facilities at some of the smaller airports are limited but all have basically accessible terminals and most have lifts for passengers who cannot use steps into aircraft.

THINGS TO SEE OR DO

CairnGorm Mountain Railway
Cairngorms National Park, Aviemore, PH22 1RB

The highest railway journey in the UK with visitors travelling on a 2km trip from the base station at car park level to the Ptarmigan top station, which is 1,097m above sea level and just below the summit of the mountain itself. The Funicular Mountain Railway is fully accessible for wheelchair users with lift access to all levels and assistance available from staff if required. At the Ptarmigan top station there is lift access to all floors including the weather watching terrace. There is also wheelchair access into the Day Lodge. Wheelchairs can be made available for use on site. Within the ski area at CairnGorm Mountain there are a number of walking trails around the car park area that are suitable for wheelchair use. During the winter skiing season the ground conditions can be difficult under foot and it is strongly recommend checking weather conditions before planning visits in the winter months.
- www.cairngormmountain.org
- 01479 861 261

SCOTLAND

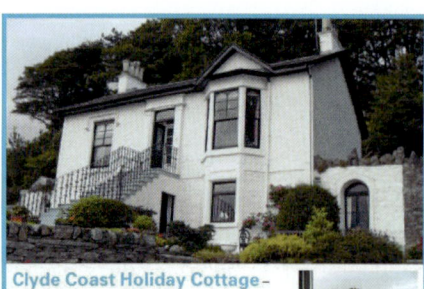

Clyde Coast Holiday Cottage – wheelchair accessible. £35 per night or £210 per week. Argyll and Bute area. Ground floor flat of a charming seaside cottage at Innellan on the Clyde Coast available to rent from August.

This property may be suitable for wheelchair users and carers can also be accommodated. There is level access to property and all rooms.

The property has one main bedroom but another bedroom may be available for carers. It also has a well equipped eating kitchen, living room with splendid sea views and a large bathroom with wheel in shower. The property has a parking space in the drive.

Please phone for further details: Jean Knox 01875 812112 or email jeanknox@hotmail.com

Wallace Caravans

Established in 1963, we are a well known and respected name within the leisure industry of North East Scotland.

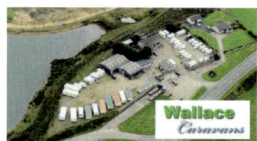

- We have access to a large number of caravan parks throughout the North East and offer a complete service from delivery, siting, site connections and repairs.
- Our workshops service and repair Motorhomes and Touring caravans and also offer a towbar fitting service.
- Storage facilities are available for Statics, Tourers and Motorhomes.
- We have a well stocked shop with leisure parts and spares.

Denhead, Mintlaw, Peterhead, Aberdeenshire AB42 4HR
Email: enquiries@wallacecaravans.com

Tel: 01771 623224
wallacecaravans.com

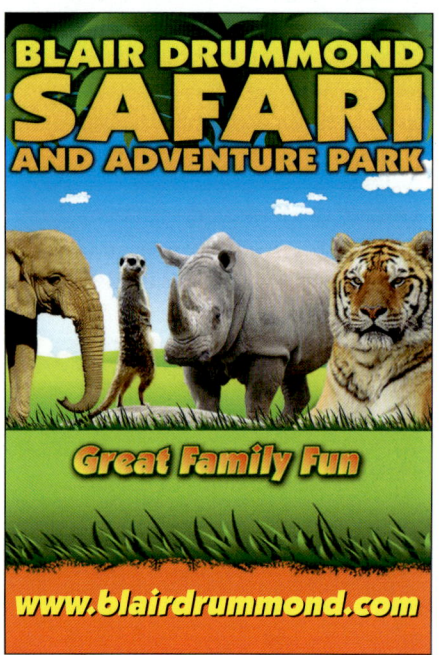

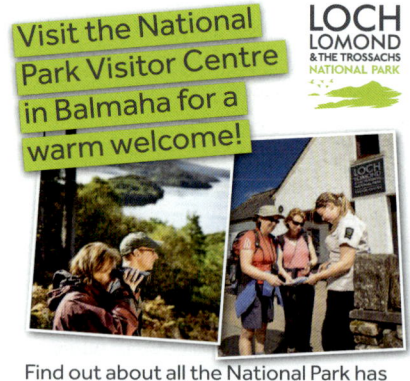

Visit the National Park Visitor Centre in Balmaha for a warm welcome!

Find out about all the National Park has to offer and what makes Loch Lomond, its shores and islands so special.

Open daily April to September and weekends all year-round (check for times)
Phone us: 01389 722100
Find us: OS grid ref NS 409909

More ideas for all abilities activities at:
www.lochlomond-trossachs.org

SCOTLAND

CalMac Ferries
The Ferry Terminal, Gourock PA19 1QP
- 0800 066 5000 (enquiries)
- reservations@calmac.co.uk
- www.calmac.co.uk

Operate a wide range of routes off the west coast of Scotland. Facilities for disabled passengers vary depending on the vessel used on the route; information is included on their website under 'The Fleet'. Anyone who may need assistance should notify the company when booking and checking in. Fare concessions for disabled drivers are available on production of appropriate documents.

NorthLink Ferries
Stromness Ferry Terminal, Ferry Road, Stromness, Orkney KW16 3BH
- Reservations 0845 6000 449
  Administration 01856 885500
- info@northlinkferries.co.uk
- www.northlinkferries.co.uk

Operate ferry services to Orkney and Shetland from Aberdeen and between Scrabster in Caithness and Stromness on Orkney, using three modern vessels. Each has toilets for disabled passengers and lifts between decks. Those used for overnight sailings have four cabins designed for disabled people of which two have enhanced facilities including hoists. Concessionary rates and special boarding arrangements are available for disabled people. There are toilets for disabled people at each of Northlink's terminals. Advance notice of passengers requiring assistance is appreciated.

Pentland Ferries
Pier Road, St Margaret's Hope, South Ronaldsay, Orkney KW17 2SW
- 01856 831226
- www.pentlandferries.co.uk

Operate car ferries on the 1-hour crossing between Gill's Bay in Caithness and the southern Orkney island of South Ronaldsay. No specific facilities are available for disabled passengers.

THINGS TO SEE OR DO

Nevis Range Mountain Gondola
Nevis Range, Torlundy, Fort Willliam, PH33 6SQ

The only one of its kind in the UK, the Nevis Range Mountain Gondola transports visitors from 300ft up to 2150ft on the north face of Aonach Mor, the eighth highest mountain in Britain. The journey takes about 12-15 minutes each way. The gondola cars are able to accommodate wheelchairs up to 60cm wide and the operators will slow or stop the gondola cycle to allow access to less able visitors, until they are onboard and fully prepared for the journey ahead. There are disabled toilets located at both the top and bottom stations and there is adequate disabled access to the Snowgoose Restaurant and the base station Café.
- www.nevisrange.co.uk/gondola-info.asp
- 01397 705 825

SCOTLAND

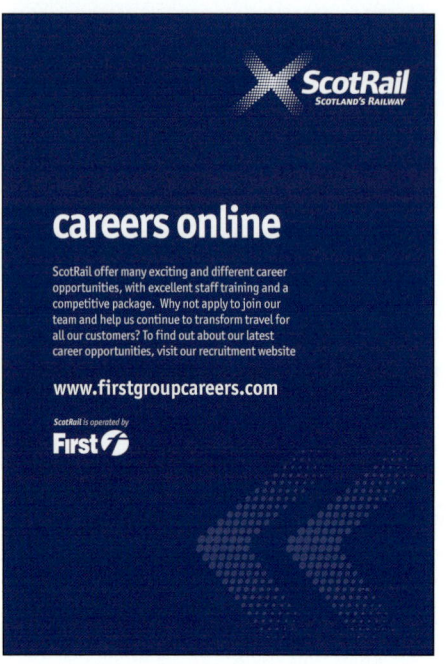

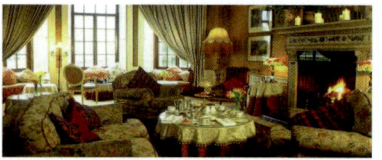

Roman Camp
Country House and Restaurant
Callander, Stirlingshire FK17 8BG
www.romancamphotel.co.uk

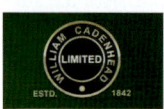

Edinburgh's best established whisky shop
'Quality, Purity, Choice'

WM Cadenhead, 172 Canongate, Edinburgh
Tel: 0131 565 5864

Ben Nevis Distillery

Lochy Bridge – Fort William - PH33 6TJ

One of the oldest licensed distilleries in Scotland, we're nestled at the foot of Britain's highest mountain – an impressive background to a traditional Scottish craft. Come and take a tour of The Legend of the Dew of Ben Nevis Visitor Centre, and then relax with a refreshment – or if you're hungry, try some of our delicious home cooking in our coffee shop and restaurant.

It will be an unforgettable treat!

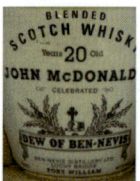

Tel: 01397 700200

www.bennevisdistillery.com

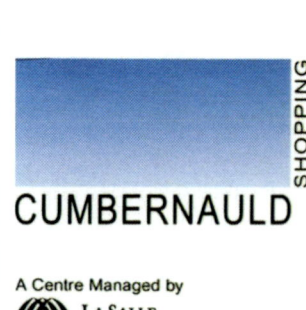

CUMBERNAULD SHOPPING

A Centre Managed by
LA SALLE
INVESTMENT MANAGEMENT

Tel: 01236 734386
Fax: 01236 720786
Email: robert.barr@EU.JLL.com

**New Disabled RADAR Toilet
NOW OPEN**

Highland Adventure Safaris
Aberfeldy, Perthshire PH15 2JQ
- 01887 820071
- info@highlandsafaris.net
- www.highlandsafaris.net

From its base at an accessible visitor centre, between Aberfeldy and Tummel Bridge, Highland Adventure Safaris use a long wheelbase Land Rover to explore the Perthshire Highlands going to areas that would otherwise be inaccessible to many people. Assistance with getting on and off the vehicle can be provided.

Mobility Assist
98 High street, Galashiels TD1 1SQ
- 01896 757075
- mobilityassist@aol.com

Operate a taxi service in the Scottish Borders area using vehicles with rear lifts.

Information & advice

Orkney Disability Forum
Power Station Offices, Great Western Road, Kirkwall KW15 1AN
- 01856 871515
- www.orkneycommunities.co.uk/ODF

Offer a Dial-a-Bus and Shopmobility service and can provide information on access in Orkney.

Equipment hire

SHOPMOBILITY
The National Federation of Shopmobility UK (NFSUK), PO Box 6641, Christchurch BH23 9DQ
- 0844 41 41 850
- info@shopmobilityuk.org
- www.shopmobilityuk.org

Scheme which lends manual wheelchairs, powered wheelchairs and powered scooters to members of the public with limited mobility to shop and to visit leisure and commercial facilities within the town, city or shopping centre. You can find the nearest Shopmobility scheme to you through their on-line directory. Contact specific Shopmobility Schemes to make equipment bookings or find out more information.

> ### THINGS TO SEE OR DO
>
> **Skara Brae Prehistoric Village**
> The best preserved prehistoric village in northern Europe, dating back 5,000 years. Just over half Orkney's ancient site is wheelchair accessible. Some external interpretation boards on the monument, the visitor centre and the ground floor of the replica house are also wheelchair friendly. The pathway linking the various buildings and sites are suitable for disabled visitors. There are two wheelchairs available for use on site at the visitor centre. Disabled toilets on site.
> - www.orkneyjar.com/history/skarabrae

SCOTLAND

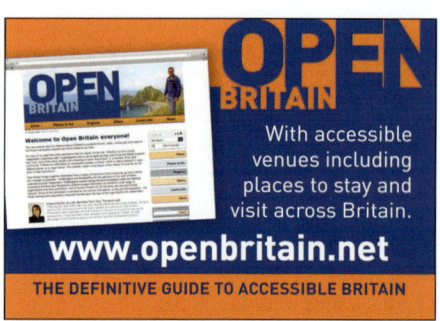

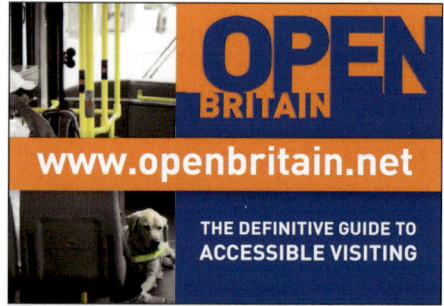

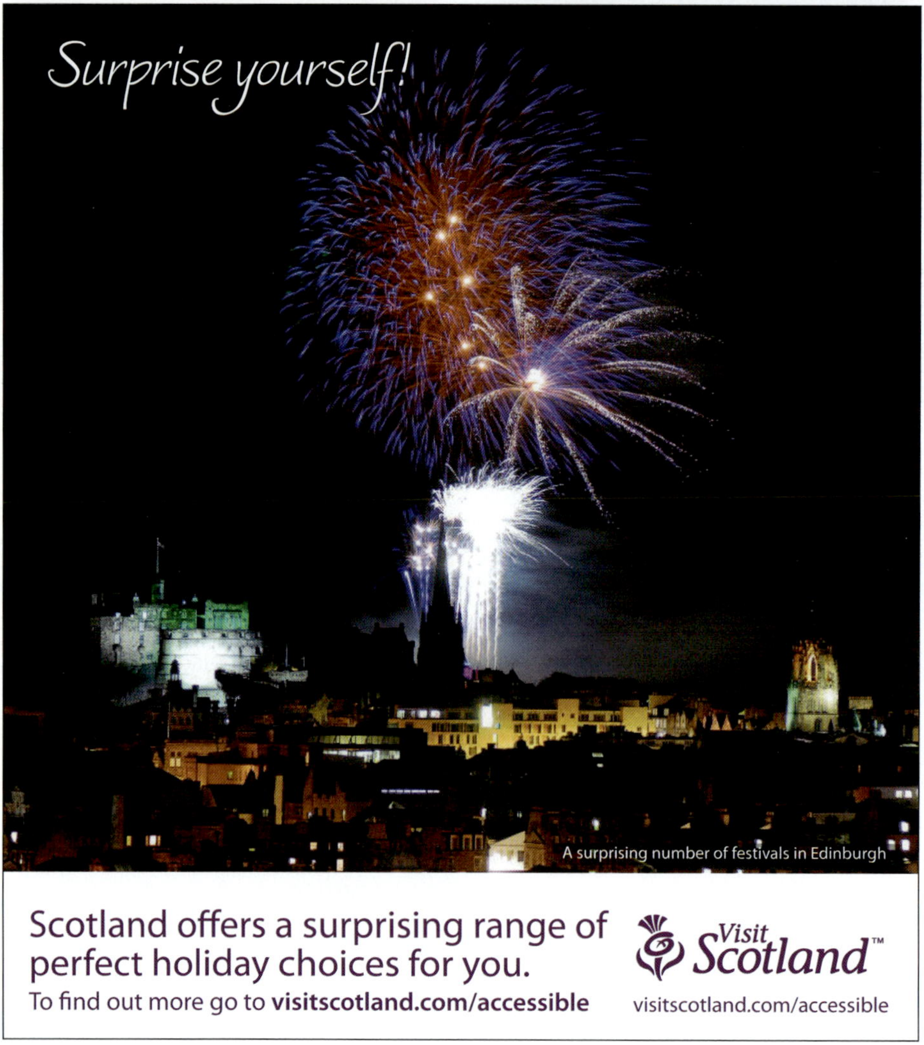

Surprise yourself!

A surprising number of festivals in Edinburgh

Scotland offers a surprising range of perfect holiday choices for you.
To find out more go to visitscotland.com/accessible

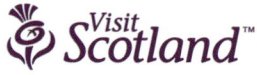

visitscotland.com/accessible

HOLIDAYS IN THE BRITISH ISLES

SCOTLAND

Publications

Historic Scotland: Access Guide
Provides information on facilities and highlights possible difficulties, for disabled people at over 70 historic buildings and sites throughout Scotland. Available free from Historic Scotland, Longmore House, Salisbury Place, Edinburgh EH9 1SH.
- 0131 668 8800
- www.historic-scotland.gov.uk

Countryside Visits: Places to visit in the Scottish Borders with some access for wheelchair users
A free booklet by the Scottish Borders Council Rangers Service with the Borders Disability Forum. Available from the. Scottish Borders Council Countryside Ranger Service, Council HQ, Newtown St Boswells, Melrose TD6 0SA.
- 01896 668578

Updated information can be found on
- www.bordersdisabilityforum/news/rangers

Online resources

Shetland Access Guide
- www.shetlandaccessguide.org.uk/AccessGuide.aspx

Site with detailed information on facilities for disabled people on inter-island ferries and some premises in Lerwick on their website.

THINGS TO SEE OR DO

Stirling Castle
Castle Esplanade, Stirling, FK8 1EJ
One of the largest and most important castles in Scotland. Its Great Hall and Palace, dating from the early 16th century, are important examples of early Renaissance architecture with a strong continental influence. Despite its location on a high volcanic crag surrounded by steep cliffs, large parts of the castle are accessible to wheelchair users. Stirling Castle has a courtesy vehicle for visitors who have difficulty with steep inclines and steps. The areas which cannot be reached in a wheelchair include the Museum of the Argyll and Sutherland Highlanders, the medieval kitchens and the Elphinstone Tower. An Access Gallery, located in the palace vaults, has been designed to enable visitors with mobility difficulties to experience areas which are inaccessible. Braille information boards are on display and a Braille guidebook is available from the gift shop. Disabled parking and toilets on site. Historic Scotland offers free entry for one-to-one carers accompanying disabled visitors.
- www.stirlingcastle.gov.uk/home.htm
- 01786 450 000

SCOTLAND

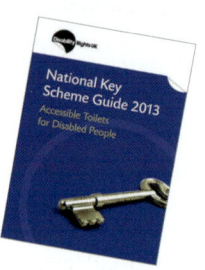

Available to order from our online shop
www.disabilityrightsuk.org

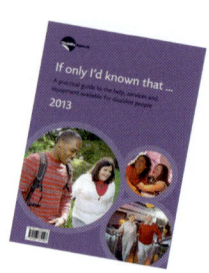

Available to order from our online shop
www.disabilityrightsuk.org

Ayrshire Railway Preservation Group

Founded in 1974 to preserve some of Scotland's industrial railway heritage, especially that of Ayrshire and south-west Scotland.

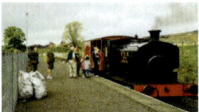

Steam Open Days 2013
Held various Sundays from May to September
For more information: http://arpg.org.uk/wp

Bringing Industrial Heritage to Life

Loch Tay Lodges
Self-catering accommodation in Perthshire

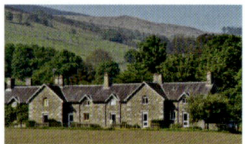

For more information contact:
James Duncan Millar, Remony Estate Partnership,
Remony, Aberfeldy, Perthshire, PH15 2HR
Tel: +44 (0) 1887 830209
E-Mail: remony@btinternet.com
www.lochtaylodges.co.uk

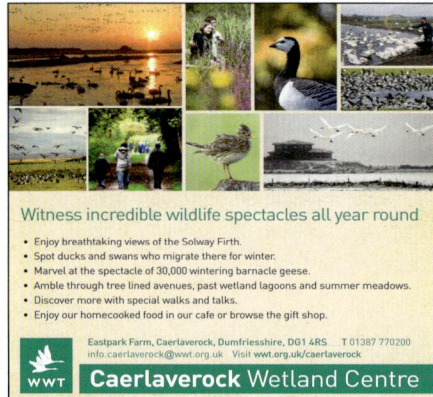

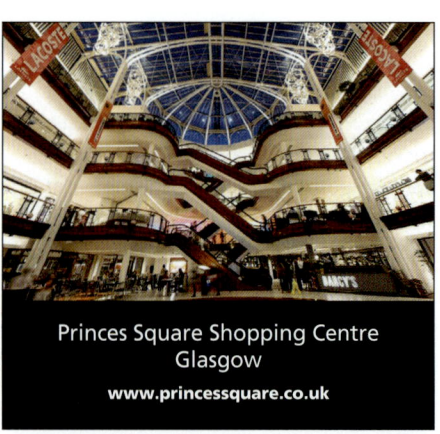

SCOTLAND

Accommodation

CRATHIE, Aberdeenshire
Crathie Opportunity Holidays
The Manse Courtyard, Crathie, Ballater AB35 5UL
- 01339 742100
- info@crathieholidays.org.uk
- www.crathieholidays.org.uk

Set within the restored Manse Courtyard of Crathie Kirk. Four wheelchair accessible self-catering holiday cottages. Each cottage has been carefully designed and furnished. Offer a range of facilities so that disabled people can enjoy a relaxing holiday in accessible accommodation. There is a fenced play area with a security gate.

CRIEFF, Perthshire
Ancaster BLESMA Home
Alligan Road, Crieff PH7 3JU
- 01764 652480
- blesma.crieff@btconnect.com
- www.blesma.org

BLESMA nursing and residential home for disabled ex-servicemen and women set on a south-facing slope of the Grampian foothills. 24 hour nursing, respite and residential care provided. Single rooms and twin bedded rooms, with en-suite facilities and colour television. Communual areas include a television lounge, games room with a full size snooker table and a 2.5 acre garden. There is entertainment in the evenings and an itinerary of up to five excursions a week is available to those who enjoy the active life. Electronic buggies and wheelchairs are available for added independence.

DIRLETON, East Lothian
Denis Duncan House
Manse Road, Dirleton
- 01787 372343
- info@thelinberwicktrust.org.uk
- www.thelinberwicktrust.org.uk

Purpose built cottage in village west of North Berwick run by a registered charity, the Lin Berwick Trust. The cottage has a twin bedroom with en-suite bathroom designed for disabled people on the ground floor where there are also living rooms, kitchen and utility room. There are also two twin bedrooms a bathroom and sitting room on the first floor.

THINGS TO SEE OR DO

Loch Katrine
Trossachs Pier, Loch Katrine, By Callander, Stirling, FK17 8HB
Situated in the heart of the Trossachs, Katrine is a freshwater loch, around 8 miles in length, surrounded by scenic woodland and mountains. The area offers a number of activities for disabled people, which can be started at Trossachs Pier by the lake. A golf buggy can be hired to explore the roadway along the northern shore of Loch Katrine, which is mainly flat and suitable for wheelchairs. The steamship Sir Walter Scott, which is wheelchair accessible, cruises the lake with live commentary.
- www.lochkatrine.com
- 01877 376 315/6

SCOTLAND

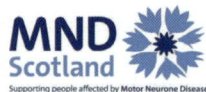

HOLIDAYS IN SCOTLAND

MND now has two holiday facilities for the MND community, both with special adaptations highly useful for people with physical disabilities.

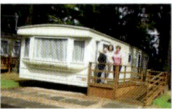 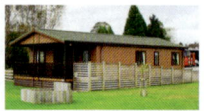

Lan Break Caravan at Craigtoun Meadows Holiday Park near St Andrews in East Scotland. An ideal spot to explore Fife and Tayside.

Holiday Chalet at Tralee Bay Holiday Park, near Oban in West Scotland. On the coast, close to lots of tourist attractions and just ten miles from the ferry terminals to take you on the short journey to stunning islands including Mull and Staffa.

Both sleep up to six and are suitable for wheelchair users. To find out more call 0141 945 1077 or visit www.mndscotland.org.uk/services/holiday-facilities

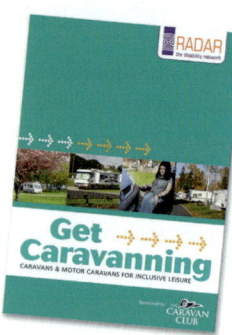

Get Caravanning

A guide to exploring caravanning from a disabled person's point of view. It provides all the information you need to start or resume this popular leisure activity.

Available to order from our online shop
www.disabilityrightsuk.org

John Gray Centre

Library   Museum   Archive

East Lothian Council's new heritage hub in Haddington!

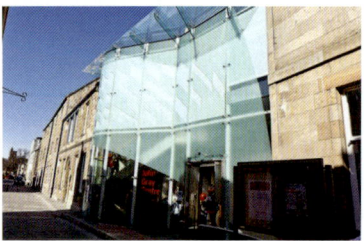

With Haddington's branch library on the ground floor, a museum gallery, a gallery for temporary exhibitions and the East Lothian Archives and Local History Centre upstairs, there's plenty to see and do here. There is free wi-fi and a computer room for public access, and we also have regular activities and events.

www.johngraycentre.org

Open from 10am Monday-Saturday; 1pm-4pm on Sundays
15 Lodge Street, Haddington, East Lothian, EH41 3DX
Telephone: Library 01620 820680   Museum 01620 820690   Local History/Archives 01620 820695

SCOTLAND

DRUMNADROCHIT, Inverness-shire
Lochletter Lodges
Balnain, Drumnadrochit, Inverness IV63 6TJ
- 01456 476313
- info@lochletter.com
- www.lochletter.com

Chalet lodges west of Loch Ness in Glenurquhart. Drumnadrochit is a nearby quiet village where there are shops and restaurants. Inverness city is about half an hours drive away. There are 4, high quality, single storey wooden lodges, one of which is specially designed for disabled guests, built so that each has its own view. They are accessed via a private road.

NORTH BERWICK, East Lothian
Leuchie House
North Berwick EH39 5NT
- 01620 892864
- enquiries@leuchie.org.uk
- www.leuchie.org.uk

This specially adapted holiday home in East Lothian provides respite care and breaks for people with long term disabilities. 24 hour nursing car available and a programme of activities and outings.

At its best, Wales is the most beguiling part of the British Isles.
Rough Guide

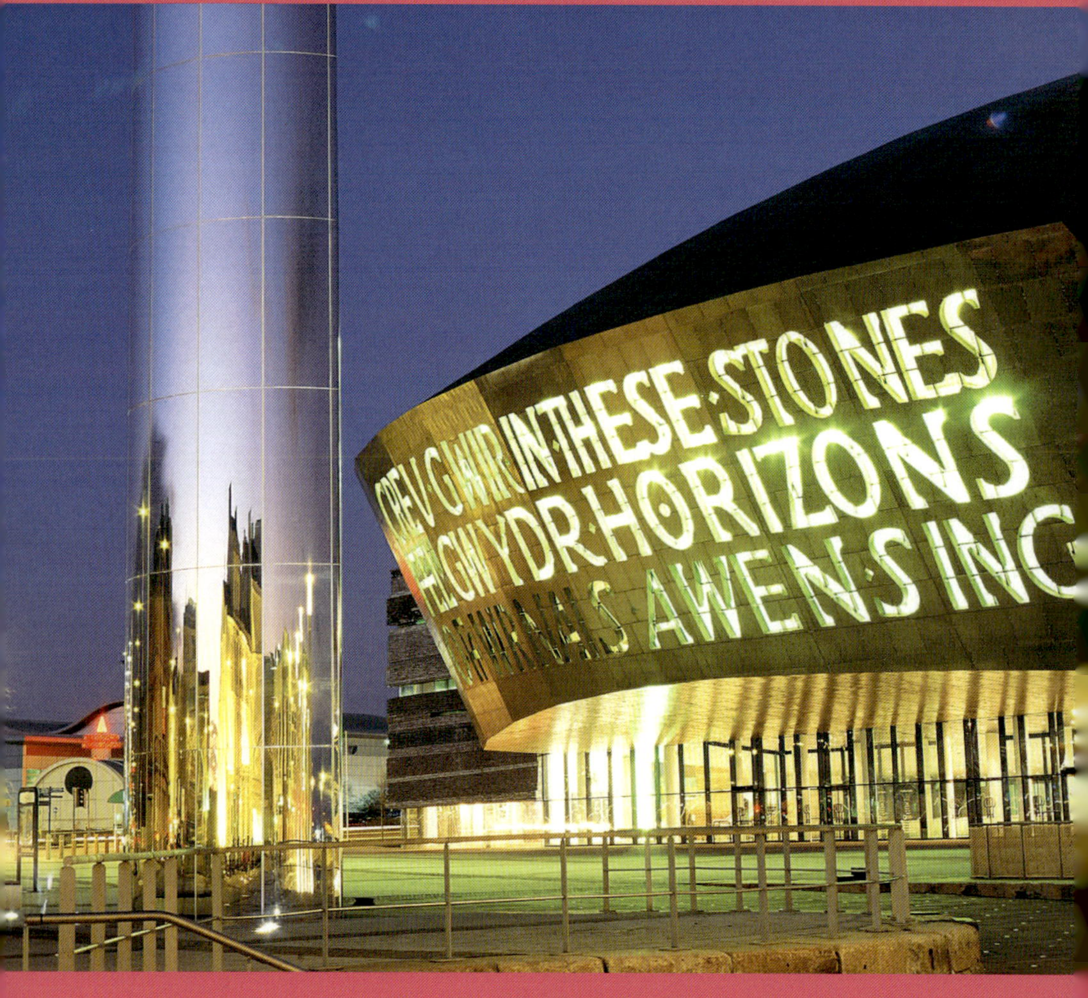

Wales

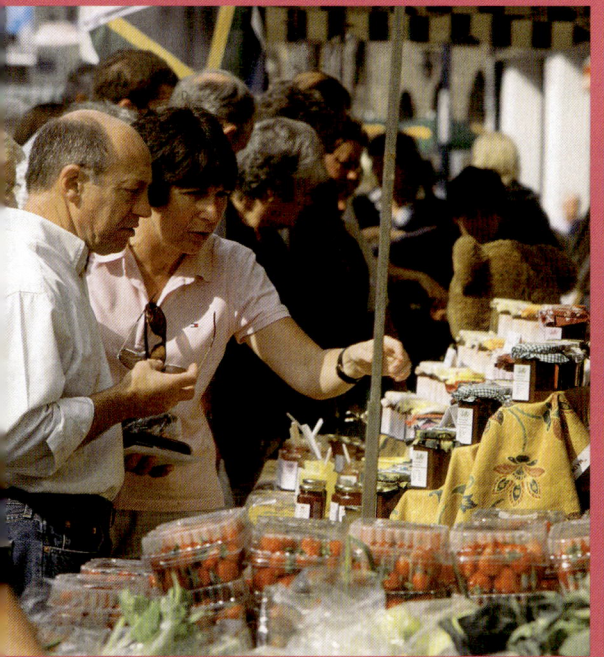

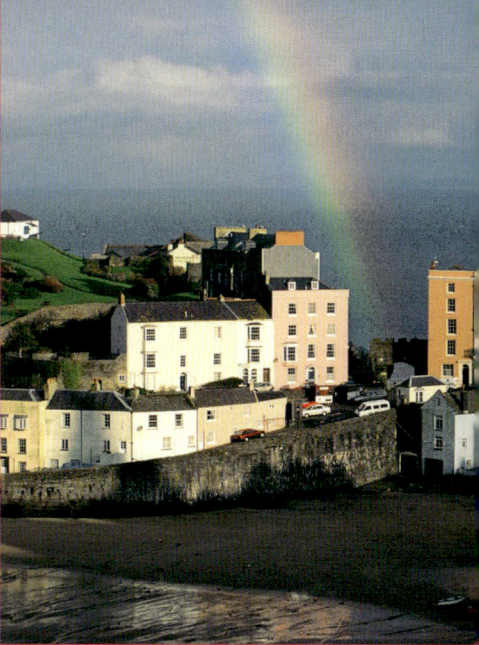

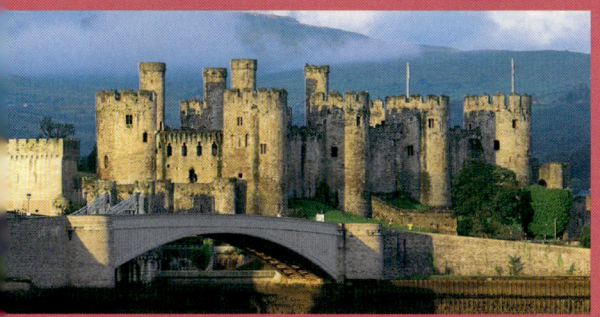

> *A place that becomes obsessive, beckoning back its visitors year after year.*
>
> **Lonely Planet**

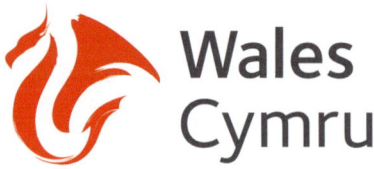

Visit Wales

We'd love to have you visit us in Wales. But then you'd expect us to say that. For travel author Mike Parker, the man given the job of compiling *The Rough Guide to Wales*, the experience of being in Wales changed his life – so much so that he upped sticks and moved to live in a Welsh valley.

"Just how much I loved the place shook me to my bones." Parker says. "It was like falling in love with a person rather than a place, with all the dizzy disorientation and heart-thumping joy and awe that accompanies it."

So what do you need to know about a country that inspires such strong feelings? Although Wales is not that far from London, it is a completely different place. Just how different can often takes first-time visitors by surprise.

Green and hilly, Wales has its own language, a distinct Celtic culture and heritage plus a self-belief that gives Wales a national spirit that resonates more strongly than ever.

Then there is the landscape. At around 8,000 square miles (close to 21,000 square kilometres) Wales is smaller than the US state of Massachusetts, but if you were to roll it out flat, it would be bigger than Texas.

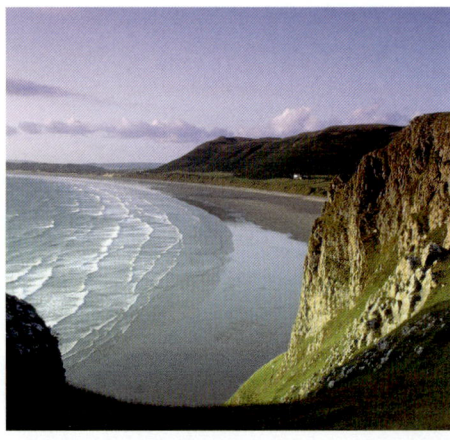

Boasting plenty of open space, Wales is around half the size of The Netherlands but compared to The Netherlands which is home to 16 million people, Wales has only 3 million.

In 2012 Wales became the first country in the world to open a dedicated path running along its entire coast – all 870 miles of it.

Wales is a country on a human-scale – somewhere where you will find more than enough space to enjoy yourself but is also a place with plenty of variety. Visitors will find something different and special around every corner. Boasting three National Parks and five Areas of Outstanding Natural Beauty the outdoors is one of Wales' greatest draws.

Not that it's just countryside. The towns and cities should definitely be on the itinerary too. There are a wide range of arts and music festivals staged in Wales throughout the year and the country has a growing reputation as a mouth-watering destination for food lovers. With 641 castles, there are countless opportunities to explore the history and heritage of this ancient land.

Travel
Many visitors come straight to Wales by air or sea, while others travel by road or train from England. It takes just two hours by train to get from London to Cardiff.

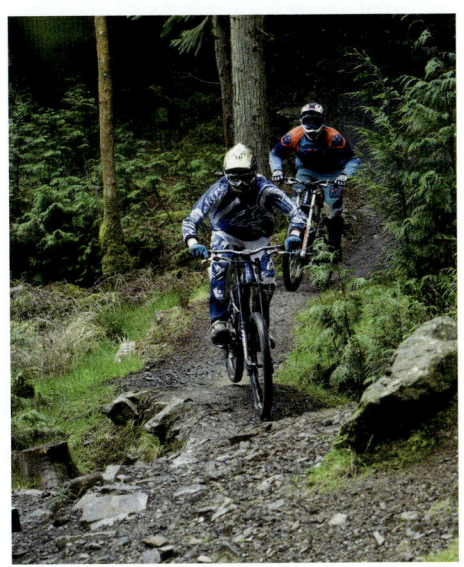

Other English cities are closer still. For example, you can drive into North Wales from Manchester Airport in less than an hour.

Visit our website
For up-to-date information on short breaks and proper holidays in Wales, go to the official Visit Wales website at:
www.visitwales.co.uk

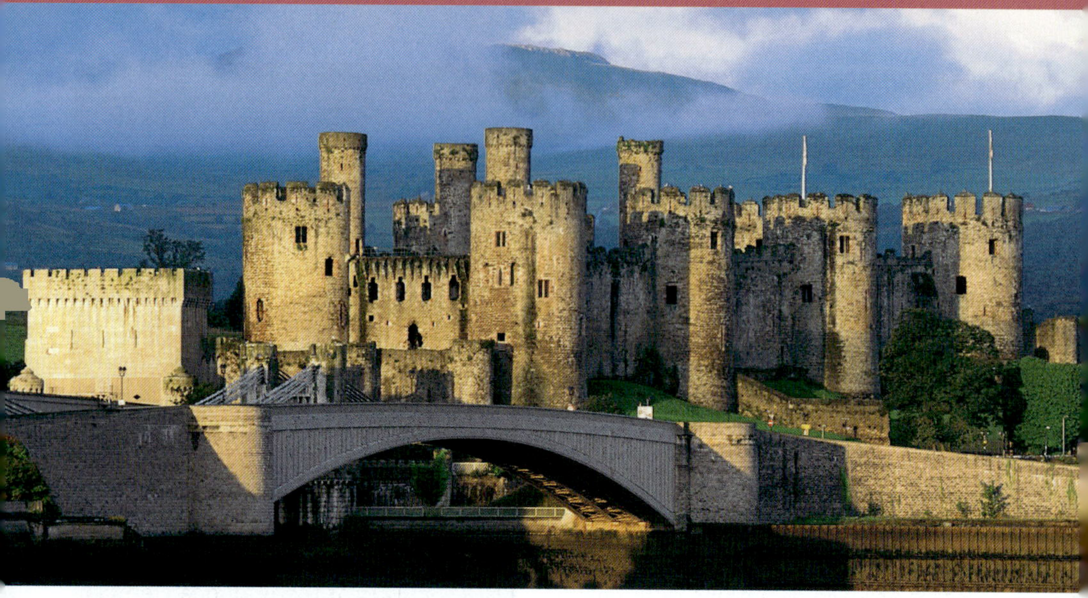

WALES

About Wales

Wales has a tourist industry that is both well established and rapidly modernising, providing opportunities for staying in traditional resorts, large cities, country towns or at more rural locations.

Well-established resorts with attractions for families and a largely level terrain are found around much of the coast. In the north these include Rhyl, Colwyn Bay and Llandudno. Aberdovey, Barmouth and Towyn are on the west coast and Tenby and Porthcawl in the south. The hillier sections of the coast have many historic towns, some with castles such as Harlech, Caernarfon and Conwy or with attractive harbours like New Quay.

Wales has three contrasting National Parks. The one covering the Pembrokeshire Coast contains some of

Britain's most dramatic coastal scenery and provides a thriving and varied wildlife habitat. The Snowdonia National Park in the north west has impressive mountains. It is possible to get to the top

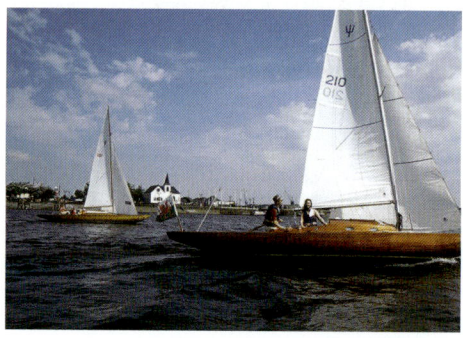

HOLIDAYS IN THE BRITISH ISLES

of Wales' highest mountain on the Snowdon Mountain Railway with advance notice. The Brecon Beacons, stretching from the top of the once industrial valleys into mid-Wales, are not as high as Snowdonia but have a countryside which feels just as remote. Facilities for disabled visitors have been developed by each of the National Park Authorities.

Rural areas with attractive scenery can be found in other parts of Wales and there are many opportunities for countryside activities. Water sports of all kinds are available on many reservoirs. The Wildfowl & Wetlands Trust has a centre near Llanelli and country parks have been developed in many areas including Ty Mawr near Wrexham and Caldicot Castle in Monmouthshire. The National Botanic Garden of Wales, including the spectacular Great Glasshouse, is at Llanarthe near Carmarthen.

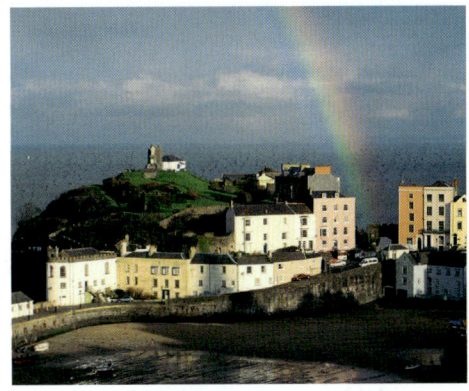

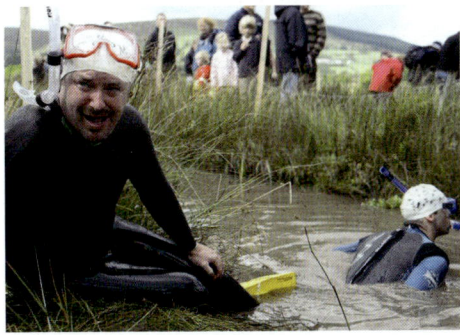

Machynlleth is the home of the Centre for Alternative Technology. Elsewhere there are re-creations of local industrial heritage, be it slate mining in Snowdonia, quarrying in Anglesey, the National Wool Museum near Newcastle Emlyn in Carmarthenshire or coal mining and heavy industry at the Rhondda Heritage Centre. Wales is notable for the number of preserved steam railways, several of which, including the Llanberis Lake Railway, can carry disabled passengers.

All the facilities expected of a major modern capital city can be found in Cardiff – shops, music, sports including the Millennium Stadium, museums, night life and much more. The regenerated Cardiff Bay area is the home of the Welsh Assembly and the Wales Millennium Centre. A similarly wide range of attractions can be found in Swansea including the Dylan Thomas Centre and the National Waterfront Museum. Smaller towns worth visiting include the Victorian spa town of Llandrindod Wells in mid-Wales, St David's with the country's smallest Cathedral, the university town of Aberystwyth on the west coast and the county towns of Cardigan, Carmarthen and Monmouth.

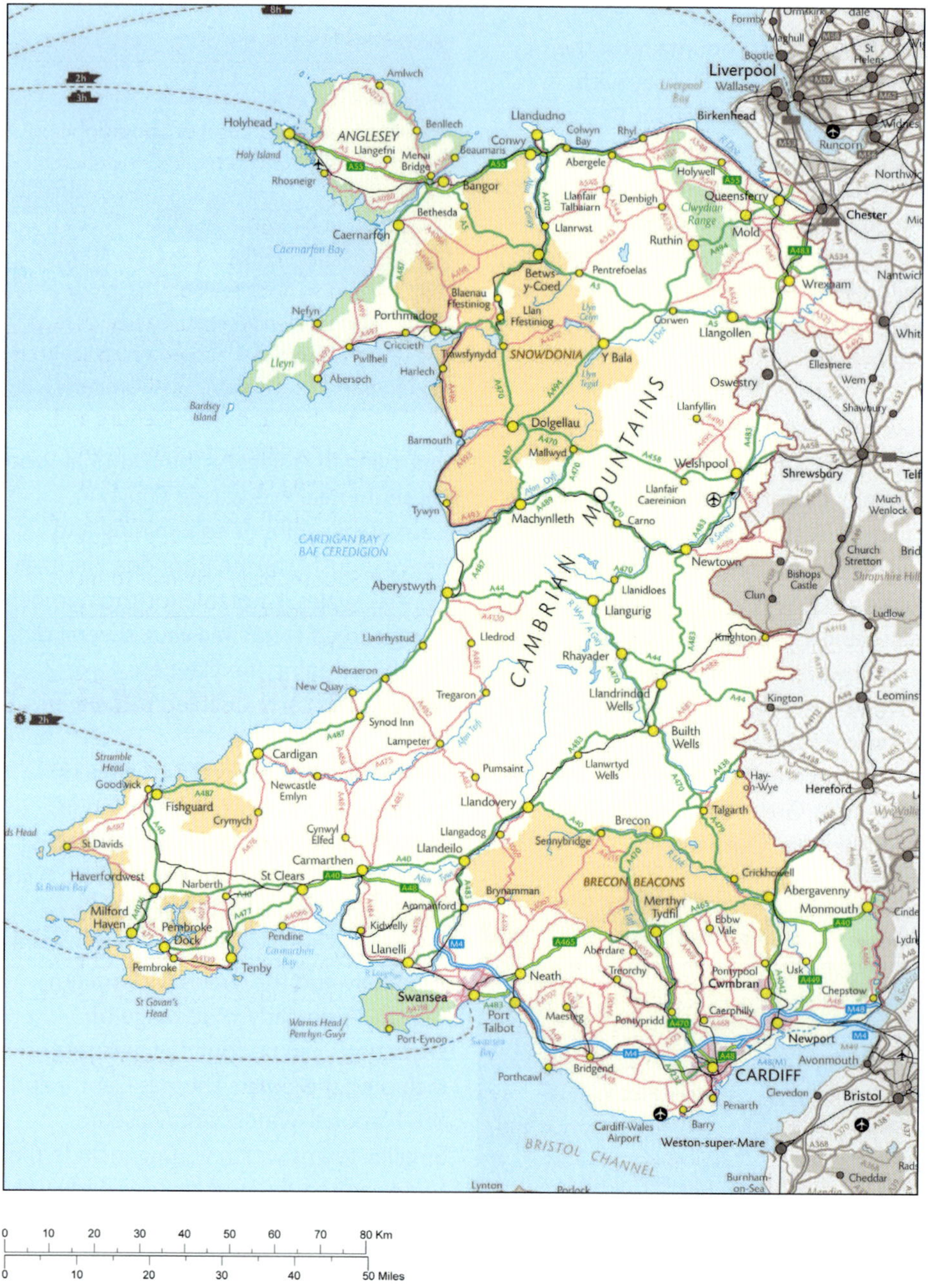

WALES

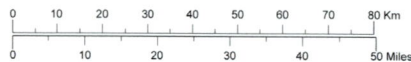

HOLIDAYS IN THE BRITISH ISLES

Resources

Tourism

Visit Wales
Visit Wales, QED Centre, Main Avenue, Trefforest Industrial Estate, Trefforest, Pontypridd, Rhondda, Cynon Taff CF37 5YR
- ☎ 08708 300 306
- ✉ info@visitwales.co.uk
- 🌐 www.visitwales.co.uk

Produce a range of general tourist literature, which indicates accommodation suitable for disabled guests.

Information & advice

Disability Wales/Anabledd Cymru
Bridge House, Caerphilly Business Park, Van Road, Caerphilly CF83 3GW
- ☎ 029 2088 7325
- 🌐 www.disabilitywales.org

Can answer enquiries by letter or phone.

DIAL
Offer free, impartial and confidential information and advice by telephone to disabled people, their relatives and professionals. Local branches of DIAL are constantly changing but at the time of writing, the following groups were members of DIAL UK and may be able to help visitors in their areas. Please call before travelling to check whether the service and organisation is still available:

Disability Advice Project, Cwmbran
- ☎ 01633 485865

Disability CAN DO
- ☎ 01495 233555

Disability Powys
- ☎ 0800 988 1691

Equipment hire

SHOPMOBILITY
The National Federation of Shopmobility UK (NFSUK), PO Box 6641, Christchurch BH23 9DQ
- ☎ 0844 41 41 850
- ✉ info@shopmobilityuk.org
- 🌐 www.shopmobilityuk.org

Scheme which lends manual wheelchairs, powered wheelchairs and powered scooters to members of the public with limited mobility to shop and to visit leisure and commercial facilities within the town, city or shopping centre. You can find the nearest Shopmobility scheme to you through their on-line directory. Contact specific Shopmobility Schemes to make equipment bookings or find out more information.

> **THINGS TO SEE OR DO**
>
> ### Barry Island
> All-terrain beach wheelchairs are available at Barry Island, giving more visitors the chance to get on to the sand at Whitmore Bay to enjoy the Blue Flag beach. Available for loan for free from the Tourist Information Centre at Barry Island throughout the summer. Contact Barry Island Tourist Information Centre on
> - ✉ barrytic@valeofglamorgan.gov.uk
> - ☎ 01446 747171

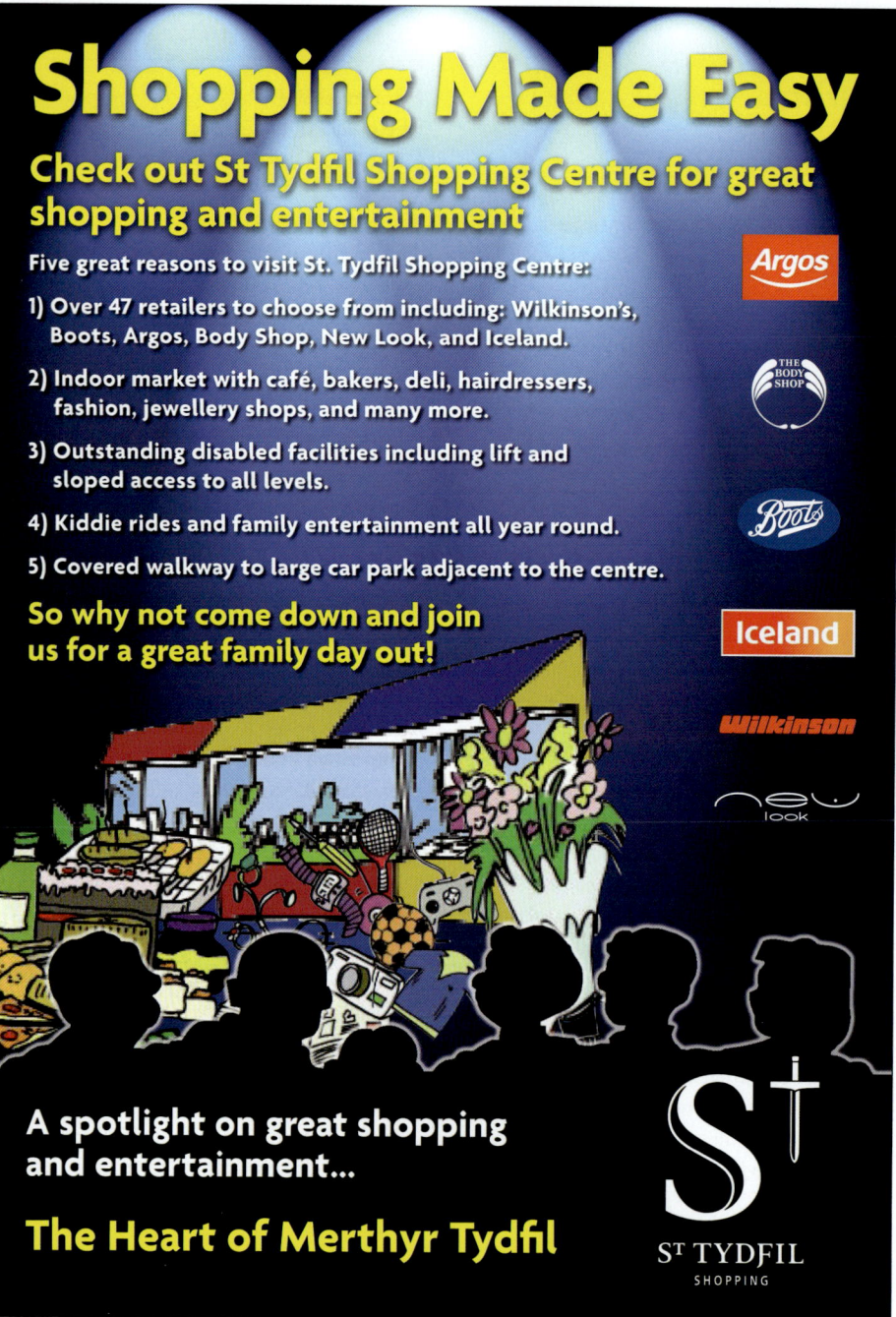

WALES

Bridgend Wheelchair Hire
Unit 23 St Theodores Way, Brynmenyn Industrial Estate, Bridgend CF32 9TZ
- 01656 661579
- info@bridgendwheelchairhire.co.uk
- www.bridgendwheelchairhire.co.uk

Manual and electric wheelchairs and scooters with a range of attachments and other equipment for hire. Repair service also offered.

CYMROD Clwb Teithio Dwyfor Travel Club
Sgwar yr Orsaf, PO Box 60, Pwllheli LL53 5WT
- 01758 614311

Wheelchairs and scooters are available for hire for disabled people on holiday in the area around Pwllheli on daily and weekly rates. They also have wheelchair accessible vehicles for use in the area that can be hired on a mileage basis. Advance enquiries requested.

Mobility Freedom Direct
Trem-Y-Gorwel, Cwmcou, Newcastle Emlyn, Ceredigion SA38 9PE
- 01239 710261
- enquiries@mobility-freedom-direct.com
- www.mobility-freedom-direct.com

Scooters and powered wheelchairs are available to hire with delivery available at additional cost.

Physically Impaired People of Pembrokeshire Association
Pembrokeshire FRAME, Unit 3, Goodwich Industrial Estate, Goodwick, Pembrokeshire SA64 0BD
- 01348 873034
- pippapembs@hotmail.co.uk

Offer a hire service for wheelchairs, scooters and bathroom equipment for visitors. Daily and weekly hire rates available. Advance bookings accepted in high season.

Publications

Places to Visit with Disabled and Easier Access
- 01874 6220451

A guide listing over 60 short trails, sites of historic, landscape or wildlife interest suitable for disabled people and anyone who just wants a nice and easy, hassle-free stroll in the Brecon Beacons. Available from National Park Information Centres, by post from Brecon Beacons National Park Authority, Plas y Ffynnon, Cambrian Way, Brecon LD3 7DP.
Or view it online at:
- www.breconbeacons.org/visit-us/easy-access

THINGS TO SEE OR DO

Pembrokeshire Coastal Path
- www.pembrokeshirecoast.org.uk

Saundersfoot to Wiseman's Bridge
Surfaced path suitable for wheelchair users. A former railway line, initially horse-powered, without obvious gradient. Uninterrupted coastal views with few exceptions over 1.2 km. Accessible toilets at Saundersfoot.

HOLIDAYS IN THE BRITISH ISLES

WALES

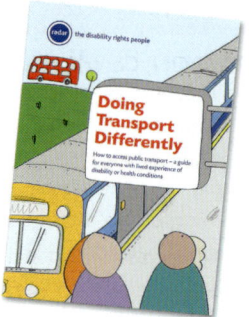

Doing Transport Differently
This guide includes information and travellers' tales to help and inspire people with lived experience of disability or health conditions to use public transport.

Available to order from our online shop
www.disabilityrightsuk.org

Bank Farm
2-bedroom disabled friendly bungalow
Lounge/dining area, kitchen and bathroom, colour television, fridge, cooker, microwave, cutlery and crockery. Heating and electricity included in the price. Dedicated parking space with ramped approach from the car park. Please call for more information, layouts, measurements and facilities.

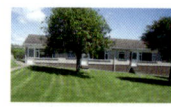

Bank Farm Leisure, Horton,
Gower, Swansea SA3 1LL
Tel: 01792 390228
bankfarmleisure@aol.com
www.bankfarmleisure.co.uk

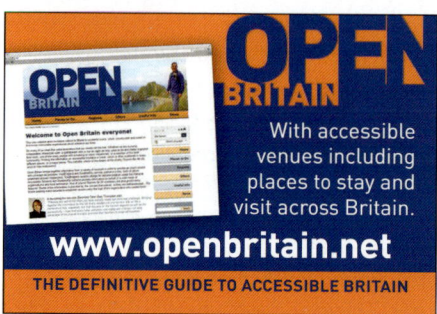

With accessible venues including places to stay and visit across Britain.
www.openbritain.net
THE DEFINITIVE GUIDE TO ACCESSIBLE BRITAIN

Gwesty'r Marine Hotel & Self-Catering Cottages
& Leisure Suite
Promenade, Aberystwyth, Ceredigion
SY23 2BX   **Tel:** 01970 612 444
www.gwestymarinehotel.co.uk & www.bryncottages.co.uk
E-mail: info@gwestymarinehotel.co.uk

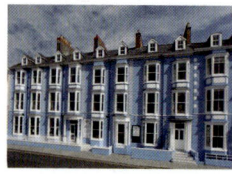
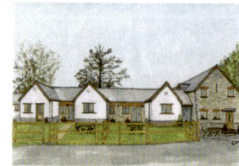

Visit Wales ***   **Visit Wales ******
A family run hotel located overlooking Ceredigion Bay
Fully accessible double room & family suite with sea-views
Sunday Carvery served every Sunday using local produce from 12.30 – 2pm

Newly converted **10 Luxury Self-Catering Cottages** - 4 & 5* Visit Wales
From 1 to 4 Bedrooms - All with en-suite and some with jacuzzi baths & wet rooms!
* Nightly or weekly bookings available *

WALES

Snowdonia for All
Information on trails, local towns and facilities for disabled people. This is available to view online in the 'Snowdonia for all' section of their website.
- 01766 770274
- parc@eryri-npa.gov.uk
- www.eryri-npa.gov.uk/visiting/snowdonia-for-all

THINGS TO SEE OR DO

Teglan Fisheries
Situated in the heart of West Wales' Aeron Valley, Teglan is a platinum award winner for disabled accessibility.
- www.teglan.net

Walks for All
National Park Centre, South Parade, Tenby, Pembrokeshire SA70 7DL
- 01834 845040
- tenby.centre@pembrokeshirecoast.org.uk
- www.pembrokeshirecoast.org.uk

The 'Walks for all' section on this website provides information on accessible trails, beaches and viewpoints. Also available is an A5 bilingual guide folder that features 17 removable easy access walks around Pembrokeshire. Includes basic maps and black and white photographs. At the rear of the booklet are sections on easy access beaches and viewpoints. Prices: from the address above.

Accommodation

ABERAERON, Ceredigion
Ty Glyn Holiday Centre
Ciliau Aeron, Near Lampeter SA48 8DE
Apply: Blaencwm, Blaenycoed, Carmarthen SA23 6ET
- 0845 0944364
- www.tyglyndavistrust.co.uk

Purpose-built centre set in the countryside for self-catering groups of children and young people with disabilities.

BONCATH, Pembrokeshire
Clynfyw Countryside Centre
Abercych, Boncath SA37 0HF
- 01239 841236
- www.clynfyw.co.uk

Contact: Jim Bowen.
Cottages designed for disabled people based on a 200 acre family-run organic farm and woodland. There are four cottages, each of which has their own distinctive character. Two of the cottages are on a single level with flat access from outside and the cottages aim to make anyone's stay as accessible as possible.

THINGS TO SEE OR DO

Janus Path
This path is a 400m long accessible wooden boardwalk through the woodland at the edge of Llyn Cwellyn, rewarding visitors with many of Snowdonia's most magnificent views of Snowdon and the surrounding mountains. Facilities include disabled parking, accessible toilet, benches and accessible picnic tables.

HOLIDAYS IN THE BRITISH ISLES

WALES

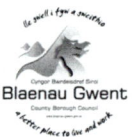

Blaenau Gwent

For more information on public facilities and access at many attractions, why not telephone before you travel?

Please telephone for all enquiries:
01495 311 556

Flintshire County Council

For more information on Public Conveniences within Flintshire please phone us on

01352 703 350

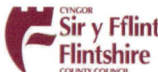

Sir y Fflint Flintshire

Laugharne Barns
Luxury accommodation in Carmarthenshire

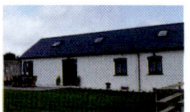

For more information contact:
The Old Cow Barn, Llansadurnen Farm House
Laugharne, Carmarthenshire SA33 4RH
T: +44 (0)1994 427241 M: +44 (0)7765 042806
enquiries@laughharnebarns.co.uk
www.laugharnebarns.co.uk

We cater for disabled and senior citizens

Amgueddfa Lloyd George Museum

Discover the life and times of the cottage bred boy who became prime minister during World War I

Open: Easter-October. Bank holiday weekends. Other times by appointment. Admission charge.
Telephone: 01766 522071
lloydgeorgemuseum@gwynedd.gov.uk
Llanystumdwy, Criccieth, Gwynedd, LL52 0SH

www.gwynedd.gob.uk/museums

Neath Port Talbot County Borough Council Directorate of Environment

Neath Port Talbot County Borough Council is committed to supporting the National Key Scheme Programme for access to all its toilets with Disabled Facilities

---

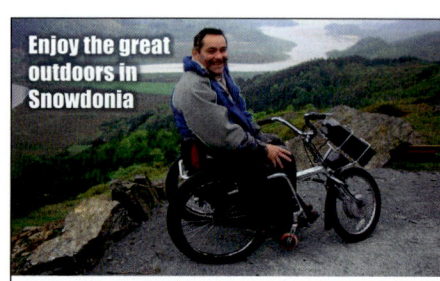

Enjoy the great outdoors in Snowdonia

Look at our website for details of 7 superb accessible walks and adventurous trails as well as lots of other useful information -
www.eryri-npa.gov.uk
01766 770274

SNOWDONIA NATIONAL PARK
one of Britain's breathing spaces

WALES

BRECON BEACONS, Powys
Brecon Beacons Holiday Cottages
Brynoyre, Talybont-on-Usk, Brecon, Powys LD3 7YS
- 01874 676446
- enquiries@breconcottages.com
- www.breconcottages.com

Offer a large selection of disability-friendly properties that have been designed with accessibility in mind. All offer stunning views of the National Park and are located in convenient places. Many properties have ramps, walk-in shower rooms, wet rooms, lifts and beds with electronic hoists and lifts for baths. The section of the website that lists accessible cottages can be found at:
- www.breconcottages.com/accessible

KIDWELLY, Carmarthenshire
Holiday Homes Trust Chalet
- 020 8433 7290
- scout.holiday.homes@scouts.org.uk
- www.holidayhomestrust.org

Adapted unit in Kidwelly, Carmarthenshire suitable for people with all levels of impairment.

LLANDUDNO, Conwy
Belmont Hotel
21 North Parade, Llandudno LL30 2LP
- 01492 877770
- belmonthotel@tiscali.co.uk
- www.royalblindsociety.org

Hotel owned by Royal Blind Society in a seafront location overlooking Llandudno Bay on the North Wales coast. Situated close to Llandudno's promenade, and local tourist attractions and within easy reach of Snowdonia. Provides specialist holiday accommodation for visually impaired people and their families and friends. Excursions with descriptive commentary are arranged and volunteers are available to accompany guests on outings.

West Shore Hotel
West Parade, Llandudno LL30 2BB
- 01492 876833
- westshore@livability.org.uk

Hotel specially adapted for disabled holiday makers run by the charity Livability. Single, twin, double and family rooms available. Entertainment and activities arranged

NARBERTH, Pembrokeshire
Caerwen
Jesse Road, Narberth SA67 7DP
Contact: The Harriet Davis Trust, Tenby Observer Offices, Warren Street, Tenby SA70 7JY
- 01834 845197
- helen@harriet-davis-trust.freeserve.co.uk

House with secure garden adapted for families with children with autism and other learning disabilities.

THINGS TO SEE OR DO

Brecon Mountain Railway
Pant, Merthyr Tydfil
Travel by narrow gauge steam train through beautiful scenery in the Brecon Beacons National Park on one of the most popular routes in Wales. One railway carriage has been designed to carry wheelchairs. There is an internal ramp from the booking office to the gift shop and platform. Disabled parking and toilets on site.
- www.breconmountainrailway.co.uk
- 01685 722 988

HOLIDAYS IN THE BRITISH ISLES

WALES

Visit our online shop for books that open doors to independent living.

www.disabilityrightsuk.org

Instantly locate your nearest toilet facility with the NKS iPhone App.

Download free from iTunes

Amroth Bay Holidays Award-winning 5-Star Holiday Park
Stunning scenery of the National Park and 5 mins drive from Amroth's golden sands

- Landscaped gardens, swimming pool and play area
- Some accommodation with ramp access, seat in shower, and grab rails
- Other aids available
- Parking next to accommodation
- Dogs welcome

Near Oakwood, Folly Farm.
Contact: amrothbay@aol.com
Tel: 01834 831259
Fax 01834 831702
www.amrothbay.co.uk

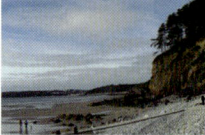
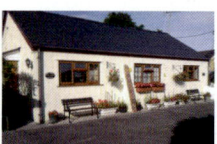
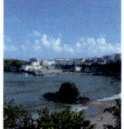

BARLOWS
Caravan Park

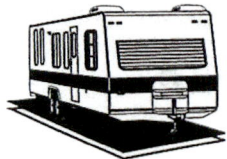

Pen-y-Cefn Road, Caerwys
North Wales CH7 5BH

Telephone 01352 720625

Bridgend County Borough Council
Passenger Transport
Co-ordination Unit

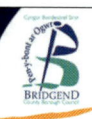

If visiting Bridgend by public transport, Bridgend Bus Station is staffed and able to provide assistance to travellers. All areas are accessible and toilets accept RADAR keys. If you require assistance please ring 01656 642591 to discuss your public transport requirements or for queries about the Welsh Government's Free Concessionary Travel Scheme. For timetable enquiries please contact Traveline Cymru 0871 200 22 33.

Should you require a little more help then why not make a booking with our Shopmobility team who can be contacted by telephone 01656 667992. Car owners with Blue Badges enjoy free parking at all Bridgend car parks.

If you intend to arrive by train, information on assistance can be obtained from Arriva Trains Wales, tel: 0845 6061 660 or
e-mail: customer.services@arrivatrainswales.co.uk

www.bridgend.gov.uk

WALES

PENALLY, Pembrokeshire
The Wheelabout
The Ridgeway, Penally, Near Tenby SA70 7RL
Contact: The Harriet Davis Trust, Tenby Observer Offices, Warren Street, Tenby SA70 7JY
- 01834 845197
- helen@harriet-davis-trust.freeserve.co.uk
- www.penally.org.uk

Purpose-designed and equipped house for families with disabled children in a quaint village in West Wales.

TENBY, Pembrokeshire
Giltar View
Southcliffe Street, Tenby
Contact: The Harriet Davis Trust, Tenby Observer Offices, Warren Street, Tenby SA70 7JY
- 01834 845197
- helen@harriet-davis-trust.freeserve.co.uk

House adapted for families with disabled children in Pembrokeshire.

Harriet's House
Castle Square, Tenby
Contact: The Harriet Davis Trust, Tenby Observer Offices, Warren Street, Tenby SA70 7JY
- 01834 845197
- helen@harriet-davis-trust.freeserve.co.uk

Flat overlooking harbour adapted for families with disabled children in Tenby.

Homeleigh Country Cottages
Homeleigh Country Cottages, Red Roses, Whitland, Carmarthenshire SA34 0PN
- 01834 831765
- enquiries@homeleigh.org
- www.homeleigh.org

Homeleigh Country Cottages are ideally situated in the peaceful Pembrokeshire countryside within a few minutes drive to many blue flag beaches including Amroth, Saundersfoot, Tenby and many more. They offer a warm welcome to guests who need a little extra help to make their holiday perfect. All doors are extra wide with level entry. Shower rooms are laid out for carefree use in the wetroom style. Disabled aids include electric beds, hoists, shower chairs, commodes etc. Call or email to request a brochure.

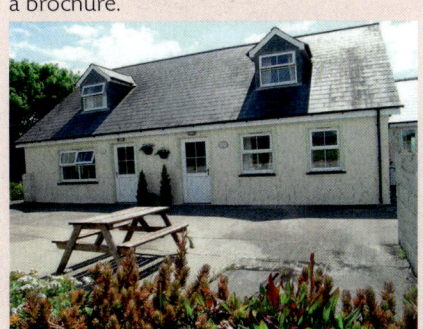

HOLIDAYS IN THE BRITISH ISLES

IRELAND

" Our coastal beauty is the stuff of legends, with shorelines trimmed by golden sands and rocky outcrops. "

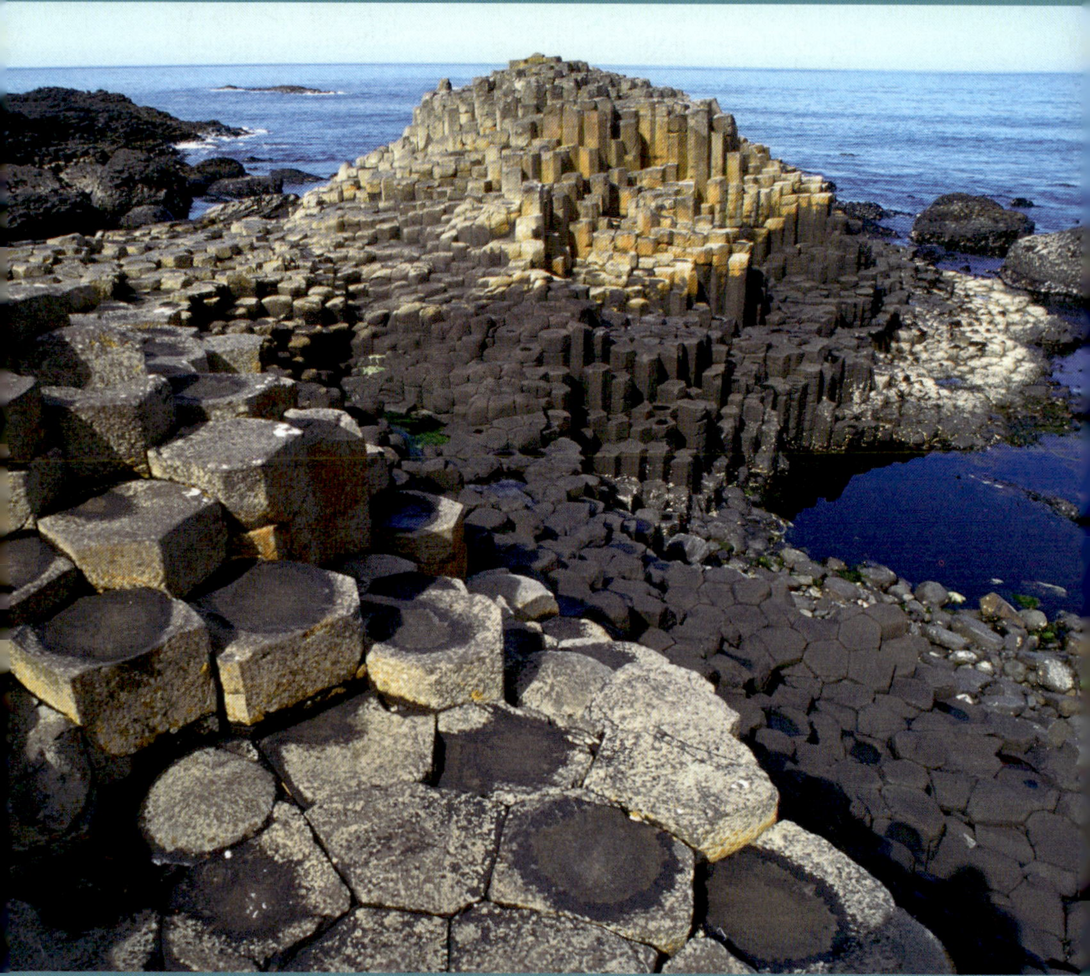

Ireland

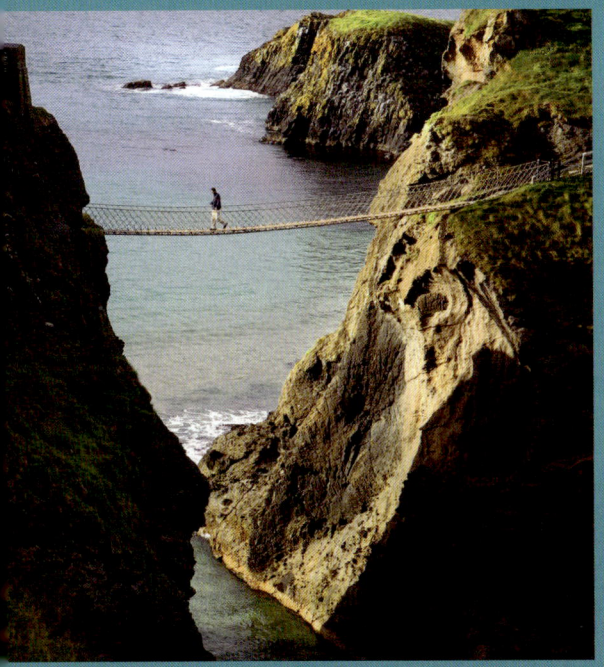

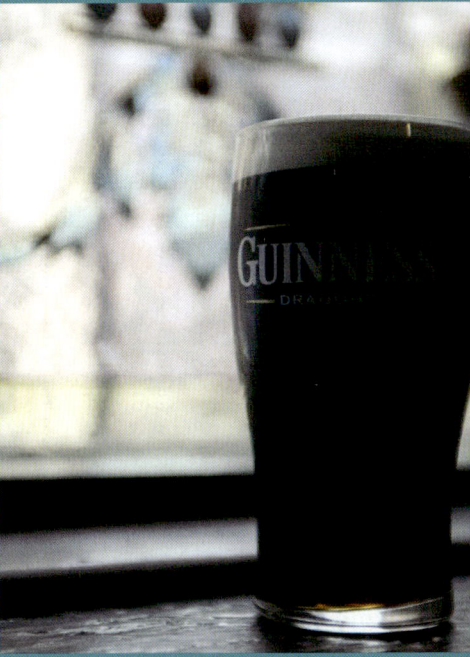

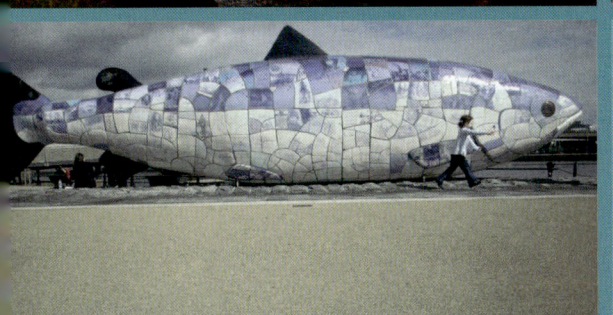

 Just go where the island of Ireland takes you. Guaranteed, you'll return home with memories that will last a lifetime.

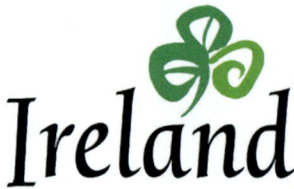

Visit the island of Ireland

Historically, Ireland is divided into four ancient provinces, Leinster, Munster, Connacht and Ulster. Politically, it is divided between the Republic of Ireland, which covers just under five-sixths of the island, and Northern Ireland, part of the United Kingdom, which covers the remainder and is located in the northeast of the island.

Perched on the northwest tip of Europe, this is the one place in the world where even time getting lost will be worthwhile ... With ancient myths and legends to uncover, amazing landscapes to explore and locals who will be more than happy to reveal our hidden gems, just go where the island of Ireland takes you. Guaranteed, you'll return home with memories that will last a lifetime.

Ireland has over 1,448km of spectacular coastline, surrounded by the Atlantic on the west and the Irish Sea on the east. As well as towering cliffs, clear fresh waters and pristine sandy beaches, the coastline enjoys lively fishing villages with some of the best seafood in the world. Inland, the lakelands and rural idylls are equally as varied as they are tranquil. You see, it's not just green on our island, it's much, much more than that ...

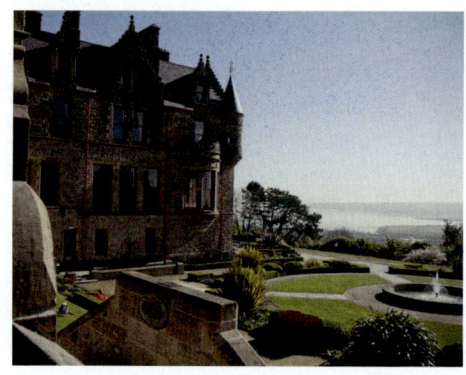

IRELAND

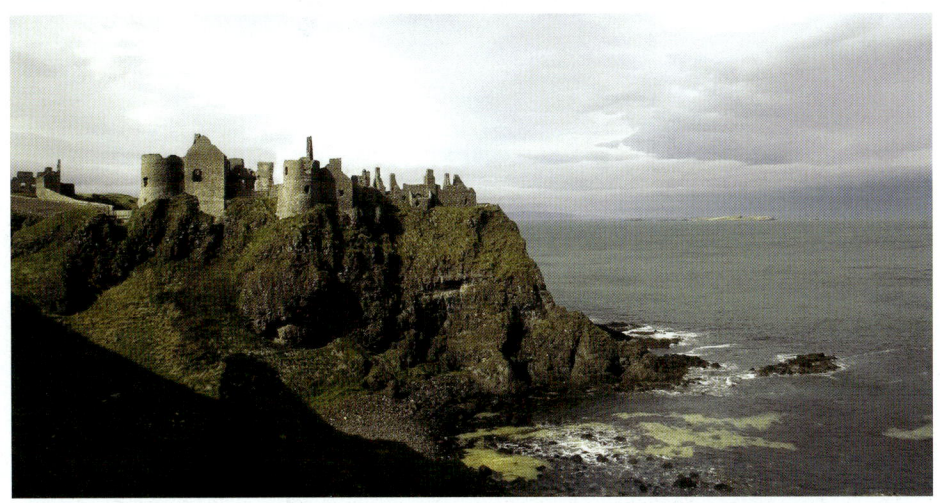

Ireland is also full or vibrant and cultural cities – in fact, the Northern Irish city of Derry-Londonderry has been named UK City of Culture for 2013. With its huge

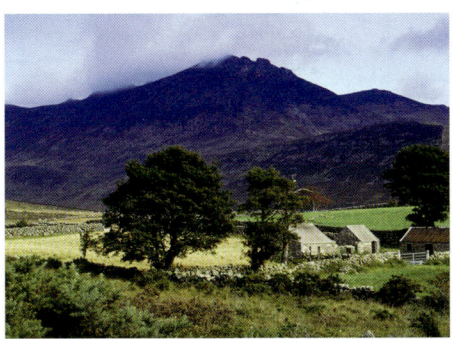

unbroken walls wrapping its cosy centre, the city is well worth a visit in 2013 as cultural celebrations take place throughout the year.

When you cross that line on the map between the Republic and Northern Ireland, the first thing you're likely to notice is that you don't notice anything different: The landscape is green and the people are friendly. From bizarre lunar landscapes and the mighty Atlantic to labyrinthine caves and crystal clear waterways, come and discover Ireland's breathtaking beauty.

For more information about Ireland:

The Island of Ireland
www.discoverireland.com
www.ireland.com

The Republic of Ireland
www.discoverireland.ie

Northern Ireland
www.discovernorthernireland.com

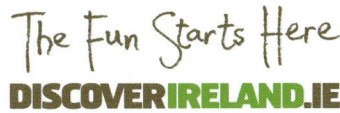

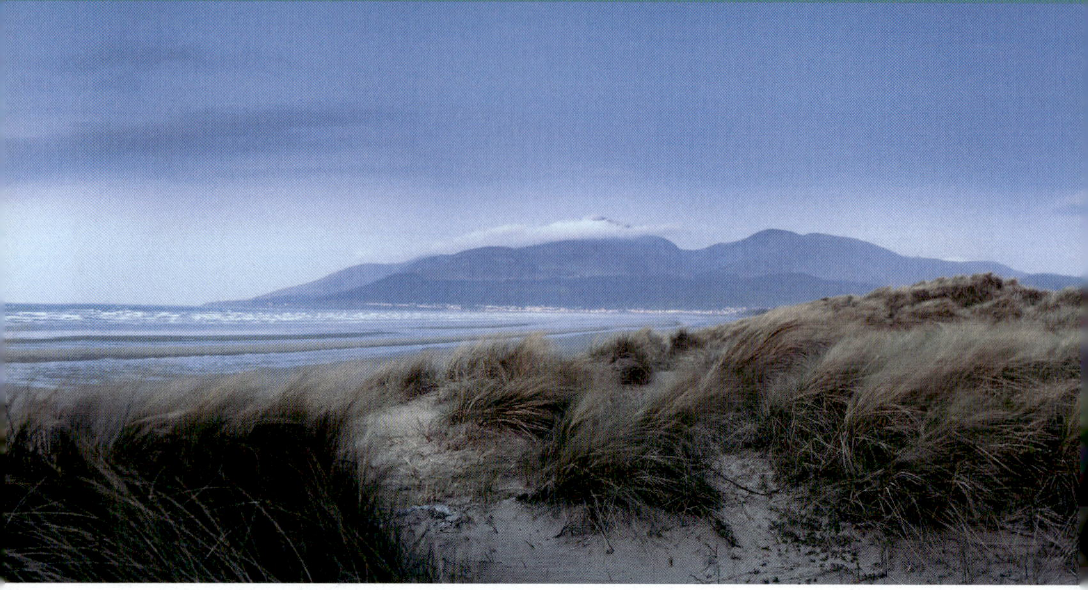

About Northern Ireland

The six counties of Northern Ireland, Fermanagh, Antrim, Down, Tyrone, Armagh and Derry provide varied countryside, dramatic coastlines, historic towns and attractive villages.

Among the most notable landscapes in the country are the Mourne Mountains on the southern coast of County Down, the Glens of Antrim on the north east coast and the Sperrin Mountains spanning counties Londonderry and Tyrone. However the most famous natural feature is Giant's Causeway on the north Antrim coast – renowned for its many-sided columns of layered basalt. A new, fully accessible Visitor Centre opened in 2012 and an accessible shuttle bus serves this World Heritage Site from the nearby town of Bushmills.

There are two major inland lakes, Lough Neagh and, in County Fermanagh, the extensive Lough Erne.

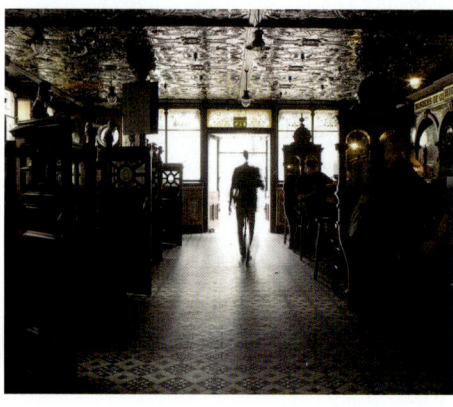

NORTHERN IRELAND

Both offer many opportunities for angling and bird watching. Boating is very popular on Lough Erne and there is the option of cruising south of the border along the re-opened Shannon-Erne waterway. The almost landlocked Strangford Lough in County Down is another mecca for birdwatchers. Near its mouth at Portaferry, a modern accessible aquarium, Exploris, displays the natural history of both the Lough and the Irish Sea.

The capital city of Belfast has an array of facilities including theatres, shops, restaurants and the Botanic Gardens, the Waterfront Concert Hall and W5, a state of the art centre to explore science. The Ulster Folk and Transport Museum, outside the city, has reconstructed buildings, one of Europe's widest ranging collections of transport history and an exhibition about the Titanic, which was built in Belfast's shipyards. Other attractions on the outskirts of the city include Colin Glen Forest Park and Belfast Zoo.

Other historic towns include the walled City of Derry-Londonderry, Armagh with its two Cathedrals and Georgian townscape, and Downpatrick which has a centre devoted to the life of St Patrick. There are great castles at Enniskillen and Carrickfergus.

Seaside resorts include Ballycastle and Portrush on the north coast and Bangor and Newcastle on the east. Tourists can

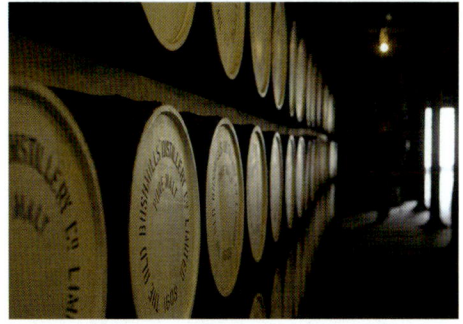

learn about the linen industry at a visitor centre and factory tour in Banbridge and visit the Ulster-American Folk Park near Omagh.

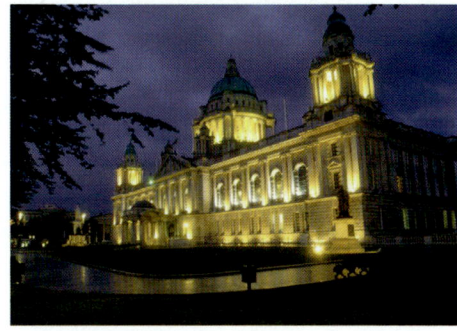

The National Trust owns several properties in Northern Ireland including Rowallane Gardens outside Belfast, Ardress House in County Armagh, the elegant Florence Court in County Fermanagh and the ornate Crown Bar in central Belfast. There are opportunities to enjoy and learn about the countryside at several of the country parks and countryside centres run by Northern Ireland Environment Agency including Roe Valley Park near Limavady and Crawfordsburn outside Bangor.

Malin Head
Tory Island
Fanad Head
Bloody Foreland
Aran Island
Buncrana
LETTERKENNY
DONEGAL
LONDONDERRY
LIMAVADY
COLERAINE
Rathlin Island
BALLYMENA
LARNE
ANTRIM
CARRICKFERGUS
BELFAST
BANGOR
NEWTOWNARDS
LISBURN
LURGAN
PORTADOWN
ARMAGH
BANBRIDGE
DOWNPATRICK
NEWRY
COOKSTOWN
OMAGH
TYRONE
ULSTER
FERMANAGH
ENNISKILLEN
MONAGHAN
CARRICKMACROSS
CAVAN
DUNDALK
Dunany Point
Clogher Head
ROSCOMMON
LONGFORD
DROGHEDA
NAVAN
MEATH
MULLINGAR
ATHLONE
BALLINASLOE
TULLAMORE
DUBLIN
Baile Átha Cliath
NAAS
BRAY
GREYSTONES
PORTLAOISE
LEINSTER
WICKLOW
Wicklow Head
0 10 20 30 40 50 60 70 80 Km
0 10 20 30 40 50 Miles

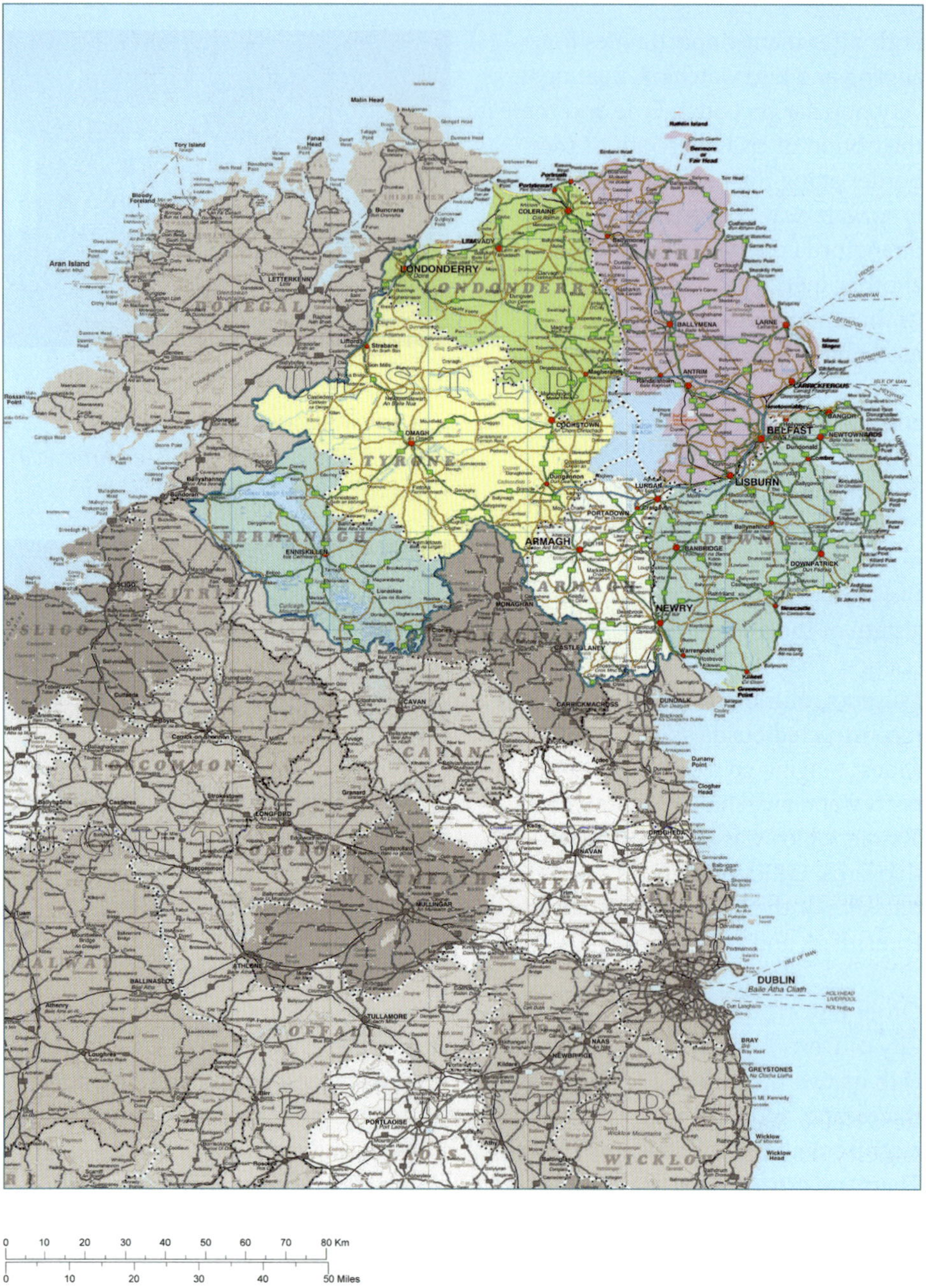

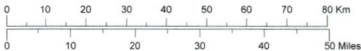

NORTHERN IRELAND

Resources

Tourism

Northern Ireland Tourist Board
59 North Street, Belfast BT1 1NB
- ☎ 028 9023 1221
  Textphone 028 9089 5512
- ✉ info@nitb.com
- 🌐 www.discovernorthernireland.com

All Northern Ireland Tourist Board publications, including guides to hotels, bed & breakfast, self-catering accommodation and attractions are available in alternative formats and can be downloaded from the website.

Transport

P & O Ferries
- ☎ 08716 64 20 20
- 🌐 www.poferries.com

Operate both fast craft and conventional ferries between Larne and Cairnryan and fast craft on a summer seasonal service between Larne and Troon. On board there are lifts between car and passenger decks and toilets for disabled passengers. Advice on the suitability of vessels is available when booking and at least 48 hours notice is requested for any assistance that may be required.

Stena Line
Stena House, Station Approach, Holyhead, Anglesey LL65 1DQ
- ☎ 08447 707070
- 🌐 www.stenaline.co.uk

Operate traditional ferry and fast-ferry services on a number of routes to Ireland. For Northern Ireland the routes are Liverpool to Belfast and Cairnryan to Belfast. These vessels are accessible to wheelchair users. Assistance can be provided at ports and on board although as much notice as possible is requested. For more information on their routes and services see their website.

> **THINGS TO SEE OR DO**
>
> **Giant's Causeway**
> This famous geological phenomenon on the North Antrim coast, renowned for its polygonal columns of layered basalt, is run by the National Trust and is the only World Heritage Site in Ireland. The causeway itself is not particularly suitable for disabled people due to uneven terrain including narrow, loose gravel paths and steep slopes. However, for people with limited mobility who would like to see the site, there are three walking trails with various levels of accessibility to choose from, including a new, all ability 'green' (easy grade) trail to Runkerry viewing point and picnic area. It provides views of the stones and, on some days, of Scotland and the Inishowen Peninsula. The visitor centre is fully accessible with ramp access to all areas. There is a loop system for hearing impaired visitors, and there are accessible toilets and parking. An accessible shuttle bus service from the visitor centre to the main Causeway operates regularly, which is chargeable (free for National Trust members).
> - 🌐 www.nationaltrust.org.uk

IRELAND

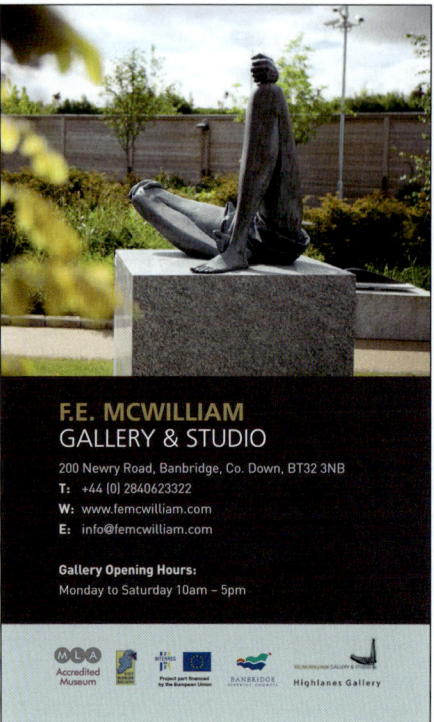

F.E. MCWILLIAM GALLERY & STUDIO

200 Newry Road, Banbridge, Co. Down, BT32 3NB
T: +44 (0) 2840623322
W: www.femcwilliam.com
E: info@femcwilliam.com

Gallery Opening Hours:
Monday to Saturday 10am – 5pm

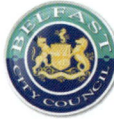

We have 14 public toilets across the City of Belfast, with disabled access available at 12 of these.

For more information call us on 0800 032 8100

www.belfastcity.gov.uk/waste

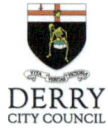

DERRY CITY COUNCIL

Council Offices, 98 Strand Road, Derry BT48 7NN
Tel: (028) 71 365 151 Fax: (028) 7126 4858
www.derrycity.gov.uk

DERRY CITY COUNCIL SUPPORT THE PROVISION OF FACILITIES FOR ALL ITS CITIZENS

Delamont Country Park

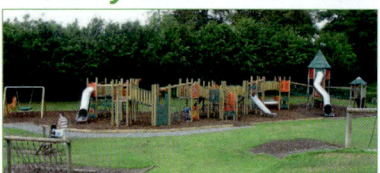

- Award winning Caravan and Camping Club
- Full Events Programme
- Delamont Miniature Railway
- Outdoor Adventure Playground
- Strangford Stone
- Boat Trips on Strangford Lough *(Booking Essential)*
- Rambler Mobility Scooters available *(Booking Essential)*
- Canoe Trail
- Ice-cream Kiosk

Open daily 9am-dusk. All events weather permitting.

For further information contact
Tel/Fax 028 44828 333
www.delamontcountrypark.com
e-mail: delamont.park@downdc.gov.uk

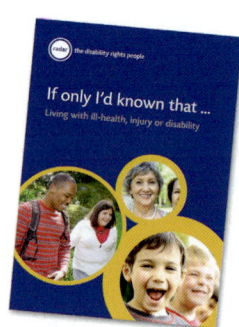

If Only I'd Known That ...

An information-packed guide to services, welfare rights, facilities and support for anyone with a disability or health condition, this guide includes resources for all ages from childhood to later years.

Available to order from our online shop
www.disabilityrightsuk.org

NORTHERN IRELAND

Translink
Central Station, Belfast BT1 3PB
- ☎ 028 9066 6630
  Textphone 028 90 38 75 05
- 🌐 www.translink.co.uk

Translink can provide information on the accessibility of train and bus transport throughout Northern Ireland. Information on access at rail and bus stations is given on their website.

Information & advice

Disability Action
Portside Business Park, 189 Airport Road West, Belfast BT3 9ED
- ☎ 028 9029 7880
  Textphone 028 9029 7882
- ✉ hq@disabilityaction.org
- 🌐 www.disabilityaction.org

Disability Action can provide general information on holiday accommodation and transport in Northern Ireland.

Diabetes UK Northern Ireland
Bridgewood House, Newforge Lane, Belfast BT9 5NW
- ☎ 028 9066 6646
- ✉ n.ireland@diabetes.org.uk
- 🌐 www.diabetes.org.uk/northernireland

An annual support holiday for children aged 8-11 years and a youth support holiday, for ages 12-17 are arranged, to help young people manage their diabetes in a holiday environment at which there is an organised programme of events and activities. The holiday is staffed by volunteers including healthcare professionals. Weekends for adults and families are also arranged.

Equipment hire

SHOPMOBILITY
The National Federation of Shopmobility UK (NFSUK), PO Box 6641, Christchurch BH23 9DQ
- ☎ 0844 41 41 850
- ✉ info@shopmobilityuk.org
- 🌐 www.shopmobilityuk.org

Scheme which lends manual wheelchairs, powered wheelchairs and powered scooters to members of the public with limited mobility to shop and to visit leisure and commercial facilities within the town, city or shopping centre. You can find the nearest Shopmobility scheme to you through their on-line directory. Contact specific Shopmobility Schemes to make equipment bookings or find out more information.

THINGS TO SEE OR DO

Ardress House
A 17th-century farmhouse, elegantly remodeled in Georgian times, is set in 40 hectares (100 acres) of countryside in County Armagh with apple orchards, woodland, riverside walks and a working farmyard and is owned by the National Trust. The majority of rooms are located on the ground floor, most of which is wheelchair accessible. Adapted toilets are located in the reception area and a wheelchair is available for loan. There are suitable routes in the grounds for wheelchair users.
- 🌐 www.nationaltrust.org.uk

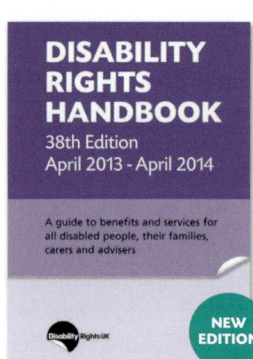

As comprehensive as ever
- How the benefit system works and how to make a claim
- Benefits for people with an illness, injury or disability
- Benefits for carers, young people and children and those looking for work, or in retirement
- Benefits for people injured at work or serving in the Armed Forces
- Challenging benefit decisions
- Getting and paying for care services

New in 2013
For people aged 16-64
- Personal Independence Payment: how to claim, what to do if you are turned down and what happens to people on Disability Living Allowance
- Extra information on Access to Work
- The new sanctions rules for Jobseeker's Allowance and Employment and Support Allowance
- The benefit cap: who will be affected and how it works

For families with disabled children
- Expanded guidance on Disability Living Allowance for children

For people 65 and over:
- Additional information on claiming Attendance Allowance

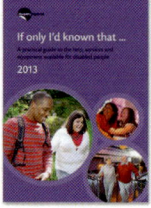

Personal Independence Payment is coming ...

From April 2013, Disability Living Allowance for people aged 16-64 will start to be replaced by a new benefit, the Personal Independence Payment. Over 2 million people will be affected.

The next two years will also see the biggest changes to the benefits system since the introduction of the welfare state. In this period of unprecedented change and benefits cuts, keeping up with the new rules is crucial.

Information and advice you can trust
The new edition of our Disability Rights Handbook, fully updated for 2013, provides in-depth information on the entire benefits system and comprehensive guidance on these critical changes.

The must-buy edition – out May 2013
Disability Rights Handbook 2013-2014 (38th Edition)
£29.99 inc P&P (£15.00 for people claiming benefits)
Order online at www.disabilityrightsuk.org

Stay informed – know your rights
This year's Handbook explains Personal Independence Payment and includes new additional guidance on Disability Living Allowance for children and Attendance Allowance (for people 65 and over) with tactics and tools to help make a successful claim.

It introduces Universal Credit which will replace several income-related benefits and tax credits and is planned to be phased in from April 2013.

All benefits explained in one book
Written in plain English by benefits specialists and legally referenced, it's the only user-friendly benefits guide designed specifically for both claimants and their advisers. It has the answers you need to help ensure the quality of your advice or to claim what you are entitled to.

Keep your Handbook up to date all year
Become a member of Disability Rights UK and we'll keep you up-to-date throughout the year with 'Disability and Welfare Rights Updates' our bi-monthly PDF magazine. 20+ pages of news and page-by-page Handbook updates. Download a free sample copy from our website.

If only I'd known that ...
Our companion guide, 'If only I'd known that a year ago' provides practical advice on accessing the help, services and equipment available for disabled people of all ages. See overleaf for more information.

Order your copy now at www.disabilityrightsuk.org

NORTHERN IRELAND

McElmeel Mobility Services
15 Ballyscandal Road, Armagh BT61 8BL
- 028 3752 5333
- info@mobility-services.com
- www.mobility-services.com

Vehicle adaption company that hires both cars fitted with hand controls and those that can carry passengers in wheelchairs.

THINGS TO SEE OR DO

Lagan Towpath
The Lagan Towpath, which dates back to the late 18th century and is home to a variety of wildlife, takes visitors along the river and canal system through a variety of wetland, riverside meadows and mixed woodland from Belfast to Lisburn. The path is off-road, quiet and has a hard surface suitable for manual wheelchairs. The entire path is 11 miles long, but it can be completed in sections. Facilities are located at the nearest town, Stranmillis. A leaflet on the towpath and Lagan Valley Regional Park is available from local Tourist Information Centres and libraries.
- www.walkni.com

Accommodation

KILKEEL, Co. Down
Mourne Activity Centre
42 Ballinran Road, Kilkeel BT34 4JA
- 028 4176 5727
- info@inclusionmatters.org

Holiday & Conference Centre near the Mourne Mountains. Special interest tours, festival breaks, craft and traditional skills courses are available. Offer multi-activity breaks, such as walking, cycling, horse riding, golf, falconry, fishing, adventure outdoor activities, team building and painting breaks many of which are suitable for disabled visitors.

LISNASKEA, Co. Fermanagh
Share Holiday Village
Smith's Strand, Lisnaskea BT92 0EQ
- 028 6772 2122
- www.sharevillage.org

Holiday and Activity Centre designed for use by disabled people based on Smith's Strand near Lisnaskea in County Fermanagh. Waterside location. Accommodates people from all backgrounds in large numbers. Share is a charity that works for the inclusion of disabled and non-disabled people by providing opportunities for all to participate in a wide range of creative, educational and recreational programmes through over 30 different arts, land and water activities.

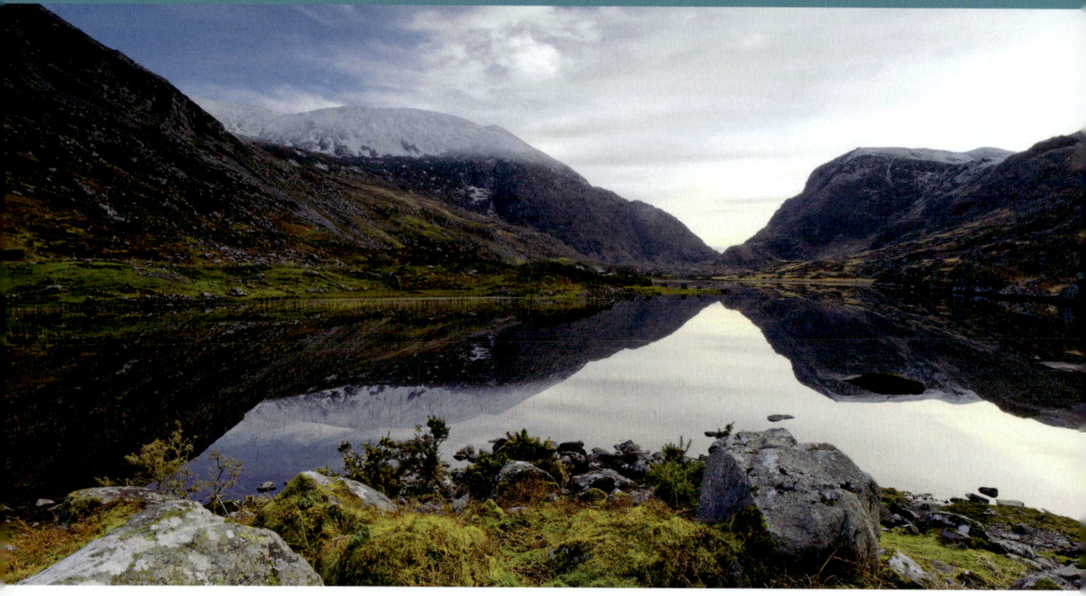

IRELAND

About the Republic of Ireland

The 26 counties of the Republic: Carlow, Cavan, Clare, Cork, Donegal, Dublin, Galway, Kerry, Kildare, Kilkenny, Laois, Leitrim, Limerick, Longford, Louth, Mayo, Meath, Monaghan, Offaly, Roscommon, Sligo, Tipperary, Waterford, Westmeath, Wexford and Wicklow provide a varied and rich holiday opportunity.

The ancient heritage is all around and the Republic is full of myths and legends. Turn off a motorway and you'll find standing stones, fairy forts, stone circles, burial mounds and dolmens that have intrigued travelers for centuries. The Celtic love of arts and song is alive in modern Ireland, where a taste for theatre, music, literature and history are key to the national identity.

You could spend days in the Boyne Valley, visiting the World Heritage Neothlithic site of Brú na Bóinne and archaeological wonder of the Hill of Tara. Or take a trip to an island: the Iron

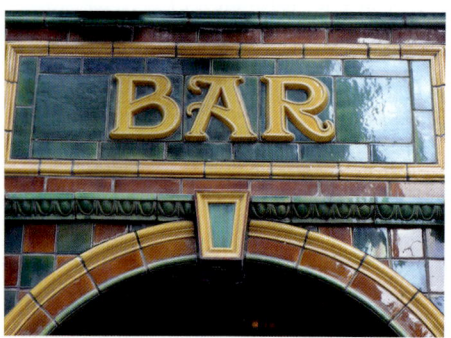

HOLIDAYS IN THE BRITISH ISLES

Age fort, Dun Aengus, has survived on Inis Mór for 2000 years, while Skellig Michael, off the Kerry coast, dates from the 7th century. This monastic complex perched on a rock is also a World Heritage Site.

You could check out the Bronze Age stone circles in Cork and Kerry or the Céide Fields in North Mayo, the most extensive Stone Age site in the world.

Or visit the National Museum in Dublin to see the greatest collection of prehistoric gold objects in Western Europe. The sun shining through the passage tomb at Newgrange at the winter solstice was one of the wonders of the ancient world.

The capital city, Dublin, offers an eclectic mix of city, countryside and coastline. Temple Bar, on the south bank of the River Liffey is Dublin's cultural quarter, with a medieval street pattern and

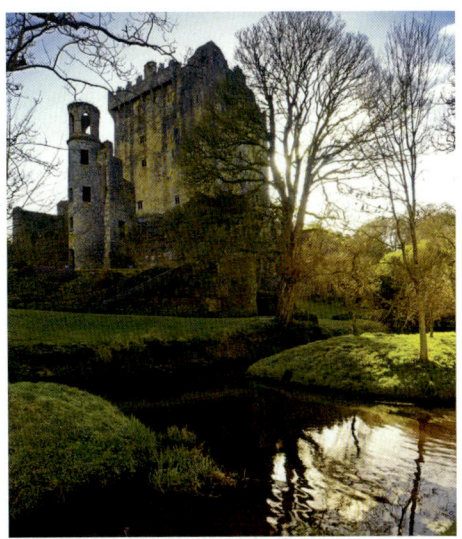

narrow cobbled streets. It has many pubs, a regular book market, a lively nightlife and a popular shopping area. It is also the location of many Irish cultural institutions including the Irish Photography Centre, the Ark Children's Cultural Centre, the Irish Film Institute, incorporating the Irish Film Archive, the Temple Bar Music Centre and the Arthouse Multimedia Centre. In addition, it houses the Irish Stock Exchange and the Central Bank of Ireland.

Visit Kilmainham Gaol, one of the largest unoccupied gaols in Europe. Or Dublin castle, originally built on the orders of King John of England in 1204 on a site previously settled by the Vikings. For fun, try the National Wax Museum at Foster Place.

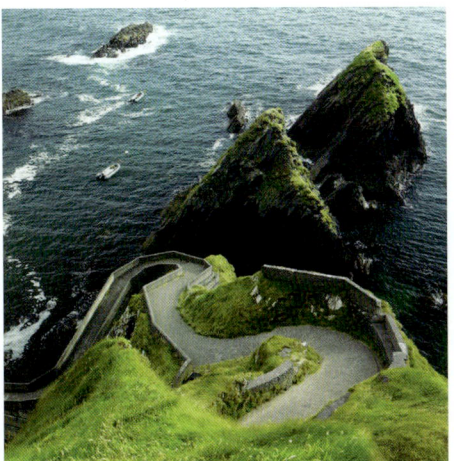

IRELAND

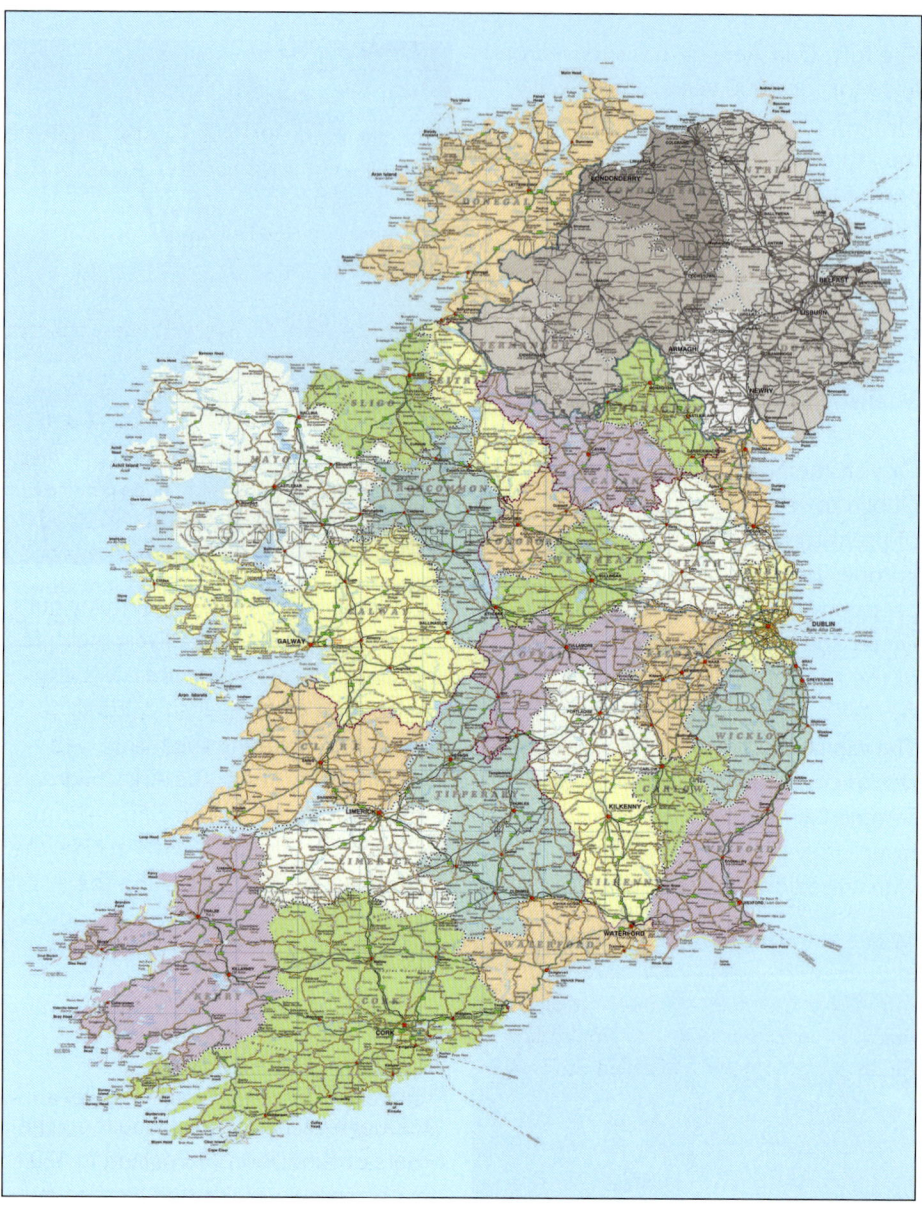

REPUBLIC OF IRELAND

Resources

Tourism

Tourism Ireland Ltd
Head Office, 5th Floor, Bishop's Square, Redmond's Hill, Dublin 2
- +353 (0)1 476 3400
- www.tourismireland.com

UK Office: Nations House, 103 Wigmore Street, London W1U 1QS
- 0800 039 7000
- info.gb@tourismireland.com

National tourist Board who holds some information on accessible accommodation. Suitable properties are indicated in their annual *Guide to Guest Accommodation* and *Guide to Self-Catering Accommodation* and on their website although the information is not readily searchable.

Office of Public Works
Visitor Services, Office of Public Works, Unit 20, Lakeside Retail Park, Claremorris, Co. Mayo
- +353 1 647 6592
- info@heritageireland.ie
- www.heritageireland.ie

Manage a wide range of heritage sites including monuments and historic buildings throughout the country. Their annual visitor Information leaflets include an indication of the extent of access for disabled visitors.

Transport

Irish Ferries
Contact Centre, PO Box 19, Alexandra Road, Ferryport, Dublin 1
- 0818 300400
- info@irishferries.com
  disabilityofficer@irishferries.com
- www.irishferries.com

UK office: Corn Exchange, Brunswick Street, Liverpool L2 7TP
- 08717 300 400

Operate car ferry services on the Holyhead-Dublin and Pembroke-Rosslare routes and also a fast ferry service between Holyhead and Dublin. All vessels have facilities for disabled passengers and at all four ports terminals have been built to be accessible. Advance notification at the time of booking is requested if passengers feel they have specific requirements. Much information for disabled passengers can be found on their website under 'special needs' and anyone with more specific information should contact the Disability Officers through the Contact Centre or via the disability officer email address above.

Irish Railways – Iarnród Eireann
- +353 (0)1890 77 88 99
- access@irishrail.ie
- www.iarnrodeireann.ie

General information on access and services for disabled passengers as well as information on the accessibility of individual stations is available on the website. Choose 'Travel and Station Information' and then 'Accessibilty'. Requests for assistance should be made in advance, preferably at least 24 hours, to the station from which the journey is starting or to the Mobility Liaison Office, Iarnród Eireann, Connolly Station, Dublin 1.

IRELAND

P&O Ferries
- 08716 64 20 20
- www.poferries.com

Car ferry services are operated to Dublin from Liverpool but the vessels used do not have lifts between the car deck and the main passenger areas. Advice on the suitability of vessels is available when booking and at least 48 hours notice is requested for any assistance that may be required.

Stena Line
Stena House, Station Approach, Holyhead, Anglesey LL65 1DQ
- 08447 707070
- www.stenaline.co.uk

Operate ferry services between Holyhead and Dun Laoghaire and Dublin and between Fishguard and Rosslare using vessels that are accessible to wheelchair users. Assistance can be provided at both port and on board although as much notice as possible is requested. There are toilets fitted with the NKS lock at the Fishguard and Holyhead terminals.

Information & advice

Irish Wheelchair Association
Áras Chúchulainn, Blackheath Drive, Clontarf, Dublin 3
- +353 1 818 6400
- info@iwa.ie
- www.iwa.ie

Voluntary organisation of people with physical disabilities. Operate an Information Resource Centre which has some information on accessible holidays in Ireland and elsewhere. It also has a holiday and respite centre in Roscommon, a small holiday centre in Kilkenny, and a respite centre in Dublin.

Equipment hire

SHOPMOBILITY IRELAND
- info@shopmobility.ie
- www.shopmobility.ie

Established over 5 years ago by the Disabled Drivers Association of Ireland to improve access to shopping in Ireland for people with limited mobility. Operate in 4 town centres across Ireland:

Cork – Mahon Point Shopping Centre
- 021 431-3033

Dublin – Dundrum Town Centre
- 01 298 982

Dublin – Liffey Valley Shopping Centre
- 01 620 8731

Newbridge, Co. Kildare – Whitewater Shopping Centre
- 04 545 0736

Advance Electrical Mobility
4 Crumlin Village, Dublin 12, Ireland
- +353 1 455 3168
- info@aemobility.com
- www.aemobility.com

Supply and maintain a wide range of mobility and other equipment with powered scooters and wheelchairs available for rent.

BOC Medispeed
BOC Home Care, Blyry Business Park, Athlone County West Meath, Ireland
- 00 800 220 20202
- healthcareinfo.ie@boc.com
- www.boconline.ie
  www.bochealthcare.ie

The major supplier of medical oxygen in Ireland can provide both domestic and ambulatory oxygen for tourists with advanced notice on arrival in the country or at their final destination.

MMS Medical Ltd
51 Eastgate Drive, Little Island, Cork, Ireland
- +353 1890 880 880
- info@mmsmedical.ie
- www.mmsmedical.ie

Company, with additional centres in Dublin and Galway, that can hire and sell a wide range of mobility and other equipment.

Motability Ireland Ltd
The Irish Mobility Centre, Unit 21, Ashbourne Industrial Park, Ashbourne, Co Meath, Ireland
- +353 1 835 9173
- sales@motabilityireland.com
- www.motabilityireland.com

Family-owned company that carryies out vehicle adaptations for disabled people. They have a fleet of hire cars including wheelchair accessible vehicles and automatic cars fitted with hand controls.

McElmeel Mobility Services
15 Ballyscandal Road, Armagh BT61 8BL
- 028 3752 5333
- info@mobility-services.com
- www.mobility-services.com

Vehicle adaption company that also hires out cars fitted with hand controls and cars that can carry passengers in wheelchairs.

Cuisle Holiday Centre
Donamon, Co. Roscommon
- +353 (0)90 666 2277
- cuisle@iwa.ie
- www.cuisle.com

A fully accessible holiday owned by the Irish Wheelchair Association and based within Donamon Castle's 50 acre site. Highly-trained staff provide supported holidays, respite care and breaks.

Accommodation

DUBLIN
Carmel Fallon Respite Centre
Blackheath Drive, Clontarf, Dublin 3
- +353 1 818 6458
- carmelfallonrespite@iwa.ie
- www.iwa.ie

Holiday and respite centre in grounds of Irish Wheelchair Association headquarters, near the coast and public transport north of City Centre.

KILCOOLE, Co. Wicklow
Trident Holiday Homes
E8 Network Enterprise Park Kilcoole, Co. Wicklow
- +353 1 201 8440
- reservations@tridentholidayhomes.ie
- www.tridentholidayhomes.ie

Represent a range of self-catering accommodation in many parts of Ireland. Their brochure indicates those that have some facilities for disabled people.

KNOCK, Co. Mayo
Knock House Hotel
Ballyhaunis Road, Knock, Co. Mayo
- +352 94 93 88088
- info@knockhousehotel.ie
- www.knockhousehotel.ie

Modern hotel minutes from the famous Knock Shrine. 20 minutes from Ireland West Airport Knock and 10 minutes from Claremorris Train Station. The hotel provides a courtesy coach pick up & drop off service and has 68, of which six have been specially designed to cater for wheelchair users. Many rooms have views of the countryside of County Mayo.

CHANNEL ISLANDS

> "Guernsey is a special place, a thriving community that welcomes its visitors and leaves a lasting impression on all who set foot there."

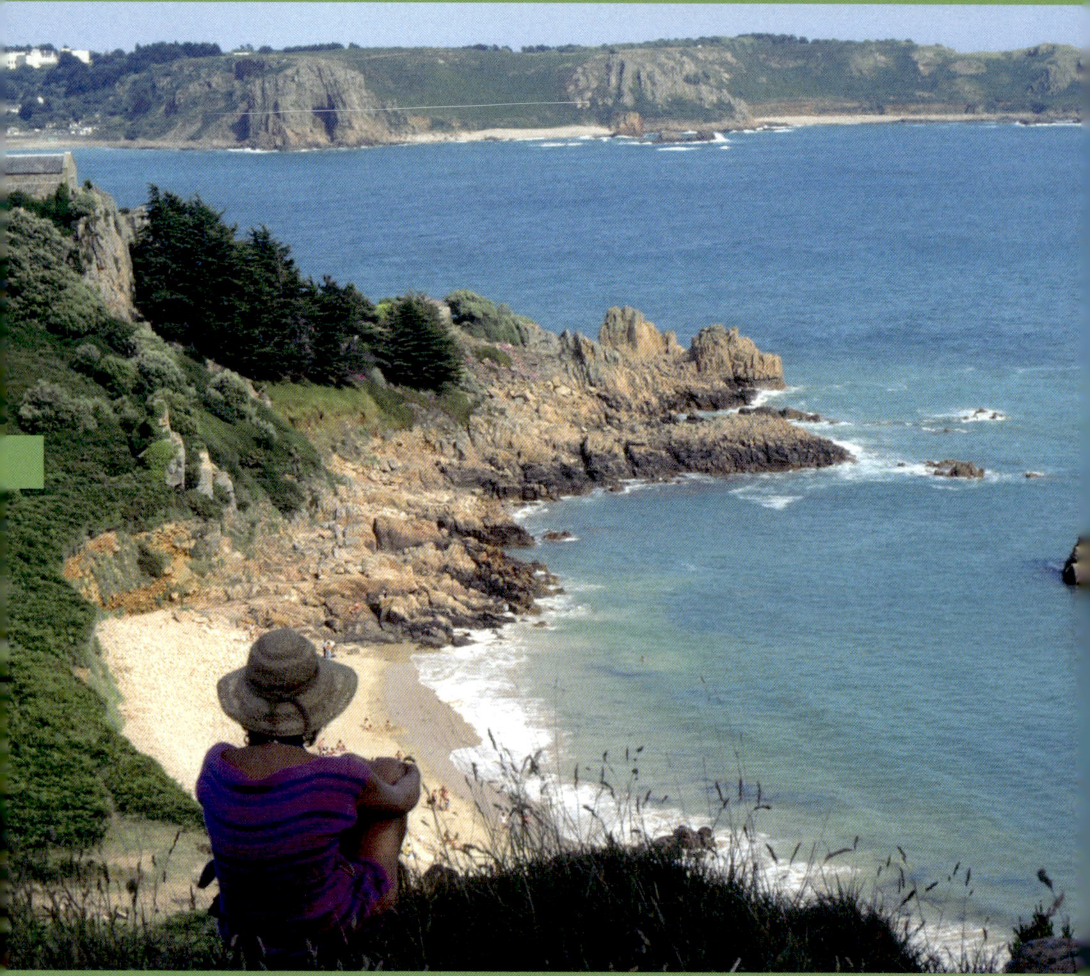

Channel Islands

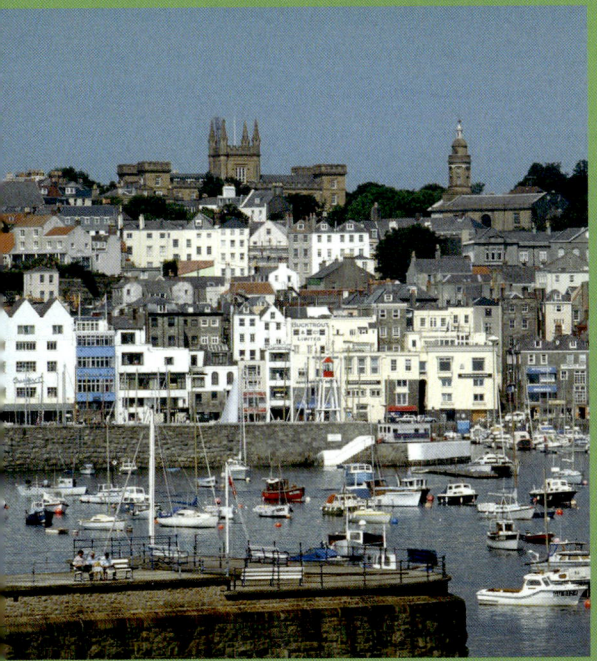

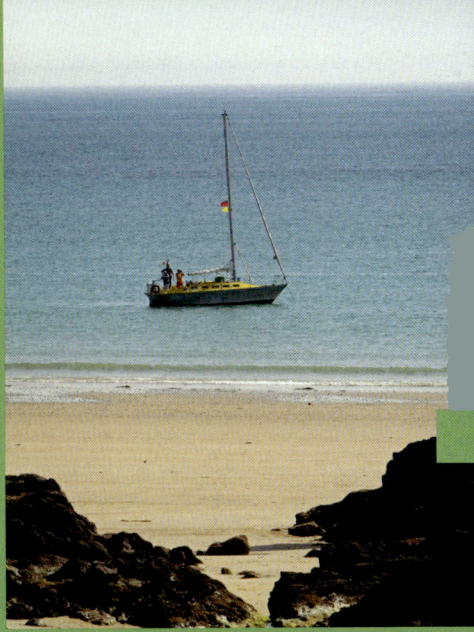

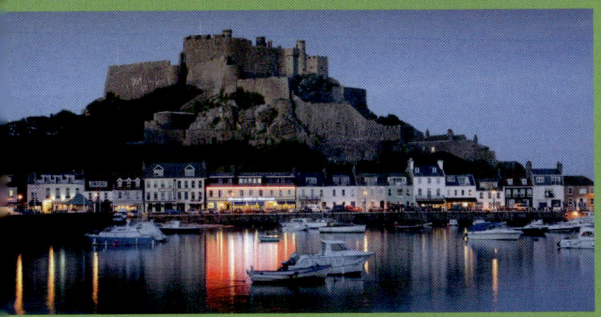

" *There are no cars, giving Sark an enchantment which is quite unique; its spell draws visitors back for their holidays, year after year.* "

CHANNEL ISLANDS

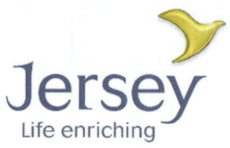 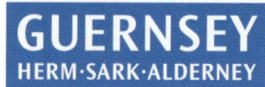

Visit the Channel Islands

Welcome to the Channel Islands, where British and French influences meet and where an unexpected mix of stunning scenery, rich heritage and varied lifestyles are waiting to be discovered.

Jersey

With its unspoiled landscape and unique blend of British and French influences, Jersey really is a place where you can get away from it all. Lose yourself in the Island's winding lanes or on its breathtaking coast. English is spoken and sterling is the currency – yet the streets are named in French. Jersey is reassuringly familiar to visitors from both sides of the Channel.
www.jersey.com

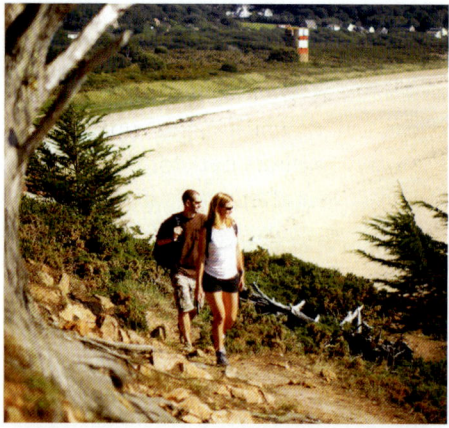

Guernsey

A heady mix of stunning scenery and the best of contemporary living, Guernsey is the perfect destination. Inspiring walks along the cliff paths, or lazy days on the island's beautiful beaches, Guernsey has it all.

St Peter Port, the island's capital, is a bustling harbour town, a tapestry of architectural styles that tell the story of the region's changing fortunes. Ask anyone who's been here. Guernsey is a special place, a thriving community that welcomes its visitors and leaves a lasting impression on all who set foot there.
www.visitguernsey.com

Alderney

Alderney, the third largest of the Channel Islands invites you to travel to and discover one of the few unspoiled, peaceful and natural British Isles. The island enjoys a mild climate and

CHANNEL ISLANDS

independence, with its own government and a fledgling off-shore finance and e-commerce sector. Despite being only eight miles from mainland France and 30 miles from Jersey, Alderney has avoided mainstream tourism.

Visit Alderney and you will discover an oasis with an ancient and varied history, an abundance of flora and fauna, beautiful beaches, an enviable lifestyle with that unique, contagious phenomenon known as 'the Alderney Feeling'.
www.visitalderney.com

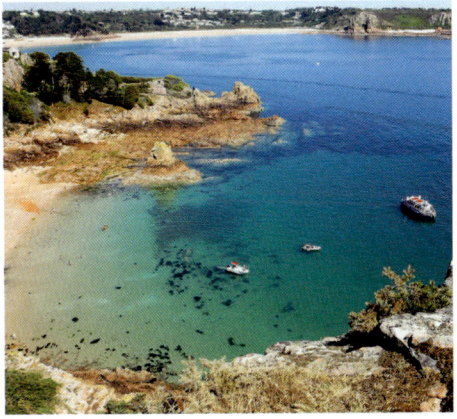

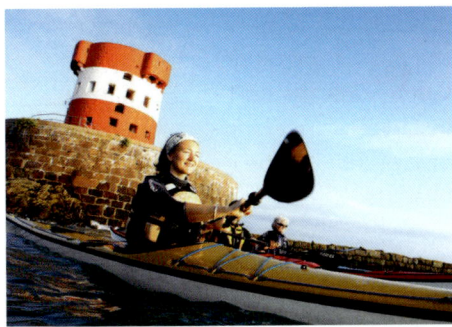

Herm
Herm is three miles from the coast of Guernsey and the perfect place to stay for a truly relaxing island holiday; ideal for families and anyone wanting to 'get away from it all'. Enjoy our beautiful unspoilt beaches and safe, clean pollution-free environment. There are no cars, no crowds and definitely no stress.

You can visit Herm for the day or choose to stay on the Island where we can offer a variety of accommodation to suit all tastes. You could stay in one of our comfortable self catering cottages or be pampered at The White House Hotel, the only hotel on the Island, where there are no telephones, televisions or clocks. You can also camp with glorious views across the French coast.
www.herm.com

Sark
Sark is the smallest of the four main Channel Islands, located 80 miles off the south coast of England. It boasts 40 miles of what must be one of the most picturesque coastlines anywhere in the world. There are no cars, giving Sark an enchantment which is quite unique; its spell draws visitors back for their holidays, year after year.
www.sark.co.uk

Find out more information about the Channel Islands at:
www.visitchannelislands.com

CHANNEL ISLANDS

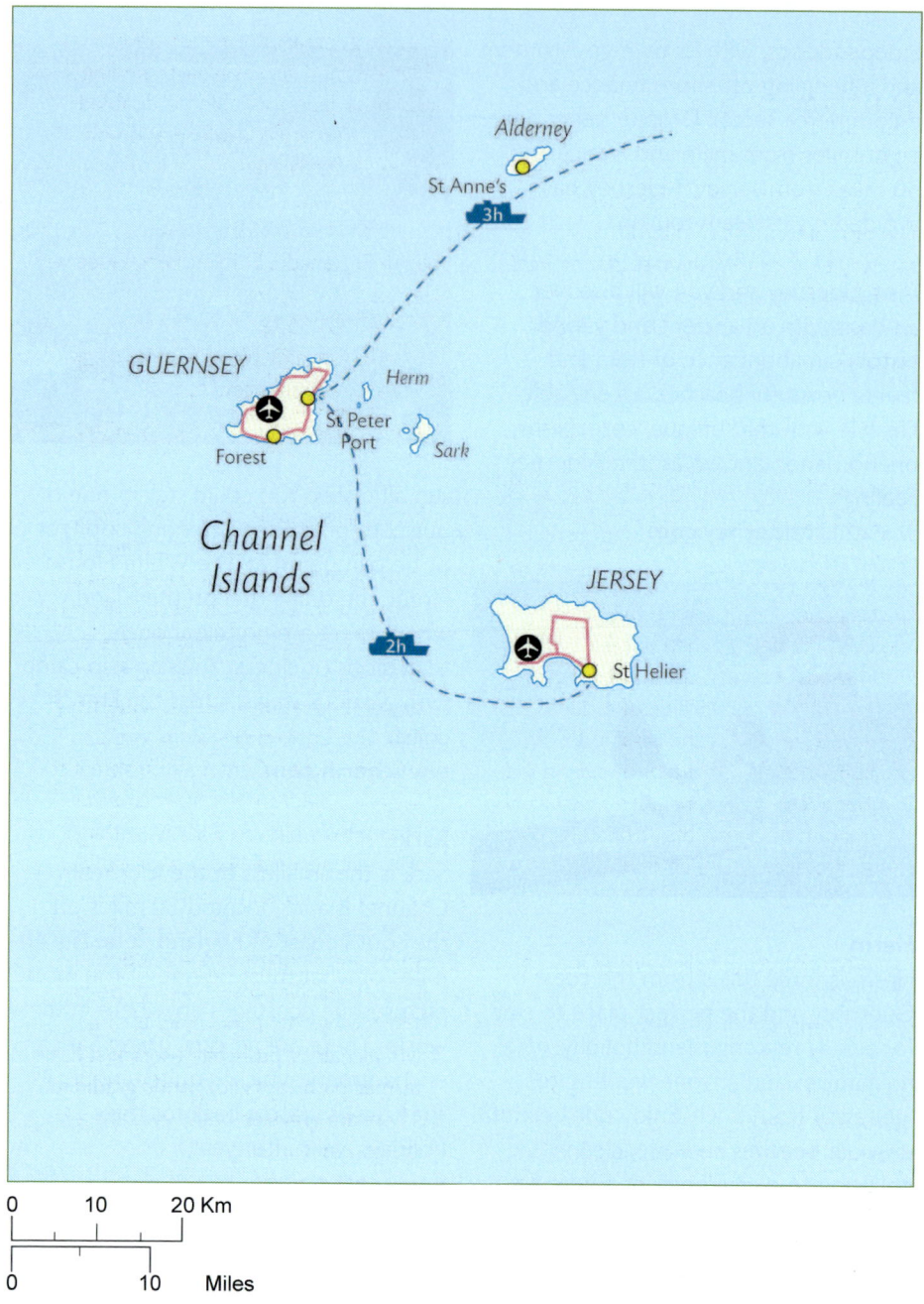

CHANNEL ISLANDS

Resources
Tourism

Visit Channel Islands
- www.visitchannelislands.com

The official tourist board information gateway to all of the Channel Islands. You can find information and resources on visiting Jersey, Guernsey, Alderny, Herm and Sark.

JERSEY
Jersey Tourism
Liberation Square, St Helier, Jersey JE1 1BB
- 01534 500777
- info@jersey.com
- www.jersey.com

Supply general information for tourists and can provide information on accessible accommodation, attractions, transport, equipment hire and facilities. Produce A Guide to Jersey for the Disabled available on their website or by calling the number above, which includes a wealth of information on accessible attractions, places to stay, travel and parking on the island.

Jersey Information Centre
Liberation Place, St Helier, Jersey JE1 1BB
- 01534 448877
- info.centre@jersey.com

GUERNSEY
Visit Guernsey
Information & Accommodation Services, PO Box 23, St Peter Port, Guernsey GY1 3AN
- 01481 723552
- enquiries@visitguernsey.com
- www.visitguernsey.com

Provide general information about Guernsey and also assist with finding accommodation suitable for disabled visitors. Also provide information on Alderney for tourists.

Guernsey Information Centre
North Esplanade, St Peter Port, Guernsey GY1 2LQ
- 01481 723552
- info.centre@cultureleisure.gov.gg
- www.visitguernsey.com

THINGS TO SEE OR DO

Saumarez Park
The largest public park in Guernsey, located in the centre of the island in the Castel Parish. The Park is open all year round from dawn until dusk and is free of charge. Features include a large adventure playground for toddlers to teens, the National Trust of Guernsey Folk and Costume Museum and a Walled Kitchen Garden. Refreshments are available from the Saumarez Park Tearooms which are located within the park near the National Trust Folk Museum. Public toilets are located near the tearooms. There is an NKS toilet and ramps into the tearooms for wheelchair access. Two car parks are nearby. The park is suitable for wheelchair or pushchair users as it has tarmac pathways with gentle gradients. There are graveled pathways through the formal gardens.
- www.gov.gg/ParksandGardens

HOLIDAYS IN THE BRITISH ISLES

CHANNEL ISLANDS

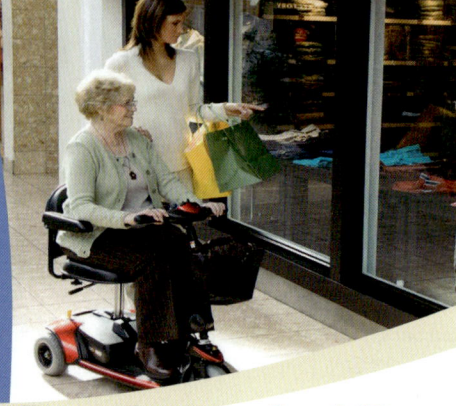

Completing the package for an easier holiday.

A wide range of Health care, mobility and Access products

TECHNICARE

Contact **01534 888975** or
www.technicare-jersey.com

Products *for* Hire

- Mobility scooters
- Powered or manual wheelchairs
- Ramps
- Walking frames
- Adjustable beds
- Lift & recline armchairs
- High seat chairs
- Hoists
- Bath lifts

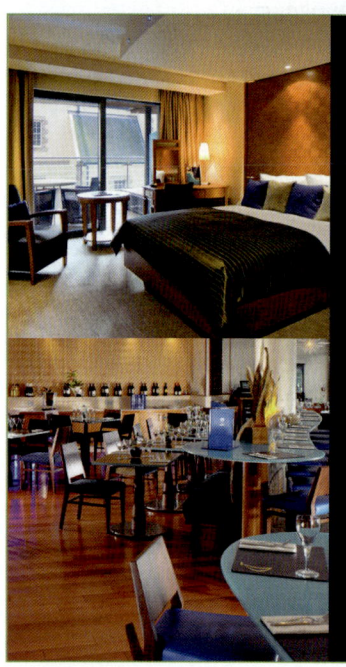

Visit Jersey
And stay at the exquisite Royal Yacht

Situated in St Helier, The Royal Yacht is a modern luxury hotel offering fabulous restaurants, bars and an award winning spa. All Rooms are decorated to an extremely high standard and include all the latest modern facilities.

For further information visit our website or email reception@theroyalyacht.com

★★★★
THE ROYAL YACHT
HOTEL · SPA · RESTAURANTS

WWW.THEROYALYACHT.COM · TEL 01534 720511

CHANNEL ISLANDS

ALDERNEY
Alderney Tourism Office
- 01481 822811
- www.visitalderney.com

Provide information on attractions and access for disabled visitors on the island of Alderney.

HERM
Herm Island Administration Office
Administration office, Herm Island, Guernsey GY1 3HR
- 01481 750000
- reservations@herm.com
- www.herm.com

Herm Island's administration office can be contacted to provide information on available accommodation and events. Their website provides useful information on getting to the island and things to do there.

SARK
Sark Tourism
Administration office, Herm Island, Guernsey GY1 3HR
- 01481 832 345
- office@sark.co.uk
- www.sark.co.uk

The official website for Sark, the smallest of the Channel Islands that provides information on places to stay, things to do and how to get there and travel around (note, Sark is completely free of vehicles).

Transport

Air services
There are flights to both Jersey and Guernsey from many airports and regular inter-Island flights and ferries. You can also get a ferry to Jersey and Guernsey if you'd prefer. Consult your travel agent and request assistance in advance if needed. Airlines offering scheduled services include:

Aer Arann
- 0800 587 2324
- www.aerarann.com

Aer Lingus
- 0870 876 5000
- www.aerlingus.com

Aurigny Air Services
- 01481 822886
- www.aurigny.com

Blue Islands
- 08456 202122
- www.blueislands.com

BmiBaby
- 0905 8282828
- www.bmibaby.com

British Airways
- 0844 4930787
- www.britishairways.com

British Midland
- 0844 8484888
- www.flybmi.com

FlyBE
- 0871 7000535
- www.flybe.com

HOLIDAYS IN THE BRITISH ISLES

CHANNEL ISLANDS

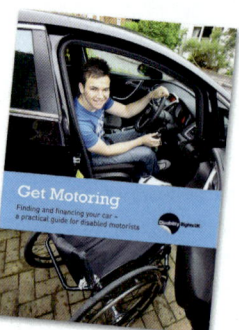

Get Motoring
A practical guide for disabled motorists to help find and finance a car. New 2012 edition.

Available to order from our online shop
www.disabilityrightsuk.org

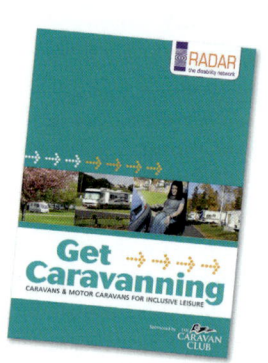

Get Caravanning
A guide to exploring caravanning from a disabled person's point of view. It provides all the information you need to start or resume this popular leisure activity.

Available to order from our online shop
www.disabilityrightsuk.org

LES ROCQUETTES
GUERNSEY

Originally a country mansion, Les Rocquettes is now a thriving hotel providing accommodation of a high standard. The hotel has 51 ensuite bedrooms 3 of which have wheelchair access.

Situated on the outskirts of St Peter Port within walking distance of the town centre it is well served by the local bus service as well as a courtesy bus which operates from May to October.

Our Oak Restaurant has been awarded a rosette by the AA and guests will find a great atmosphere and food in the Oak Bar, a great favourite with locals! The Mulberry Health Suite has wheelchair access and has an indoor pool, a children's pool, sauna, Jacuzzi, state of the art gym and a beauty therapist.

Open all year round.
★★★

Les Rocquettes Hotel, St Peter Port, Guernsey
Telephone: 01481 722146

www.lesrocquettesguernsey.com

Enjoy Jersey with carefree holidays for disabled people and their carers at Maison des Landes Hotel

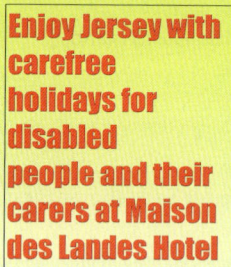
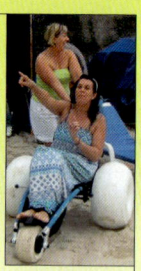

Maison des Landes is a hotel catering exclusively for disabled guests and their families or carers in accommodation which has been specially designed to meet their needs. Set in glorious unspoiled countryside overlooking a major international heritage area

- Heated indoor pool with ramps and hoists
- En-suite facilities including walk-in showers
- Extensive gardens with magnificent views
- Licensed lounge
- Pétanque (a version of bowls ideal for players in wheelchairs!)
- Daily Island tours in specially adapted minibuses
- The hotel is open from the beginning of April to the end of October

RATES per person per day include full board accommodation, daily excursions and transfers to harbour and airport and return.

NOW WITH A SELF CATERING OPTION. ASK FOR DETAILS

CONTACT US NOW FOR A BROCHURE
St Ouen, Jersey JE3 2AA
Tel: 01534 481683 Fax 01534 485327
Email: contact@maisondeslandes.co.uk
Website: www.maisondeslandes.co.uk

CHANNEL ISLANDS

Thomsonfly
- 0871 2314787
- www.thomsonfly.com

Ferry services

The main ferry provider is:

Condor Ferries
- reservations@condorferries.co.uk
- www.condorferries.co.uk

Operate fast car ferry services to Guernsey and Jersey all year round from Weymouth and from Poole from spring to October. A traditional ferry service is also operated all year from Portsmouth. The ferry terminals have accessible toilets, cafes, bars and shops and assistance can be requested when making a booking for your whole journey. All fast ferries have accessible toilets with an alarm and a lift from the car deck to the main passenger deck. You can also arrange for Shopmobility to leave powered wheelchairs and scooters with the ferry companies for use on board.

For port enquiries contact:

Weymouth
- 01305 763003

Poole
- 01202 207215

Guernsey
- 01481 729666

Jersey
- 01534 601000

JERSEY

Bus services

There are a number of accessible buses and coaches in use across the island, the following two companies are particularly useful.

Connex Public Buses
- 01534 877772
- www.mybus.je

Half of this public bus fleet is now wheelchair accessible with powered ramps, low floors and special 'kneeling' suspension which allows the buses to be lowered to pavement level. You should contact the information office on the number above to ask when an accessible bus will be on your route and to help you plan your journey.

Tantivy Blue Coaches
- 01534 706706
- www.jerseycoaches.com

Coach fleet that can offer assistance to disabled passengers but can only carry collapsible wheelchairs.

> **THINGS TO SEE OR DO**
>
> **St Brelade's Bay Beach**
>
> Jersey's wheelchair accessible beach. Very popular due to its scenic surroundings, golden sands and clear blue water, as well as restaurants and cafes. There are a number of public toilets along the length of the bay with access to the beach without crossing roads. There is a promenade along the beach and various parks and gardens. The beach carries a recommendation of the Marine Conservation Society for 2012. Parking is available; however, it can get busy in summer. The beach is well served by a bus service throughout the year, making it a credible alternative to queuing for parking spaces. Currently, half of the bus fleet is wheelchair-friendly – for accessible bus timetable information please contact
> - www.mybus.je

CHANNEL ISLANDS

Taxis

In addition to accessible taxis that can be hired from taxi ranks, the following companies have private hire cars that can carry wheelchair users:

Luxicabs
- 01534 887000

Have seven cars that have been adapted to carry wheelchairs. Accessible car should be requested on booking.

Citicabs
- 01534 499999

Have three cars that have been adapted to carry wheelchairs. Accessible car should be requested on booking.

Andy Tague
- 07797 721476

A specially adapted taxi with a raised back and viewing windows which allows wheelchairs and scooters to be wheeled into the rear of the vehicle. Can accommodate three passengers and a wheelchair.

GUERNSEY
Island Coachways

The Tramsheds, Les Banques, St Peter Port, Guernsey GY1 2HZ
- 01481 720210
- www.icw.gg

Operate bus services on Guernsey and is introducing new low floor vehicles with ramps and space for a wheelchair user. Contact the company for information on routes and schedules.

ALDERNEY
Bumblebee Boat Cruises

Weighbridge, St Peter Port, Guernsey
- 01481 720200
- skipper@bumblebee.gg
- www.bumblebee.gg

Opened in 2012, these boats carry up to 12 passengers and offer regular crossings from Guernsey to Alderney with no need to check in. Wheelchair users should contact before bookings. The configuration of Bumblebee normally makes it impractical to carry wheelchair-bound passengers without forward planning. If you are able to move from a wheelchair to a seat, staff will be happy to help you. If boarding at the right state of tide, it is possible to board 1 or 2 wheelchairs. This normally works for charters where we can change the time to suit you but seldom for scheduled services. Wheelchairs must not be more than 800mm wide.

HERM
Herm Island Ferry

Weighbridge, St Peter Port, Guernsey
- 01481 721379

The only way to access Herm is to get a ferry from Guernsey. The ferry sails daily and assistance is required for a wheelchair user to be able to gain access as there are uneven surfaces and is no level access.

SARK
Isle of Sark Shipping Company
- 01481 724049

Provide a passenger ferry service between Guernsey and Sark with several ferries travelling daily during peak season.

CHANNEL ISLANDS

Equipment hire

SHOPMOBILITY
The National Federation of Shopmobility UK (NFSUK), PO Box 6641, Christchurch BH23 9DQ
- 0844 41 41850
- info@shopmobilityuk.org
- www.shopmobilityuk.org

Scheme which lends manual wheelchairs, powered wheelchairs and powered scooters to members of the public with limited mobility to shop and to visit leisure and commercial facilities within the town, city or shopping centre. You can find the nearest Shopmobility scheme to you through their on-line directory. Contact specific Shopmobility Schemes to make equipment bookings or find out more information.

JERSEY
Channing's Mobility
- 0779 7743381

Supply toilet and walking aids and manual and electric wheelchairs and mobility scooters. Free delivery.

Guardian Nursing Services
3 Savile Street, St Helier
- 01534 732335

Supply wheelchairs, commodes and bathing equipment. Can deliver and collect.

Mercury Medical Jersey
Augres Garage Complex, La Route de la Trinite, Trinity
- 01534 610055

Hire out manual lightweight wheelchairs, rise and recline chairs, profile beds, static and active mattresses, portable hoists, commode chairs and ramps. Free delivery.

SGB Hire Shop
Millbrook, St Lawrence
- 01534 873699

Manual wheelchairs are available to hire but must be booked at least one week in advance.

Technicare
Doué House, Longueville Road
- 01534 888975

Scooters, manual wheelchairs, walking and bathing aids, hoists and other equipment are all available to hire.

THINGS TO SEE OR DO

Hamptonne Country Life Museum
St Lawrence, Jersey

This open air museum in St Lawrence explores close to 300 years of Jersey's rural heritage with a collection of farm buildings and meadows. Dating back to the 15th century, the house and farm are brought to life with characters from the Island's past, some of whom demonstrate by-gone skills, such as cider making. There are also guided tours and plenty of small animals. Newly added features include a woodland walkway, a wildlife pond and a wildflower garden. There is disabled parking and reasonable access to most of the site for wheelchair users and people with mobility impairments. Due to re-open in summer 2013.
- www.jerseyheritage.org

HOLIDAYS IN THE BRITISH ISLES

GUERNSEY

St John's Ambulance & Rescue Service
Healthcare Equipment Centre, Rohais, St Peter Port, Guernsey GY1 1YN
☎ 01481 729268
Offer a range of equipment, including wheelchairs, for sale or hire. Early booking of hired equipment is recommended. Spare parts are stocked and repairs can be carried out.

Publications

JERSEY
A Guide to Jersey for the Disabled
🌐 jersey.com/english/aboutjersey/disabledinformation
This guide has been compiled in association with the Jersey Access Group to assist disabled visitors to the Island. It includes a listing of accessible toilets and details of local activities. It can be found in the Disabled Information area of the 'About Jersey' section of the tourist board website.

Gentle Wanders: Access to Nature in Jersey
Gives details of 15 wildlife sites that can be accessed by wheelchair users is available from Jersey Tourism (see contact details at the beginning of this section).

Information & advice

GUERNSEY
Guernsey Information Exchange
☎ 01481 707470
A member of DIAL, they offer a free, impartial and confidential service of information and advice by telephone to disabled people, their relatives and professionals.

ALDERNEY
Alderney Information Exchange
☎ 01483 824823
A member of DIAL offering free, impartial and confidential information and advice by telephone to disabled people, their relatives and professionals.

Accommodation

JERSEY
For accommodation descriptions see the Stay Guide produced by Jersey Tourism:
☎ 01534 448888
🌐 www.jersey.com/crs

ST HELIER, Jersey
Jersey Cheshire Home
Eric Young House, Rope Walk, St Helier JE2 4UU
☎ 01534 285858
✉ welcome@jerseycheshirehome.je
🌐 www.jerseycheshirehome.je
Offer a respite suite attached to a purpose-built residential/nursing home for disabled people suitable for severely disabled people. Use of the suite entitles visitors to use the homes other facilities including a hydrotherapy pool.

Grand Hotel
Esplanade, St Helier JE2 3QA
☎ 01534 722301
✉ enquiries@grandjersey.com
🌐 www.grandjersey.com
Five-star hotel that has two rooms specially designed for disabled people. These rooms have walk in showers with hand rails and help cords. Spacious bar, dining room and lounge are all on one level and there's a life to access all floors.

CHANNEL ISLANDS

ST MARTIN, Jersey
Westlea Centre for the Visually Impaired
Rue de Huquet, St Martin
- 01534 864689
- westleacentre@jerseymail.co.uk

Permanent base of the Jersey Blind Society. Hotel situated in the heart of the countryside offering both holiday and respite bed and breakfast accommodation.

ST OUEN, Jersey
Maison Des Landes Hotel
La Route des Landes, St Ouen, Jersey JE3 2AA
- 01534 481683
- contact@maisondeslandes.co.uk
- www.maisondeslandes.co.uk

Charitable Trust set up by the Lions Club of Jersey to provide holidays in Jersey specifically for disabled people. The Hotel caters for disabled guests and their families, in accommodation which has been specially designed to meet the needs of disabled people. The hotel is situated nine miles from St. Helier on the gorse and heather covered headlands of Les Landes, with panoramic views of St. Ouen's Bay and the Atlantic. The hotel has a large heated indoor pool, with special wheelchairs and ramped sides for easy access. Hotel staff are on hand to assist guests into the pool.

GUERNSEY
ST PETER PORT, Guernsey
Les Rocquettes Hotel
La Gravees, St Peter Port, Guernsey GY1 1RN

Hotel on the outskirts of St Peter Port, Guernsey's capital that was once a country mansion. Three of the superior rooms allow wheelchair access into the bathrooms, along with ample turning space in the bedrooms.

The Royal Yacht Hotel
The Royal Yacht Hotel is a new, modern, luxury Jersey hotel situated in St. Helier, Jersey, Channel Islands. Within the hotel there are several bars with live entertainment, a luxury spa, 'Spa Sirène', a fully equipped gym and indoor heated swimming pool plus three restaurants with alfresco dining and gourmet cuisine in the brasserie Café Zephyr and fine-dining in the Restaurant Sirocco.

All our hotel rooms and accommodation are decorated and finished to a high standard with a warm modern style. Many rooms have a balcony or terrace and benefit from the latest hotel facilities. Whether your visit to Jersey in the Channel Islands is for a short stay, weekend break, luxury holiday, business trip, conference, wedding or honeymoon.

The Royal Yacht Hotel, Spa, and Restaurants will ensure your holiday in Jersey is fun, relaxing and luxurious.

www.theroyalyacht.com

ISLE OF MAN

> *The long history of the Isle has much to show. Ancient stone-age monuments such as Cashtal Yn Ard abound.*

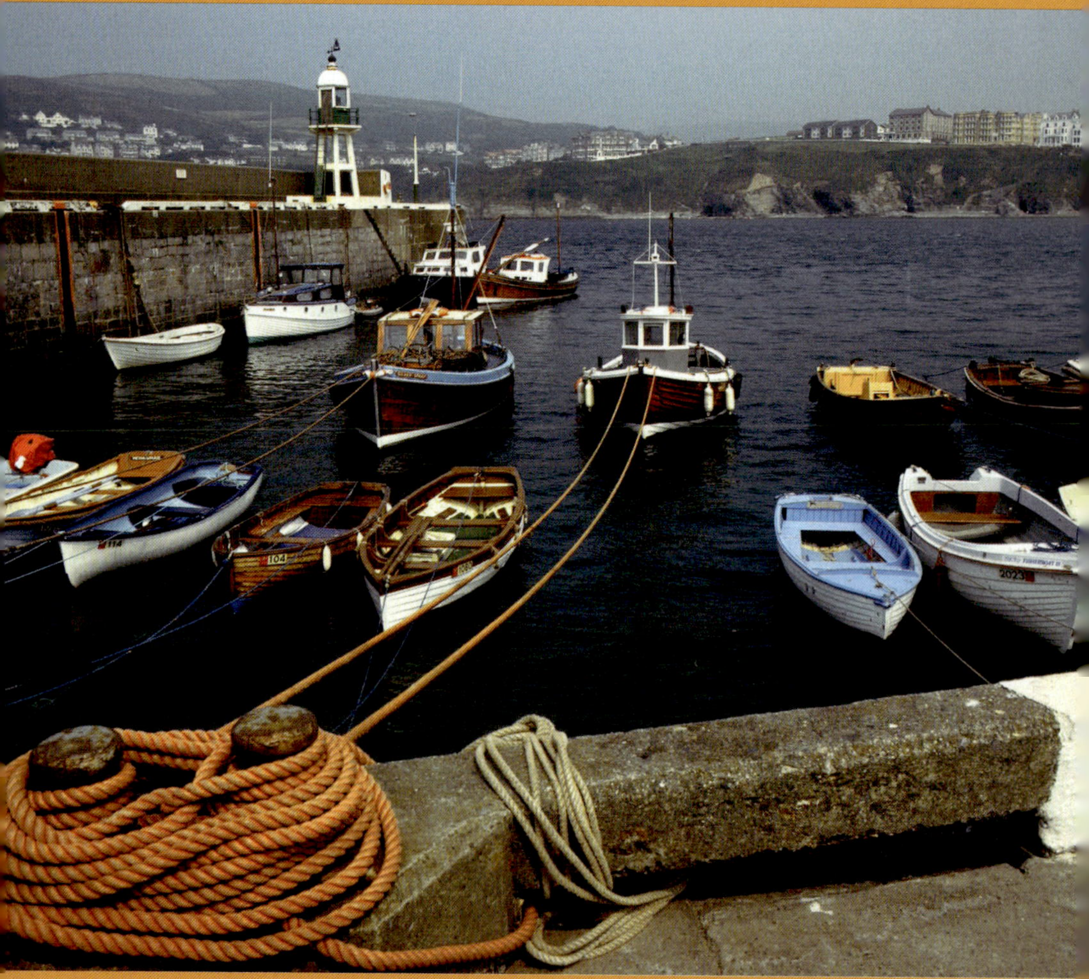

Isle of Man

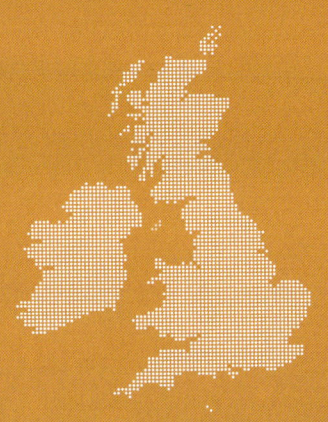

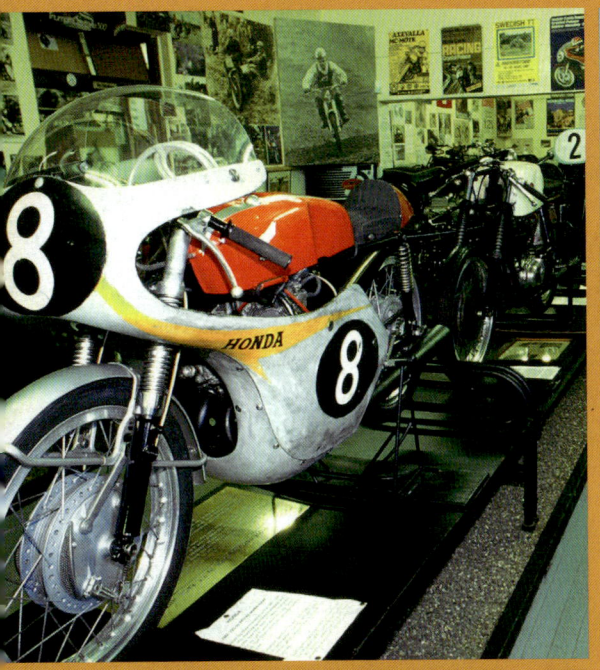

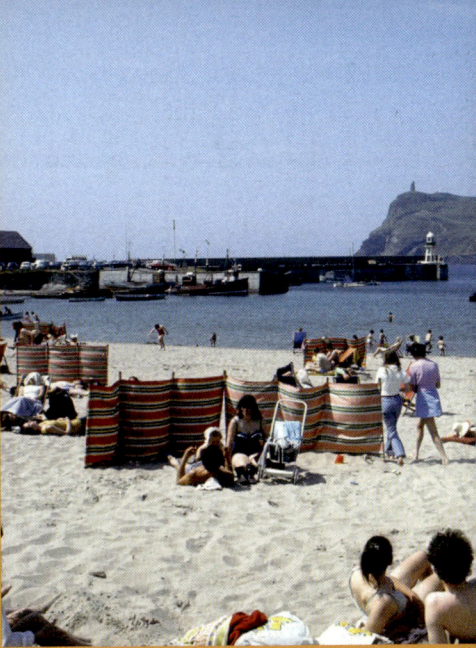

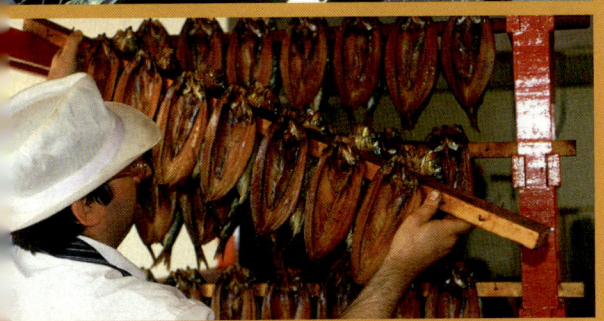

> Sometimes, the best discoveries are right under your nose. Lying right at the heart of the British Isles, the Isle of Man is both familiar and a world apart.

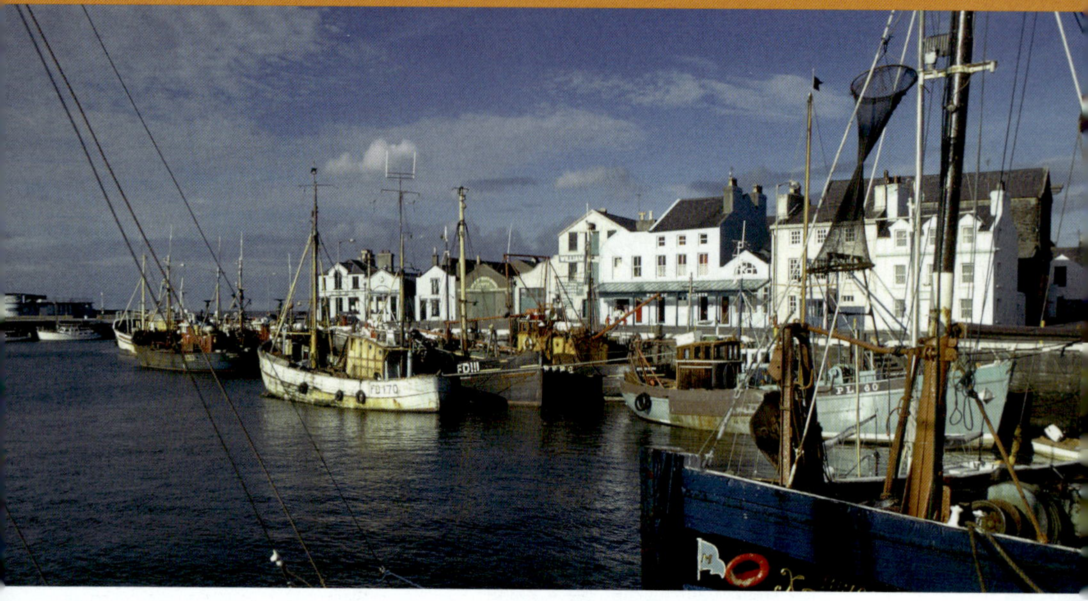

Visit the Isle of Man

The Isle of Man is as lovely as it is odd. Sitting in the middle of the Irish Sea, between England, Ireland, Wales and Scotland, you'll find our beautiful Island. Blessed with an extensive coastline, stunning natural landscapes and unspoilt beaches, it's the perfect holiday destination.

We are an entirely separate nation (we aren't even in the European Union). We have our own language, the engaging Manx, an ancient Celtic tongue. We have our own government, the Tynwald, which has ruled continuously for a thousand years (longer than any other). The cats have no tails and the sheep have got four horns. It is home to the hugely popular and wonderfully dangerous TT races.

The landscape is surprisingly dramatic for such a small place. High hills rise up along the length of the island. The highest is Snaefell; best climbed in the comfort of a Victorian tram. From the top you can see six kingdoms (heaven

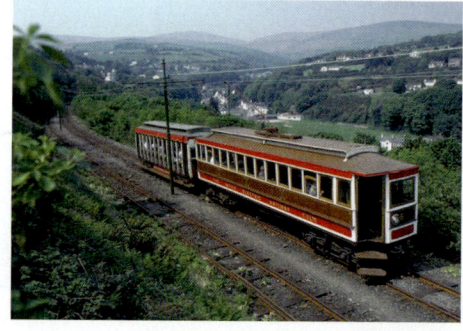

ISLE OF MAN

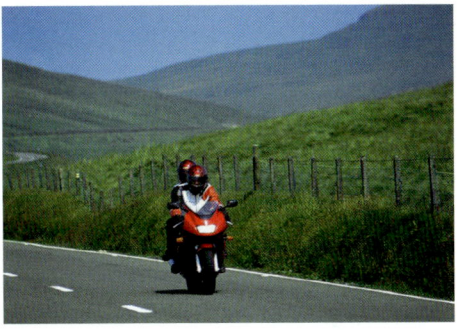

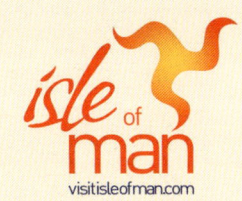

Explore the Isle of Man

Sometimes, the best discoveries are right under your nose. Lying right at the heart of the British Isles, the Isle of Man is both familiar and a world apart. Timelessly beautiful, with a character and spirit all of its own.

Explore the Isle of Man and you will find a place full of beguiling contrasts and character. Many people fall under its spell and return year after year – perhaps you will be next.

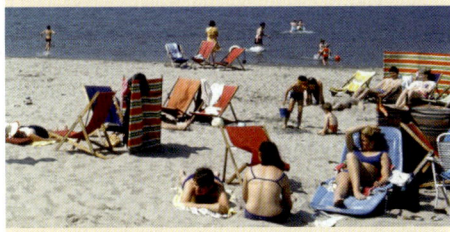

included!); on a good day you can easily make out the mountaintops in the countries edging the Irish Sea. Where the mountains of the island meet the sea to the west, great sea cliffs rise up. The landscape has an Irish feel (it stood in for Ireland in the comedy film *Waking Ned*). Where the island's streams and becks meet the coast, verdant glens are formed, thick with ferns.

The long history of the Isle has much to show. Ancient stone-age monuments such as Cashtal Yn Ard, abound. Celtic and Viking crosses can be found in churchyards across the island. It has two wonderful castles, Castle Rushen in the old capital Castletown is one of Europe's best preserved, Peel Castle on its own island, one of the most romantic. The Victorian age has given it elegant resorts such as Douglas, and the world's largest waterwheel at Laxey.

The food is rather good too. Kippers, a Manx specialty. And queen scallops or 'queenies'. The seagulls at Peel like queenies too, dropping them onto the cliffs to get at their succulent flesh!

"I can't tell you how brilliant it was – it is so pretty, the pace so chilled and relaxed, and everyone was so friendly and helpful. I'm definitely going back".

Find out more information about the Isle of Man at:
www.visitisleofman.com
www.gov.im/tourism

ISLE OF MAN

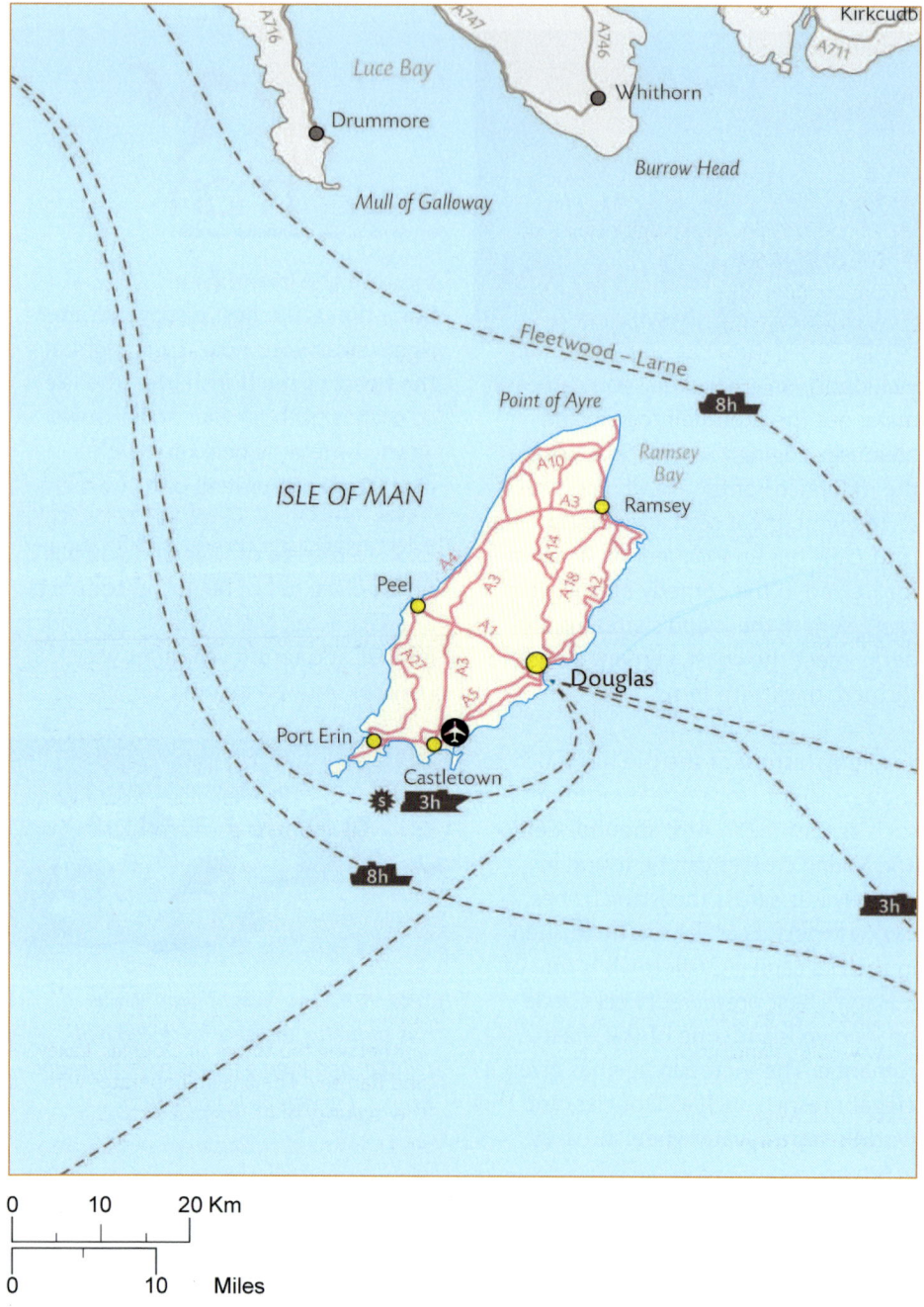

Resources
Tourism

Isle of Man Department of Tourism & Leisure
Sea Terminal Buildings, Douglas IM1 2RG
- 01624 686766
- tourism@gov.im
- www.visitisleofman.com

The annual holiday guide to the Isle of Man gives details of accommodation, events and attractions. An accessible accommodation leaflet lists a number of serviced and self-catering places to stay meeting the criteria of the Isle of Man Accessible Scheme.

Transport

Air services
There are flights to the Isle of Man from many mainland airports. Consult your travel agent and request assistance in advance. Among the airlines offering scheduled services are:

Aer Arann
- 0800 587 2324
- www.aerarann.com

Blue Islands
- 08456 20 21 22
- www.blueislands.com

Eastern Airways
- 08703 669100
- www.easternairways.com

FlyBE
- 0871 522 6100
- www.flybe.com

Loganair
- 0871 700 2000
- www.loganair.co.uk

Manx2
- 0871 200 0440
- www.manx2.com

Ferry services
Isle of Man Steam Packet Co.
Imperial Buildings, Douglas, Isle of Man IM1 2BY
- 08722 992 992
- www.steam-packet.com

Operate services to Douglas from Heysham all year, from Liverpool seasonally, and from Belfast and Dublin late March to September. The 'Ben-my-Chree' ferry on the Heysham route has a lift to all decks and two cabins adapted for disabled passengers. The winter weekend service from Liverpool increases to twice daily in summer. The seasonal Belfast and Dublin services use a fast Superseacat which is adapted for disabled passengers. Notify the company about any assistance required when making a reservation.

> **THINGS TO SEE OR DO**
>
> **Manx Electric Railway**
> www.manxelectricrailway.co.uk
> This historic railway, built 1893-1899 is on the eastern coast of the Isle of Man connecting the towns of Douglas, Laxey and Ramsey. The line still operates with the majority of its original Victorian and Edwardian rolling stock in daily use along some of the most scenic stretches of railway in the British Isles. The railway has one wheelchair accessible vehicle that is used by special request only and needs to be booked in advance.

ISLE OF MAN

Space donated by

**Roger Harper
Isle of Man**

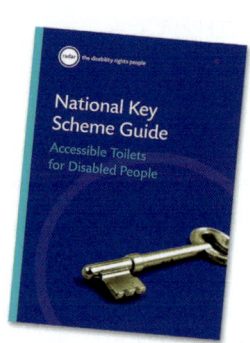

National Key Scheme Guide

Updated every year, this guide lists the location of 9,000 NKS toilets around the UK. It shows opening times, provider name and whether the toilet is unisex.

Available to order from our online shop
www.disabilityrightsuk.org

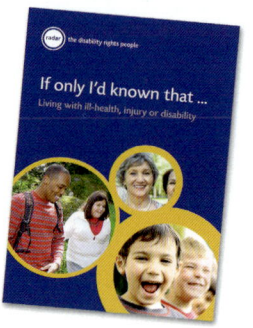

If Only I'd Known That ...

An information-packed guide to services, welfare rights, facilities and support for anyone with a disability or health condition, this guide includes resources for all ages from childhood to later years.

Available to order from our online shop
www.disabilityrightsuk.org

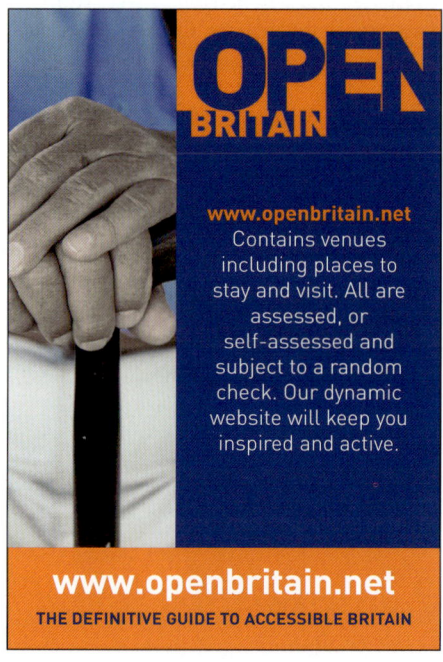

Bus services

Bus services run between the airport and Douglas and other major towns. Low floor buses are being introduced and information on these, and on arrangements for disabled passengers on their railways, can be obtained from:

Isle of Man Transport

Banks Circus, Douglas IM1 5PT
- 01624 662525
- info@busandrail.dtl.gov.im
- www.iombusandrail.info

THINGS TO SEE OR DO

Manx Museum

This museum in the island's capital Douglas contains artefacts and treasures unique to the Isle of Man and presents the story of the island through films, galleries and interactive displays. The museum is fully accessible and provides disabled parking spaces. Lifts for public use are available to access the Lower Folk Gallery, Temporary Exhibition Gallery, Library and Archive and the Bayroom restaurant. Guided tours can be arranged for visually impaired and blind visitors and large format information about the site can be provided. Registered assistance dogs welcome.
- www.gov.im

Information & advice

Crossroads Care, Isle of Man

35-36 Derby Square Douglas, Isle of Man IM1 3LW
- 01624 673103
- isleofman@crossroads.org.uk
- www.crossroadsiom.org

Accommodation

You can search for accessible accommodation on the Isle of Man Department of Tourism & Leisure's website:
- www.visitisleofman.com

You will also find accessible accommodation and facilities throughout the Isle of Man on:
- www.disabledgo.com
- www.openbritain.net

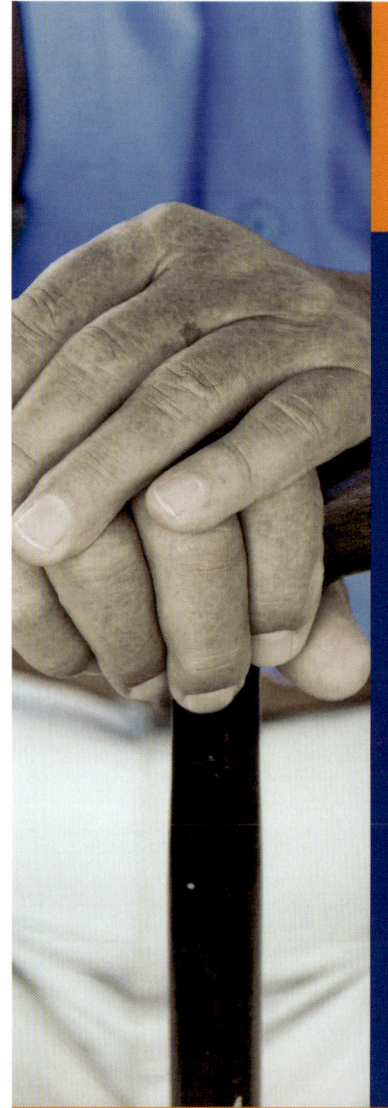

Index of advertisers

Disability Rights UK thanks all its advertisers for supporting the publication of our books for disabled people.

A

ABDO	14
Ability Aware	88
ABTA	34
Accor UK	Inside back cover
Adapt-Ability	118
Amroth Bay Holidays	316
Anglia Square Shopping Centre	206
Archery World	78
Arjo Wiggins Fine Papers	14
Arley Hall and Gardens	248
AT Graphics Ltd	14
ATOC	Outside back cover
Ayrshire Railway Preservation Group	298

B

Bank Farm	312
Barlows Caravan Park	316
Bath-Knight	26
Bedford Borough Council	206
Belfast City Council	326
Belford Hoist Ltd	54
Ben Nevis Distillery	294
Blaenau Gwent County Council	314
Blair Drummond Safari and Adventure Park	292
Bluebell Railway	150
Bocaddon Holiday Cottages	194
Brading Roman Villa	164
Bridgend County Borough Council	316
Bridgestone UK Ltd	110
Brig-Ayd Controls Ltd	52
Bristol City Council	174
British Pepper & Spice	26, 72
Brookfields Bed & Breakfast	192
Brotherwood Automobility	180
Bruce Wake Charitable Trust	72

C

C & S Seating Ltd	54, 118
Cadenhead's Whisky Shop	294
Calvert Trust Exmoor	64
Chartwell Insurance	52
Chester Zoo	252
Chris Elliott Adaptions Ltd	72, 206
City of London	142
Cliff House Holiday Park	208
Clyde Coast Holiday Cottage	292
Cotswold Charm	176
Crelling Harnesses	64
Cumbernauld Shopping Centre	294
Currall Lewis and Martin Construction Ltd	240
Currys	26

D

D & HB Associates Ltd	240
D Beevers – Disabled Apartment	224
David Kellett & Partners	238
Delamont Country Park	326
Derry City Council	326
Derwentside Homes	278
Des Gosling Mobility Ltd	226
Double-Gate Farm	174
Drybeck Farm	252

E

Elms Farm Cottages	220
England and Wales Cricket Board	26, 80

F

F.E. McWilliam Gallery and Studio	326
FIC UK	192
First ScotRail	294
Fittleworth	120

INDEX OF ADVERTISERS

Fleet Air Arm Museum	162
Flintshire County Council	314
Forest Laboratories Ltd	26
Forestry Commission	78

G

General Estates Co Ltd	150
GM Coachwork	116
Grosvenor Centre	222
Guildford Cathedral	150
Gwesty'r Marine Hotel	312

H

H Kemp & Son Ltd	226
Heads Up Holidays	110
Houses of Parliament	138

I

Imago at Burleigh Court	220
Isle of Wight Railway Co Ltd	162

J

Julian Ellis Chartered Accountant	208

K

K&B Marketing Ltd	164
KC Computers	152
Kilbowie Outdoor Centre	64
Kings Lodge	152
King's Lynn and West Norfolk Borough Council	208
Knight James Commercial	154

L

Labelon Ltd	208
Lancashire County Council	250
Laugharne Barns	314
Lee Valley Boat Centre	138
Lee Valley Regional Park Authority	138
Leigh Adams LLP	142
Les Rocquettes Hotel	344
Liberty's Owl, Raptor and Reptile Centre	162
Lincoln Cathedral	222
Livability	34, 98
Lloyd George Museum	314
Loch Lomond and The Trossachs Park National Park	292
Loch Tay Lodges	298

M

Maison des Landes Hotel	344
Majestic Transformer Co	164
Medpac	122
Mel House Cottages	270
MIC Hotel and Conference Centre	138
Milestones Trust	174
Minki Balinki	178
MND Scotland	300
Motability	Inside front cover, 6
Musmate Ltd	118

N

National Maritime Museum Cornwall	190
National Theatre	140
Neath Port Talbot Borough Council	314
Norfolk County Council	206
North West Trading Co	14
Northumberland National Park	278

O

Old Stables	178
Oldham Council (Castleshaw Centre)	250

P

P A Meecham	164
PCM Risk Solutions	142
Pekes Manor House & Cottages	154
Pelican Flooring Ltd	140
Penrose Burden Holiday Cottages	194
Plantcraft Limited	224
Polux Ltd	14
Poole's Cavern and Country Park	222
Prescription Footwear Associates Ltd	122
Princes Square Shopping Centre	298

INDEX OF ADVERTISERS

Q

Quartis Ltd	14

R

Ratcliffe Disabled Holidays	266
Redwings Horse Sanctuary	206
Rhodia UK Ltd	110
Roger Harper & Co	358
Roman Camp Hotel	294
Rother District Council	150
Royal Borough of Kensington & Chelsea	140
Royal Military Police Museum	162
Royal School for the Deaf Derby	222
Royal Signals Museum	174
Royal Yacht Hotel	342

S

SETS	154
Shamba Holidays Ltd	164
Sharp & Nickless Ltd	64
Shell UK	56, 248
Shewee Ltd	88
Snowdonia National Park Authority	314
South Somerset District Council	178
St Tydfil Shopping Centre	310
Steering Developments Ltd	116

T

Tamarack Lodge	178
Tate Britain	78
Tavern Snacks	140
Techni Care	342
Teleflex	122
Tersus Consultancy Ltd	238
Thanet District Council	154
The Coppleridge Inn	178
The Cornish Collection	194
The Cottage By The Pond	224
The John Gray Centre	300
The Octogon Shopping Centre	240
The Waterways Trust	78
Ticino Bakery Ltd	142
Torbay Council	194
Trenona Farm Holidays	192

V

VisitEngland	362
VisitScotland	296
Visit York	266
Vulco Spring & Presswork Ltd	240

W

Wallace Caravans	292
West Somerset Railway	176
Westminster Abbey	140
Wheelchair Travel Ltd	152
Wheely Boat Trust	72
Wilson & Scott Ltd	164
Wollaston Mini	54
Wooda Farm Holiday Park	194
WWT Arundel Wetland Centre	152
WWT Caerlaverock Wetland Centre	298

Y

Yorkminster Cathedral	266

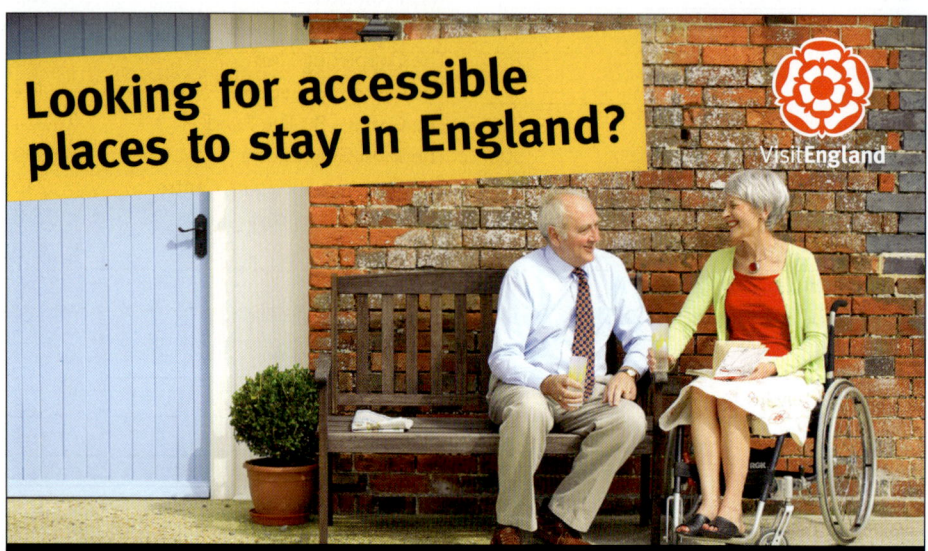

Use the National Accessible Scheme

Operators of accommodation taking part in the **National Accessible Scheme (NAS)** have gone out of their way to ensure a comfortable stay for guests with hearing, visual or mobility needs.

Using the **NAS** could make the difference between a good holiday and a perfect one!

NAS means:
• Accommodation is independently assessed by trained assessors against demanding criteria

• Facilities such as handrails, ramps, level-access showers, hearing loops and colour contrast

• Members of staff will be aware of what assistance you may need

For tips and advice on holiday travel in England and to find NAS accredited accommodation, go to
www.visitengland.com/accessforall

INDEX OF ACCOMMODATION

ACCOMMODATION & NAS RATING

LONDON

Accommodation	Page								
BROMLEY Best Western Bromley Court Hotel	144	•	•	•			•		•
DOCKLANDS Radisson Blu Edwardian Providence Wharf	144	•	•	•					
HOLBORN SACO London – Holborn	144	•					•		•
KENSINGTON Copthorne Tara Hotel	145								
KENSINGTON Meininger Hotel London Hyde Park	145	•							
TOWER HILL Mint Hotel Tower of London	145	•							•
ROTHERHITHE YHA London Thameside	145	•							
WESTMINSTER Tune Hotel – Westminster	145	•							•
WESTMINSTER YHA London Central	145	•							

SOUTH EAST

Accommodation	Page								
BOGNOR REGIS Farrell House	156								
BOGNOR REGIS Invicta Warren	156								
BOGNOR REGIS Russell Hotel	156								
BRACKLESHAM BAY Tamarisk	157								
BRACKLESHAM BAY VASD Holiday Chalet	157								
BRIGHTON Jurys Inn Brighton Hotel	153	•	•				•		•
BRIGHTON Myhotel Brighton	153	•	•						
CANTERBURY Iffin Farmhouse	153	•	•						
CHICHESTER Bishop Otter Campus – University Of Chichester	153	•	•		•				
CHICHESTER Chichester Park Hotel	153	•							
CHICHESTER Eastmere House	153	•							
CHICHESTER George Bell House	153	•	•						
CHIDDINGSTONE Hay Barn & Straw Barn	155	•							
EAST PRESTON Bradbury Hotel	157								
EASTBOURNE Best Western York House Hotel	155	•							
EASTBOURNE Hydro Hotel	155	•							
EASTRY The Old Dairy	155	•							
FARNHAM High Wray	155	•	•						

HOLIDAYS IN THE BRITISH ISLES

INDEX OF ACCOMMODATION

ACCOMMODATION & NAS RATING

Accommodation	Page	1	2	3	4	5	6	7	8
FELPHAM **Beach Lodge**	157								
FOLKESTONE **Shuttlesfield Barn**	155	•	•						
HASTINGS **Seaspray**	155	•					•		•
HERNE BAY **Strode Park Foundation**	157								
HORLEY **Brambles MS Respite Care Centre**	157								
MAIDSTONE **Coldblow Farm**	155	•	•						
MAIDSTONE **Village Maidstone**	155	•	•						
MARDEN **Pitlands Barns**	155	•							
MARDEN **West Marden Farm**	155	•							
PEACEHAVEN **Little Haven**	155	•							
PLUMPTON GREEN **Heath Farm**	156	•	•						
ROBERTSBRIDGE **Poppinghole Farm Cottages**	156	•	•						
ROYAL TUNBRIDGE WELLS **Alconbury Guest House**	156	•							•
SOUTH NUTFIELD **Kings Lodge Centre for Complex Needs**	157								
STANWELL **The Stanwell**	156	•	•				•		•
TENTERDEN **Little Silver Country Hotel**	156	•	•	•					
TUNBRIDGE WELLS **Smart and Simple Hotel**	156	•							
WADHURST **Bardown Farm**	156					•		•	•

SOUTHERN ENGLAND

Accommodation	Page	1	2	3	4	5	6	7	8
ABINGDON **Abbey Guest House**	166	•	•				•		•
ABINGDON **Kingfisher Barn**	168								
BORTHWOOD **Borthwood Cottages**	166	•	•						
BRACKNELL **SACO Bracknell**	166	•					•		•
BRIGHSTONE **Yafford Mill Barn**	166	•	•	•	•				
COGGES **Swallows Nest**	166	•	•						
EAST BOLDRE **Ivy Roost Cottage**	167	•							
FRESHWATER **Brambles Chine Bungalow**	168								
HAMPSTEAD NORREYS **Manor Farm Courtyard Cottages**	167	•	•	•	•				

INDEX OF ACCOMMODATION

ACCOMMODATION & NAS RATING	Page	1	2	3	4	5 (Exceptional)	6 (Exceptional)	7 (1)	8 (2)	9 (1)	10 (2)
LECKHAMPSTEAD **Weatherhead Farm**	167	•									
LISS **The Jolly Drover**	167	•									
LYMINGTON **Garden Bench, Bench Cottage & Little Bench**	168										
MAIDENHEAD **Holiday Inn Maidenhead**	167	•									
MARLOW **Granny Anne's**	167	•									
MILTON KEYNES **South Lodge**	167	•	•								
NEW MILTON **Holiday Homes Trust Caravans**	168										
NEW MILTON **Smugglers View Chalets**	168										
NEWCHURCH, NEAR SANDOWN **Mulberry Rest**	167	•									
OXFORD **YHA Oxford**	167	•									
SANDOWN **Fort Holiday Park**	167	•								•	
SANDOWN BAY HOLIDAY PARK **No 6 & No 113**	167	•									
SHANKLIN **Sunny Bay Apartments**	168	•									
SHANKLIN **The Marine Villa**	168	•	•								
SOUTHAMPTON **Vitalise Netley Waterside House**	169										
STOKE MANDEVILLE **Olympic Lodge**	168	•	•		•						
WEST COUNTRY											
AWRE NEAR NEWNHAM ON SEVERN **Priory Cottages**	177	•									
BATH **Carfax Hotel**	179	•	•								
BATH **SACO Bath**	177	•							•		•
BATH **University of Bath**	179	•	•		•						
BEAMINSTER **Stable Cottage**	179	•	•								
BLANDFORD FORUM **The Ellwood Centre**	184										
BOOKHAM, ALTON PANCRAS **Bookham Court**	179	•	•								
BOURNEMOUTH **BOD**	179	•	•	•					•		•
BRISTOL **SACO Bristol – Broad Quay**	179	•							•		•
BURNHAM-ON-SEA **BPF Bungalow**	184										

HOLIDAYS IN THE BRITISH ISLES

INDEX OF ACCOMMODATION

ACCOMMODATION & NAS RATING

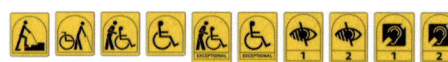

Accommodation	Page	1	2	3	4	5	6	7	8	9
BURNHAM-ON-SEA Scout Holiday Homes Trust Caravan	184									
BURTON BRADSTOCK Norburton Hall	179	•								
CHEDDAR YHA Cheddar	179	•								
CHEW MAGNA Woodbarn Farm Cottages	179	•								
CHICKERELL The Lugger Inn	179	•	•							
CHICKERELL Tidmoor Self Catering Cottages	179	•	•							
CHRISTCHURCH Number 31, Christchurch, Dorset	184									
CORFE CASTLE Mortons House Hotel	179	•	•		•				•	
DORCHESTER Aquila Heights	181	•	•							
EXFORD Westermill Farm	181	•								
FERNDOWN Birchcroft	181	•	•				•		•	
GLOUCESTER Deerhurst Cottages	181	•								
GODNEY Double-Gate Farm	181	•	•	•	•					
GORWELL Gorwell Farm Cottages	181	•	•							
HIGH LITTLETON Greyfield Farm Cottages	181	•								
HORSINGTON Half Moon Inn	181	•	•	•			•		•	
HUNTWORTH Lakeview Holiday Cottages	181	•	•							
LANGTON HERRING / RODDEN Character Farm Cottages	181	•	•							
LITTLEDEAN Orchard Barn & Meadow Byre	181	•								•
LONG BREDY Stables Cottage	182	•	•							
LYDNEY 2 Danby Cottages	182		•							
LYDNEY The Lodge	182	•	•							
LYTCHETT MINSTER South Lytchett Manor Caravan & Camping Park	182	•							•	
MALMESBURY Best Western Mayfield House Hotel	182	•	•							
MINEHEAD Promenade Hotel	184									
MINEHEAD Woodcombe Lodges	182	•	•							

366   HOLIDAYS IN THE BRITISH ISLES

INDEX OF ACCOMMODATION

ACCOMMODATION & NAS RATING		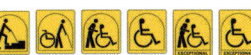								
NEWENT **Leadon View Barn**	182		•							
NEWENT **The Moorhens**	182	•	•							
POOLE **Holton Lee**	184									
POOLE **Orton Rigg Hotel**	184									
POOLE **Holiday Homes Trust Caravan**	184									
POOLE **The New Beehive Hotel**	182	•								
RADSTOCK **The Garden House**	182	•	•							
SALISBURY **Old Stables**	182									
SALISBURY **Websters**	185									
SOUTH BARROW **The Stables**	182	•								
STOKE ABBOTT **Lewesdon Farm Holidays**	182	•	•							
TAUNTON **Holly Farm Cottages**	183	•	•							
TINCLETON **Tincleton Lodge and Rose Cottage**	183				•					
TYTHERINGTON **The Lighthouse**	183	•	•							
UPWEY **Millspring**	183	•								
WEST MILTON **Lancombes House**	183	•								
WESTON-SUPER-MARE **Spreyton Guest House**	183	•								
WESTON-SUPER-MARE **The Royal Hotel**	183	•	•	•	•				•	
WESTON-SUPER-MARE **The Lauriston Hotel**	185									
WEYMOUTH **Anchor House**	185									
WEYMOUTH **Jubilee View Apartment**	183	•								
WEYMOUTH **Wimborne & Ferndown Lions Club Caravans**	185									
WINFORD **Winford Manor Hotel**	183	•	•		•					
WINSLEY **Church Farm Country Cottages**	183	•	•							
WOOLLAND **Ellwood Cottages**	183	•	•		•					
DEVON & CORNWALL										
AXMINSTER **Goodlands**	195	•								
BARNSTAPLE **Calvert Trust Exmoor**	195	•	•	•	•			•	•	
BEAWORTHY **Blagdon Farm Country Holidays**	199									

HOLIDAYS IN THE BRITISH ISLES

INDEX OF ACCOMMODATION

ACCOMMODATION & NAS RATING

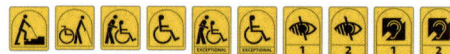

Accommodation	Page	🚶	🦽	♿	♿ Exc	♿ Exc	👂1	👂2	👂3	👂4
BODMIN **Lanhydrock Hotel and Golf Club**	195	•	•							
BOSCASTLE **Reddivallen Farmhouse**	195	•								
BOSCASTLE **The Old Coach House**	195	•	•							
BRAUNTON **Phoenix Retreat**	195			•						
BUCKLAND BREWER **West Hele**	195	•	•		•	•				
BUDLEIGH SALTERTON **Badgers Den**	195	•	•							
CHAPEL AMBLE **The Olde House**	195	•								
CREDITON **Creedy Manor**	195			•						
CROWS-AN-WRAY **Tredinney Farm Holiday Cottage**	196	•								
DAVIDSTOW **Pendragon Country House**	196	•								
EXETER **Hue's Piece**	196	•	•							
EXMOUTH **Holiday Homes Trust Caravans**	201									
GOLANT **South Torfrey Farm**	196	•	•	•						
GOLANT, CORNWALL **Penquite Farm**	196	•	•							
GOLBERDON, NEAR CALLINGTON **Berrio Mill**	196	•								
GUNNISLAKE **Todsworthy Farm Holidays**	196	•	•	•						
HARLYN BAY **Yellow Sands Cottages**	196	•								
HAYLE **Rowan Barn**	196		•							
HOLCOMBE ROGUS **Whipcott Water Cottages**	196	•	•		•					
HONITON **Stonehayes Farm Cottages**	196	•								
ILFRACOMBE **Mullacott Farm**	196	•								
ILFRACOMBE **Wildercombe House**	197	•	•	•			•		•	
IVYBRIDGE **Hannah's at Ivybridge**	201									
KILKHAMPTON **Forda Lodges & Cottages**	197	•	•	•	•					
LANREATH, LOOE **Bocaddon Holiday Cottages**	197	•	•	•						
LIZARD, CORNWALL **YHA Lizard Point**	197	•								
LOOE **Lesquite**	197	•	•	•						
MORETONHAMPSTEAD **Budleigh Farm**	197	•								
MORVAL **Tudor Lodges**	197	•	•	•	•					

INDEX OF ACCOMMODATION

ACCOMMODATION & NAS RATING	Page	1	2	3	4	5	6	7	8	9
MOUNT HAWKE Ropers Walk Barns	197	•	•	•	•					
MYLOR Mylor Yacht Harbour – Admiralty Apartments	197	•								
NEWQUAY The Park	197	•	•							
NORTHLEIGH Smallicombe Farm	197	•	•							
OKEHAMPTON Beer Farm	197	•	•							
PAIGNTON Holiday Homes Trust Caravan	201									
PENZANCE Hotel Penzance	198	•								
PILLATON Kernock Cottages	198	•	•	•						
POLZEATH Manna Place	198	•	•							
PORTHTOWAN Rose Hill Lodges	198	•								
PORTREATH Gwel an Mor Lodges	198			•						
PORTSCATHO Pollaughan Cottages	198	•	•							
REDMOOR Chark Country Holidays	198	•	•	•						
RUAN HIGH LANES Trenona Farm Holidays	198	•	•							
SANDFORD Ashridge Farm	198	•	•	•						
SIDMOUTH Boswell Farm Farm Cottages	198	•								
ST AUSTELL Holiday Homes Trust Caravans	201									
ST BREWARD Penrose Burden Cottages	199									
ST CLETHER Ta Mill	198		•							
ST ENDELLION Tolraggott Farm Cottages	198	•	•							
ST MARTINS Bucklawren Farm	199	•	•							
ST MARY'S Isles of Scilly Country Guest House	199	•								
ST MARY'S The Atlantic	199	•	•							
ST VEEP A Little Bit Of Heaven	199	•	•		•					
STRATTON, BUDE Oak Lodge Bed and Breakfast	199	•	•							
TEIGNMOUTH Cliffden	201									
TORQUAY Atlantis Holiday Apartments	199	•	•				•		•	
TORQUAY Crown Lodge	199	•	•		•					
WHITNAGE West Pitt Farm	199	•	•	•				•		•

HOLIDAYS IN THE BRITISH ISLES

INDEX OF ACCOMMODATION

ACCOMMODATION & NAS RATING

Accommodation	Page	1	2	3	4	5	6	7	8	9
WIDECOMBE-IN-THE-MOOR Wooder Manor Holiday Homes	199	•	•							
WOOLACOMBE Lions Bungalow	201									
EASTERN ENGLAND										
ALDEBURGH The Brudenell Hotel	209	•	•							
ASHDON Hill Farm Holiday Cottages	209	•								
AYLMERTON Roman Camp Inn	209		•							
BACTON Castaways Holiday Park	209	•							•	
BACTON Primrose Cottage	209	•	•							
BECCLES The Lodge	209	•	•	•	•					
BEESTON Holmdene Farm	209	•	•							
BLAXHALL YHA Blaxhall	209	•	•							
BOXFORD Sherbourne Lodge Cottages	210	•	•							
BURGH NEXT AYLSHAM North Farm Cottages	210	•								
BURGH ST PETER Waveney River Centre	210	•	•							
CARLTON COLVILLE, LOWESTOFT Ivy House Country Hotel	210			•						
CASTLE HEDINGHAM The Lodge at Hedingham Castle	210							•		
CHELMSFORD Boswell House Hotel	210	•								
CHIGWELL Vitalise Jubilee Lodge	215									
CLACTON-ON-SEA Groomshill	215									
CRATFIELD School Farm Cottages	210	•								
EAST HARLING Berwick Cottage	210	•	•		•	•		•		•
EAST RUNTON Incleborough House Luxury Self Catering	210	•	•							
EDGEFIELD Wood Farm Cottages Ltd	210	•								
ELM The Elm Tree Inn	210	•	•							
ELY Little Downham Anchor	210	•	•			•		•		
FOXLEY WOOD Moor Farm Stable Cottages	211	•								
FRITTON Decoy Barn	211	•								
GREAT BARTON Wylene	211	•	•						•	

INDEX OF ACCOMMODATION

ACCOMMODATION & NAS RATING

Accommodation	Page	♿1	♿2	♿3	♿4	♿E1	♿E2	👁1	👁2	👂1	👂2
GREAT FINBOROUGH **Jack Bridge Cottage @ Jack Bridge Farm**	211	•									
GREAT SNORING **Vine Park Cottage**	211	•	•	•							
GREAT YARMOUTH **The Holiday Homes Trust Caravan**	215										
HAPPISBURGH **Boundary Stables**	211	•	•								
HAUGHLEY **Red House Farm**	211	•	•								
HENLEY **Damerons Farm Holidays**	211	•	•		•						
HITCHAM **The White Horse Inn**	211	•									
HOLT **Norfolk Country Cottages**	215										
HORNING **Heron Cottage**	211	•									
HORNING **King Line Cottages**	211	•	•								
HORNING **Norfolk River Cottages**	211	•	•								
HOVETON **Broomhill**	215										
HUNSTANTON **Caley Hall Hotel**	212		•								
HUNSTANTON **Foxgloves Cottage**	212	•	•								
KELLING **The Pheasant Hotel**	212	•	•								
LITTLE DOWNHAM **Wood Fen Lodge**	212	•									
LITTLE SNORING **Jex Farm Barn and Stable**	212	•	•								
MAUTBY **Lower Wood Farm Country Cottages**	212		•								
METHWOLD **Next Door at Magdalen House**	212		•								
MICKFIELD **Read Hall Cottage**	212		•								
MIDDLEWOOD GREEN **Leys Farmhouse Annexe**	212	•									
NAYLAND **Gladwins Farm**	212	•	•								
NORWICH **Prince's Barn**	212	•									
NORWICH **Spixworth Hall Cottages**	212	•		•							
PAKEFIELD **Pakefield Caravan Park**	213	•							•		•
PULHAM MARKET **The Old Bakery**	213	•									
REYDON, SOUTHWOLD **Newlands Country House**	213	•	•	•	•						

INDEX OF ACCOMMODATION

ACCOMMODATION & NAS RATING	Page	Mobility impaired	Visually impaired	Wheelchair accessible	Wheelchair exceptional	Hearing impaired exceptional	Hearing 1	Hearing 2	Visual 1	Visual 2
SAINT OSYTH **Lee Wick Farm Holiday Cottages**	213	•	•							
SANDRINGHAM **Park House Hotel**	213				•					
SANDY **Fullers Hill Cottages**	213	•	•							
SHERINGHAM **Sheringham Cottages**	213			•			•		•	
SHERINGHAM **YHA Sheringham**	213	•	•							
SHOTLEY **Orwell View Barns**	213	•	•							
SIBTON **Park Farm Sibton**	213	•								
SISLAND **Owl Barn at Sisland Tithe Barn**	213	•						•		
SOUTH WALSHAM **Break-O-Day**	213		•							
SWILLAND **Swilland Mill**	214									•
THORPE-LE-SOKEN **Lifehouse Spa & Hotel**	214	•	•							
TITCHWELL **Titchwell Manor Hotel**	214		•							
TRIMINGHAM **Woodland Leisure Park**	214	•	•							
WALTHAM CROSS **YHA Lee Valley Village**	214	•	•							
WALTON-ON-THE-NAZE **Bufo Villae Guest House**	214	•	•							
WATTISFIELD **Jayes Holiday Cottages**	214	•	•	•						
WATTISHAM **Wattisham Hall Holiday Cottages**	214	•								
WELLS-NEXT-THE-SEA **YHA Wells-next-the-Sea Youth Hostel**	214	•	•							
WENDLING, NR DEREHAM **Greenbanks**	214	•	•							
WEST RUDHAM **Oyster House**	214	•								
WEYBOURNE **Home Farm Holiday Cottages**	214	•								
WISBECH ST MARY **Common Right Barns**	215	•	•							
WISSETT **The Old Stables, Wissett Lodge**	215		•							
WORTHAM **Ivy House Farm**	215		•							

EAST MIDLANDS

ALDERWASLEY **Wiggonlea Stable and Fletchers Barn**	223	•								
ALFORD **Half Moon Hotel and Restaurant**	223		•							

372   HOLIDAYS IN THE BRITISH ISLES

INDEX OF ACCOMMODATION

ACCOMMODATION & NAS RATING

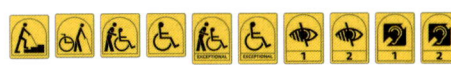

Accommodation	Page									
ASHBOURNE **Callow Hall Country House Hotel & Restaurant**	223	•								
ASHBOURNE **Ravenscliffe Farm Holidays**	223	•								
ASHBY-CUM-FENBY **Hall Farm Hotel & Restaurant**	223	•	•							
BAMFORD **Ladybower Apartments**	223								•	
BAMFORD **Yorkshire Bridge Inn**	223								•	
BICKER **Supreme Inns**	223	•								
BLYTH **The Courtyard at Hodsock Priory**	223		•							
BLYTON **Blyton Ponds**	223	•								
BOSTON **Special Needs Activity Centre Lincolnshire**	231									
BRASSINGTON **Hoe Grange Holidays**	223	•	•	•				•		•
BURGH ON BAIN **Bainfield Lodge**	225								•	
BUXTON **Alpine Lodge Guest House**	225								•	
CHURCH BROUGHTON **Oaklands Country Lodges**	225	•	•							
CLOPTON **Nene Valley Cottages**	225					•				
CLUMBER PARK, WORKSOP **Clumber Park Hotel & Spa**	225	•								
DISEWORTH **Lady Gate Guest House**	225						•			
EARL STERNDALE **Wheeldon Trees Farm**	225		•							
EAST BARKWITH **The Grange Holiday Cottages**	225	•								
EDWINSTOWE **Forest Lodge Hotel**	225	•								
EDWINSTOWE **YHA Sherwood Forest**	225	•								
GOULCEBY, LOUTH **Bay Tree Cottage**	225	•								
GRAINTHORPE **Canal Farm Cottages**	225	•								
GUILSBOROUGH **Coton Lodge**	227	•								
HALLGATES, CROPSTON **Horseshoe Cottage Farm**	227	•							•	
HAREBY **Meridian Retreats**	227	•								
HARPSWELL **The Old Stables**	227	•								
HELSEY, NR HOGSTHORPE **Helsey House Cottages**	227	•								

HOLIDAYS IN THE BRITISH ISLES

INDEX OF ACCOMMODATION

ACCOMMODATION & NAS RATING	Page	Mobility 1	Mobility 2	Mobility 3	Mobility 4	Mobility Exceptional	Visual Exceptional	Visual 1	Visual 2	Hearing 1	Hearing 2
HINCKLEY **Barceló Hinckley Island Hotel**	227	•	•		•			•		•	
HINCKLEY **Sketchley Grange Hotel**	227	•									
HUBBERTS BRIDGE, NR BOSTON **Elms Farm Cottages**	227	•	•					•		•	
INGOLDMELLS **Ingoldale Park**	227	•	•	•							
LEICESTER **Belmont Hotel**	227	•									
LEICESTER **Hilton Leicester**	227	•						•		•	
LEICESTER **Leicester Marriott Hotel**	227	•	•		•			•		•	
LOUGHBOROUGH **Imago at Burleigh Court**	229	•	•		•			•		•	
LOUTH **Brackenborough Hall Coach House Holidays**	229	•						•		•	
LOUTH **Nursery Cottage, The Granary, Millhouse & The Stables**	229	•	•								
MARKET HARBOROUGH **The Angel Hotel & Restaurant**	229									•	
MARTIN **The Manor House Stables**	229	•									
MARTON **Black Swan Guest House**	229	•									
MILFORD **The Ebenezer Chapel**	231										
MOIRA **YHA National Forest**	229	•	•								
MOULTON EAUGATE, NR SPALDING **Stennetts Farm Cottages**	229	•									
NEWARK **Dairy Cottage**	229	•									
NEWHAVEN **Old House Farm Cottages**	229	•	•								
NORTH CARLTON **Cliff Farm Cottage**	229	•	•	•	•						
NORTH WILLINGHAM **The Old Dairy Cottage**	229			•							
OAKHAM **Lodge Trust Country Park**	230	•	•								
OLD BRAMPTON **Chestnut Cottage and Willow Cottage**	230	•									
OUNDLE **Oundle Cottage Breaks**	230	•									
PARTNEY, NR SPILSBY **The Red Lion Inn**	230	•	•								
SKEGNESS **Chatsworth**	230	•									
SOUTH SCARLE **Greystones Guest Accommodation**	230	•									

INDEX OF ACCOMMODATION

ACCOMMODATION & NAS RATING	Page	♿ pusher	♿ companion	♿ assisted	♿ independent	♿ exceptional assisted	♿ exceptional independent	👁 1	👁 2	👂 1	👂 2
STAINFIELD **Rural Roosts**	230	•									
SWADLINCOTE **Forest Lodges**	230		•								
SWEPSTONE **Church View Barn**	230									•	
THORGANBY **Thorganby Hall Farm Cottages, Little Walk and Marris**	231	•	•		•						
THORPE ST PETER **Ings Barn**	231	•									
THRUSSINGTON **Walton Thorns Farm Holiday Cottages**	231										•
WOODHALL SPA **Bluebell Retreat**	231	•									
WOODHALL SPA **Petwood Hotel**	231	•									
WOODHALL SPA **Village Limits Country Pub, Restaurant and Motel**	231	•									
WORKSOP **Browns**	231	•									
WYCOMB **Stonepits Farm Bed & Breakfast**	231									•	

WEST MIDLANDS

BAGNALL **Cordwainer Cottage**	239									•	
BIRMINGHAM **SACO Livingbase**	239	•							•		•
BRIDGENORTH **The Malthouse**	239	•	•								
BROMYARD **Durstone Cottage**	239		•								
COALPORT **YHA Coalport**	239	•									
DIDDLEBURY **Goosefoot Barn Cottages**	239		•								
DILHORNE **Little Summerhill Cottages**	239	•									
EATON-UNDER-HEYWOOD **Eaton Manor**	239	•									
GRAFTON **Anvil Cottage, Apple Bough and Cider Press**	239	•	•								
HEREFORD **Poston Mill Park**	239	•									
HINDLIP **The Manor Coach House**	239	•									
ILAM **Beechenhill Cottage and The Cottage by the Pond**	241	•	•		•						
ILAM **The Orchards**	241									•	
ILAM **YHA Ilam Hall**	241	•									
KINETON **Long Ground Barn**	241	•	•								
KNIGHTCOTE **Knightcote Farm Cottages**	241	•	•		•						

INDEX OF ACCOMMODATION

ACCOMMODATION & NAS RATING

Accommodation	Page	🚶	♿	♿ EXC	♿ EXC	👂1	👂2	👁1	👁2
LEDBURY The Old Kennels Farm	241	•							
LEOMINSTER The Wain House	241	•	•				•		•
LEOMINSTER YHA Leominster	241	•	•						
LIGHTHORNE Church Hill Farm B&B	241	•							
LUDLOW Ludlow Mascall Centre	241	•	•						
LUDLOW Mocktree Barns Holiday Cottages	241	•							
MALVERN Hidelow House Cottages	241	•	•		•		•		•
MICHAELCHURCH ESCLEY Holt Farm	243	•							
ROSS-ON-WYE Flanesford Priory	243	•							
ROSS-ON-WYE Merton House Hotel	243								
ROSS-ON-WYE Trevase Granary	243		•						
ROSS-ON-WYE Tump Farm	243	•							•
SHREWSBURY Lyth Hill House	243	•							
STANSHOPE Church Farm Cottage & Ancestral Barn	243	•							•
TRETIRE Penblaith Barn	243		•						
WHITCHURCH Portland House Guest House	243		•						
WROXETER, NR SHREWSBURY Wroxeter Hotel	243	•	•						
NORTH WEST ENGLAND									
ACTON BRIDGE Wall Hill Farm Guest House	254		•						
AINSDALE, SOUTHPORT Willowbank Holiday Home and Touring Park	254		•			•			
ALSTON, LONGRIDGE Proven House	254		•			•			•
ALTRINCHAM Best Western Cresta Court Hotel	254		•						•
AMBLESIDE Nationwide Bungalow	260								
AMBLESIDE Rothay Manor	254	•	•						
ARNSIDE YHA Arnside	254	•	•						
ASHTON WITH STODDAY Ashton Hall Cottages	254	•							
BASSENTHWAITE Sandhills Farm	254	•	•						

376   HOLIDAYS IN THE BRITISH ISLES

INDEX OF ACCOMMODATION

ACCOMMODATION & NAS RATING

Accommodation	Page							
BLACKFORD, CARLISLE Mount Farm B&B	254	•	•					
BLACKPOOL Ashley Victoria	254		•					
BLACKPOOL Beachwood Guest House	255	•						
BLACKPOOL Big Blue Hotel	254	•						
BLACKPOOL Century Hotel	260							
BLACKPOOL Coast Apartments	255	•						
BLACKPOOL Elizabeth Frankland Moore Home	260							
BLACKPOOL Holmsdale	255	•						
BLACKPOOL The Address	255		•					
BLACKPOOL The Beach House	255	•						
BLACKPOOL The Berkeley	255		•					
BLACKPOOL The Lawton	255	•						
BLACKPOOL The Willow Tree House	255							
BLEASDALE Bleasdale Cottages	255	•	•					
BLITTERLEES, SILLOTH Rose Cottage	255	•						
BOSLEY Strawberry Duck Cottage	255	•						
BOWNESS ON SOLWAY The Old Chapel	255	•						
BOWNESS-ON-WINDERMERE Windermere Manor	260							
BROUGHTON-IN-FURNESS The Kepplewray Centre	261							
BURSCOUGH Martin Lane Farmhouse Holiday Cottages	255				•			
CARLISLE Old Brewery Residences	256	•	•					
CASTLE CARROCK, BRAMPTON Tottergill Farm Cottages	256	•	•					
CATLOWDY, LONGTOWN Bessiestown Farm Country Guesthouse	256	•	•					
CATON 4 The Croft (Ground floor apartment)	256		•				•	
CHESTER Brookside Hotel	256	•						
CHESTER The Chester Abode Limited	256		•					
CONGLETON Sandhole Farm	256	•						
CONGLETON Ladderstile Retreat	256	•	•					

HOLIDAYS IN THE BRITISH ISLES

INDEX OF ACCOMMODATION

ACCOMMODATION & NAS RATING	Page	c1	c2	c3	c4	c5	c6	c7	c8	c9	c10
CROOK **Lake District Disabled Holidays**	256				•						
DOWNHOLLAND **Cross Farm Cottages**	256	•									
EDGWORTH **Clough Head Farm**	257		•								
EDGWORTH **Meadowcroft Barn B&B**	256	•	•								
FRODSHAM **Lady Heyes Caravan Park**	257	•									
GARSTANG **Barnacre Cottages**	257	•									
GRANGE OVER SANDS **Netherwood Hotel**	257	•									
GRASMERE **Rothay Lodge & Rothay Lodge Apartment**	257		•								
GREAT STRICKLAND **Strickland Manor**	257	•	•								
ISEL, COCKERMOUTH **Linskeldfield Tarn Holiday Cottages**	257	•									
KIRKOSWALD **Howscales**	257	•	•								
LANGHO **Best Western Mytton Fold Hotel and Golf Complex**	257		•								
LIVERPOOL **Ibis Hotel**	257		•								
LIVERPOOL **YHA Liverpool**	257	•									
LONGTHWAITHE, BORROWDALE **YHA Borrowdale**	257	•	•	•	•						
LORTON, COCKERMOUTH **Southwaite Green**	258	•	•								
LYTHAM ST ANNES **Avondale**	258	•									
LYTHAM ST ANNES **St Annes Hotel**	261										
LYTHAM ST ANNES **The Langdales Hotel**	258	•									
MACCLESFIELD **Kerridge End Holiday Cottages**	258	•		•							
MANCHESTER **Bewleys Hotel, Manchester Airport**	258		•								
MANCHESTER **Hilton Manchester Deansgate**	258				•						•
MANCHESTER **Lancashire County Cricket Club & Old Trafford Lodge**	258		•				•				•
MANCHESTER **The Midland – Manchester**	258		•								
MANCHESTER **YHA Manchester**	258	•	•								

HOLIDAYS IN THE BRITISH ISLES

INDEX OF ACCOMMODATION

ACCOMMODATION & NAS RATING

Accommodation	Page	🧑‍🦯	♿	♿	♿ ex	♿ ex	🦻	🦻	👁 1	👁 2
MORECAMBE **Eden Vale Luxury Holiday Flats**	258	•								
MUNGRISDALE **Bannerdale**	258	•								
NANTWICH **The Wingate Centre**	261									
NEWTON-IN-BOWLAND **Stonefold Holiday Cottage**	258		•							
PULFORD **Grosvenor Pulford Hotel and Spa**	259		•				•		•	
QUERNMORE, LANCASTER **Knotts Farm Holiday Cottages**	259	•	•							
REDMAIN, NEAR COCKERMOUTH **Redmain Hall Farm**	259	•								
RIBCHESTER **Riverside Barn Bed & Breakfast**	259		•							
ROCHDALE **Fernhill B&B**	259	•								
SALFORD, MANCHESTER **The Lowry Hotel**	259	•	•							
SCALES **Scales Farm Country Guest House**	259	•								
SCORTON **Cleveley Mere Boutique Lodges**	259	•								
SEBERGHAM **Monkhouse Hill Cottages**	259	•								
SEDBERGH **Hebblethwaite Hall Farm**	259	•								
SOUTHPORT **Salfordian Hotel**	261									
SOUTHPORT **Sandy Brook Farm**	259	•	•							
SOUTHPORT **Vitalise Sandpipers**	261									
ST BEES **Springbank Farm Lodges**	259		•				•		•	
STAVELEY **Avondale**	260	•								
THURSTONFIELD **The Tranquil Otter**	260	•	•							
WEST KIRBY **Herons Well**	260		•							
WHINFELL, KENDAL **Top Thorn Farm**	260	•								
WINDERMERE **Hawksmoor Guest House**	260	•								
WINDERMERE **Linthwaite House Hotel**	260	•								

YORKSHIRE

Accommodation	Page									
BALIFF BRIDGE, BRIGHOUSE **The Lodge at Birkby Hall**	268	•	•							

HOLIDAYS IN THE BRITISH ISLES

INDEX OF ACCOMMODATION

ACCOMMODATION & NAS RATING

Accommodation	Page	M1	M2	M3e	M3e	H1	H2	V1	V2
BEAMSLEY The Beamsley Project	272								
BEVERLEY Rudstone Walk Country Cottages	273								
BOROUGHBRIDGE Buckden Pike Loft	268	•							
BRIDLINGTON Marina Holiday Apartments	268		•						
BRIDLINGTON Pride-N-Joy	268			•					
BRIDLINGTON Providence Place	268	•	•						
BROUGH Rudstone Walk Country Accommodation	268	•							
BUCKDEN 9 Dalegarth and Heron Ghyll	268	•	•						
EASINGWOLD Thornton Lodge Farm	268		•						
EBBERSTON Cow Pasture Cottage & Swallowtail Cottage	268		•						
ELLERBY The Ellerby	268	•	•						
FLAMBOROUGH Flamborough Rock Cottages	269		•						
HARWOOD DALE The Grainary	269				•				
HELMSLEY YHA Helmsley	269		•				•		
HIGH CATTON, STAMFORD BRIDGE The Courtyard & Ruxpin Cottage	269	•	•						
ILKLEY Ilkley Moor Cottages and Apartments at Westwood Lodge	269	•	•						
KELFIELD The Dovecote Barns York	269	•	•	•					
KIRKBYMOORSIDE Partridge Cottage	269	•	•		•				
LEEDS Weetwood Hall	269		•						
LEEDS Storm Jameson Court, Charles Morris Hall	269	•	•			•	•	•	•
LOCKTON YHA Lockton	269		•						
MIDDLETON, PICKERING The Hawthornes Lodges	269	•							
NEWTON-ON-RAWCLIFFE Sunset Cottage	270	•							
NEWTON-ON-RAWCLIFFE Mel House Cottages	270	•	•	•					
NORTHALLERTON Lovesome Hill Farm	270	•							

INDEX OF ACCOMMODATION

ACCOMMODATION & NAS RATING

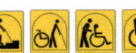

Accommodation	Page							
PICKERING **Eastgate Cottages**	270	•						
PICKERING **Keld Head Farm Cottages**	270	•						
PONTEFRACT **Tower House Executive Guest House**	270	•						
PRESTON, HULL **Little Weghill Farm**	271	•						
SANDSEND **Sandsend Bay Cottages**	271		•					
SAWDON **Basin Howe Farm Cottages**	271		•					
SCARBOROUGH **Inglenook Guest House**	271	•						
SCARBOROUGH **Scarborough Travel and Holiday Lodge**	271	•						
SEWERBY **Field House Farm Cottages**	271		•					
SKIPSEA **Holiday Homes Trust Caravan**	273							
STANNINGTON **The Cart Shed**	271	•						
STAPE **Rawcliffe House Farm**	271			•				
SUMMERBRIDGE **Helme Pasture**	271	•						
SWINTON, MALTON **Walnut Garth**	271	•						
THE BAY, FILEY **Bempton Holiday Villa**	271				•			
THIRSK **Linden Tree**	273							
THORPE BASSETT **The Old Post Office**	271	•						
WAINSTALLS **The Crossroads Inn**	272	•						
WHITBY **Captain Cook's Haven**	272		•					
WHITBY **Whitby Holiday Park**	272	•					•	
WHITBY **YHA Whitby**	272	•	•				•	•
WRELTON **Beech Farm Cottages**	272	•						
YAPHAM **Wolds View Holiday Cottages**	272	•						
YORK **Best Western Monkbar Hotel**	272		•					
YORK **Pound Cottage, Copper Cottage & Crown Cottage**	272	•	•	•				
YORK **Woodlands Respite Care Centre**	273							

NORTH EAST ENGLAND

Accommodation	Page							
ALNWICK **Holly Lodge**	279	•	•					
BAMBURGH **Outchester & Ross Farm Cottages**	279	•						
BARDON MILL **Coach House B&B**	279	•	•					

HOLIDAYS IN THE BRITISH ISLES

INDEX OF ACCOMMODATION

ACCOMMODATION & NAS RATING									
BARDON MILL **Old High Shield**	279	•							
BEAL, BERWICK-UPON-TWEED **Fenham Farm, Coastal Bed & Breakfast**	279	•							
BELFORD **Elwick Farm Cottages**	280	•							
BELLINGHAM **Brownrigg Lodges**	280	•	•						
BERWICK-UPON-TWEED **Meadow Hill Guest House**	280	•							
BERWICK-UPON-TWEED **Ord House Country Park**	283								
BERWICK-UPON-TWEED **Skylark Cottage**	280								•
BERWICK-UPON-TWEED **West Ord Holiday Cottages**	280	•							
BINGFIELD, HEXHAM **The Hytte**	280	•	•			•	•		•
BOWES **Mellwaters Barn**	280	•	•	•	•				•
BUTTERKNOWLE **Little Owl Lodge**	280	•	•						
CHATHILL **Doxford Cottages**	280		•						
CHATHILL **Doxford Hall Hotel & Spa**	280	•	•						•
COCKFIELD, BISHOP AUCKLAND **Swallows Nest**	280			•					
CORNHILL ON TWEED **The Collingwood Arms Hotel**	281	•							
CORNRIGGS, COWSHILL **Cornriggs Cottages**	281			•					•
CRAMLINGTON **Burradon Farm Cottages and Houses**	281	•		•			•		•
CRASTER **Craster Pine Lodges**	281	•	•						
DARLINGTON **River Cottage**	281								•
EDLINGHAM **Lumbylaw Cottages**	281	•							
GAINFORD **East Greystone Farm Cottages**	281		•						
GATESHEAD **Jurys Inn Newcastle Gateshead Quays**	281	•	•						
HAYDON BRIDGE **Grindon Cartshed**	281	•	•						
HAYDON BRIDGE **Shaftoe's**	281	•							
HAYDON BRIDGE **The Old Farmhouse, Grindon Farm**	281	•	•			•	•		

INDEX OF ACCOMMODATION

ACCOMMODATION & NAS RATING	Page	🧹	👤	♿ walk	♿	♿ EXCEPTIONAL	♿ EXCEPTIONAL	👁 1	👁 2	👂 1	👂 2
HIGH HESLEDEN **The Ship Inn**	281		•								
INGLETON **Mill Granary Cottages**	282	•	•								
INGRAM **Cheviot Holiday Cottages**	282	•									
KIELDER **Falstone Barns**	282	•									
KIELDER **Calvert Trust Kielder**	282	•	•	•	•					•	•
KIRKNEWTON **Crookhouse**	282	•	•								
LAMBLEY, NEAR BRAMPTON **Clover Hill Cottage**	282	•									
LONGHORSLEY **Beacon Hill Farm**	282		•								
LONGHORSLEY **Linden Hall Golf & Country Club**	282	•	•								
NEWBROUGH, HEXHAM **Carr Edge Farm**	282	•	•								
NEWCASTLE UPON TYNE **Euro Hostel Newcastle**	282	•	•							•	•
NEWCASTLE UPON TYNE **Hilton Newcastle Gateshead**	282	•	•							•	•
NORTH CHARLTON **The Reading Rooms**	282	•	•								
QUEBEC **Hamsteels Hall Cottages**	283	•									
ROCHESTER, NR OTTERBURN **Redesdale Arms**	283	•									
SHILBOTTLE **Village Farm**	283	•									
SLALEY, NR HEXHAM **The Old Byre (Rye Hill Farm)**	283		•								
SUNNISIDE, NR NEWCASTLE **Hedley Hall Country Cottages**	283	•	•	•						•	•
WARKWORTH **Garden Cottage**	283	•									
WINSTON **Alwent Mill Cottage**	283	•									
WOOLER **Fenton Hill Farm Cottages**	283	•									
SCOTLAND											
CRATHIE **Crathie Opportunity Holidays**	299										
CRIEFF **Ancaster BLESMA Home**	299										
DIRLETON **Denis Duncan House**	299										
DRUMNADROCHIT **Lochletter Lodges**	301										
NORTH BERWICK **Leuchie House**	301										

HOLIDAYS IN THE BRITISH ISLES

INDEX OF ACCOMMODATION

ACCOMMODATION & NAS RATING

WALES

ABERAERON **Ty Glyn Holiday Centre**	313
BONCATH **Clynfyw Countryside Centre**	313
BRECON BEACONS **Brecon Beacons Holiday Cottages**	315
KIDWELLY **Holiday Homes Trust Chalet**	315
LLANDUDNO **Belmont Hotel**	315
LLANDUDNO **West Shore Hotel**	315
NARBERTH **Caerwen**	315
PENALLY **The Wheelabout**	317
TENBY **Giltar View**	317
TENBY **Harriet's House**	317
WHITLAND **Homeleigh Country Cottages**	317

NORTHERN IRELAND

KILKEEL **Mourne Activity Centre**	329
LISNASKEA **Share Holiday Village**	329

REPUBLIC OF IRELAND

DONAMON **Cuisle Holiday Centre**	335
DUBLIN **Carmel Fallon Respite Centre**	335
KILCOOLE **Trident Holiday Homes**	335
KNOCK **Knock House Hotel**	335

CHANNEL ISLANDS

ST HELIER **Grand Hotel**	348
ST HELIER **Jersey Cheshire Home**	348
ST HELIER **The Royal Yacht Hotel**	349
ST MARTIN **Westlea Centre for the Visually Impaired**	349
ST OUEN **Maison Des Landes Hotel**	349
ST PETER PORT **Les Rocquettes Hotel**	349